Allergy and Immunology for the Internist

Editor

ANNE MARIE DITTO

MEDICAL CLINICS
OF NORTH AMERICA

www.medical.theclinics.com

Consulting Editor
BIMAL H. ASHAR

January 2020 • Volume 104 • Number 1

ELSEVIER

1600 John F. Kennedy Boulevard • Suite 1800 • Philadelphia, Pennsylvania, 19103-2899

http://www.theclinics.com

MEDICAL CLINICS OF NORTH AMERICA Volume 104, Number 1
January 2020 ISSN 0025-7125, ISBN-13: 978-0-323-69718-7

Editor: Katerina Heidhausen
Developmental Editor: Kristen Helm

Medical Clinics of North America (ISSN 0025-7125) is published bimonthly by Elsevier Inc., 360 Park Avenue South, New York, NY 10010-1710. Months of publication are January, March, May, July, September, and November. Business and editorial offices: 1600 John F. Kennedy Boulevard, Suite 1800, Philadelphia, PA 19103-2899. Periodicals postage paid at New York, NY, and additional mailing offices. Subscription prices are USD $295.00 per year (US individuals), $654.00 per year (US institutions), $100.00 per year (US Students), $353.00 per year (Canadian individuals), $850.00 per year (Canadian institutions), $200.00 per year for (foreign students), $100.00 per year for (Canadian students), $422.00 per year (foreign individuals), and $850.00 per year (foreign institutions). To receive student/resident rate, orders must be accompanied by name of affiliated institution, date of term, and the signature of program/residency coordinator on institution letterhead. Orders will be billed at individual rate until proof of status is received. Foreign air speed delivery is included in all Clinics' subscription prices. All prices are subject to change without notice. **POSTMASTER:** Send address changes to *Medical Clinics of North America*, Elsevier Health Sciences Division, Subscription Customer Service, 3251 Riverport Lane, Maryland Heights, MO 63043. **Customer Service: Telephone: 1-800-654-2452** (U.S. and Canada); **1-314-447-8871** (outside U.S. and Canada). **Fax: 314-447-8029. E-mail: journalscustomerserviceusa@elsevier.com** (for print support); **journalsonlinesupport-usa@elsevier.com** (for online support).

Reprints. For copies of 100 or more of articles in this publication, please contact the Commercial Reprints Department, Elsevier Inc., 360 Park Avenue South, New York, NY 10010-1710. Tel.: 212-633-3874; Fax: 212-633-3820; E-mail: reprints@elsevier.com.

Medical Clinics of North America is also published in Spanish by McGraw-Hill Interamericana Editores S. A., P.O. Box 5-237, 06500 Mexico, D.F., Mexico.

Medical Clinics of North America is covered in *MEDLINE/PubMed (Index Medicus), Current Contents, ASCA, Excerpta Medica, Science Citation Index,* and *ISI/BIOMED.*

PROGRAM OBJECTIVE
The goal of the *Medical Clinics of North America* is to keep practicing physicians up to date with current clinical practice by providing timely articles reviewing the state of the art in patient care.

TARGET AUDIENCE
All practicing physicians and other healthcare professionals.

LEARNING OBJECTIVES
Upon completion of this activity, participants will be able to:
1. Review the definition, classification, evaluation, differential diagnosis, prognosis, complications, and management of anaphylaxis.
2. Discuss the epidemiology of adult food allergy, as well as common clinical scenarios and presentations of various types of food allergies.
3. Recognize the pathophysiology, epidemiology, clinical presentation, burden, diagnosis and treatment of adult atopic dermatitis.

ACCREDITATION
The Elsevier Office of Continuing Medical Education (EOCME) is accredited by the Accreditation Council for Continuing Medical Education (ACCME) to provide continuing medical education for physicians.

The EOCME designates this journal-based CME activity for a maximum of 12 *AMA PRA Category 1 Credit*(s)™. Physicians should claim only the credit commensurate with the extent of their participation in the activity.

All other healthcare professionals requesting continuing education credit for this enduring material will be issued a certificate of participation.

DISCLOSURE OF CONFLICTS OF INTEREST
The EOCME assesses conflict of interest with its instructors, faculty, planners, and other individuals who are in a position to control the content of CME activities. All relevant conflicts of interest that are identified are thoroughly vetted by EOCME for fair balance, scientific objectivity, and patient care recommendations. EOCME is committed to providing its learners with CME activities that promote improvements or quality in healthcare and not a specific proprietary business or a commercial interest.

The planning committee, staff, authors and editors listed below have identified no financial relationships or relationships to products or devices they or their spouse/life partner have with commercial interest related to the content of this CME activity:
Bimal H. Ashar, MD, MBA, FACP; Elissa M. Abrams, MD; Derek K. Chu, MD, PhD; Linda Cox, MD; Anne Marie Ditto, MD; Mark S. Dykewicz, MD; Luz Fonacier, MD; David B.K. Golden, MD; Justin Greiwe, MD; Katerina Heidhausen; Alison Kemp; Dilawar Khokhar, MD; Fei Li Kuang, MD, PhD; Jason K. Lam, DO; Mahboobeh Mahdavinia, MD, PhD; David J. McCullagh, MB BCh BAO, DTM&H; Anil Nanda, MD; Stacy Nassau, MD; Jeyanthi Surendrakumar; Baotran B. Tran, APRN; Anita N. Wasan, MD; Susan Waserman, MD, MSc

The planning committee, staff, authors and editors listed below have identified financial relationships or relationships to products or devices they or their spouse/life partner have with commercial interest related to the content of this CME activity:
Cem Akin, MD, PhD: is a consultant/advisor for Blueprint Medicines Corporation and Novartis AG

Jonathan A. Bernstein, MD: participates in speakers bureau, is a consultant/advisor, and receives research support from AstraZeneca, CSL Behring, Genentech, Inc., Novartis AG, Pharming Group NV, Sanofi-Aventis U.S. LLC, Shire Plc, and Millennium Pharmaceuticals, Inc., a wholly owned subsidiary of Takeda Pharmaceutical Company Limited

Jonathan I. Silverberg, MD, PhD, MPH: is a consultant/advisor for AbbVie, Inc., Eli Lilly and Company, Galderma Laboratories, L.P., Kiniksa Pharmaceuticals, Ltd, LEO Pharma Inc., Menlo Therapeutics, Pfizer Inc., Realm Therapeutics, Inc., Regentys Corporation, Roivant Sciences, Ltd.; is a consultant/advisor for and receives research support from GlaxoSmithKline plc; is a consultant/advisor, receives research support, and serves on a speakers bureau for Regeneron Pharmaceuticals, Inc.

UNAPPROVED/OFF-LABEL USE DISCLOSURE
The EOCME requires CME faculty to disclose to the participants;
1. When products or procedures being discussed are off-label, unlabelled, experimental, and/or investigational (not US Food and Drug Administration [FDA] approved); and

2. Any limitations on the information presented, such as data that are preliminary or that represent ongoing research, interim analyses, and/or unsupported opinions. Faculty may discuss information about pharmaceutical agents that is outside of FDA-approved labelling. This information is intended solely for CME and is not intended to promote off-label use of these medications. If you have any questions, contact the medical affairs department of the manufacturer for the most recent prescribing information.

TO ENROLL

To enroll in the *Medical Clinics of North America* Continuing Medical Education program, call customer service at 1-800-654-2452 or sign up online at www.theclinics.com/home/cme. The CME program is available to subscribers for an additional annual fee of USD $300.00.

METHOD OF PARTICIPATION

In order to claim credit, participants must complete the following;
1. Complete enrolment as indicated above.
2. Read the activity.
3. Complete the CME Test and Evaluation. Participants must achieve a score of 70% on the test. All CME Tests and Evaluations must be completed online.

CME INQUIRIES/SPECIAL NEEDS

For all CME inquiries or special needs, please contact elsevierCME@elsevier.com.

MEDICAL CLINICS OF NORTH AMERICA

Contributors

CONSULTING EDITOR

BIMAL H. ASHAR, MD, MBA, FACP
Associate Professor of Medicine, Division of General Internal Medicine, Johns Hopkins University School of Medicine, Baltimore, Maryland, USA

EDITOR

ANNE MARIE DITTO, MD, FAAAAI, FACAAI, FACP
US Medical Expert, Respiratory, US Medical Affairs, GlaxoSmithKline, Associate Professor of Medicine, Department of Medicine, Division of Allergy–Immunology, Northwestern Medicine, Northwestern University Feinberg School of Medicine, Chicago, Illinois, USA

AUTHORS

ELISSA M. ABRAMS, MD
Department of Pediatrics, Section of Allergy and Clinical Immunology, University of Manitoba, Winnipeg, Manitoba, Canada

CEM AKIN, MD, PhD
Professor, Department of Internal Medicine, Division of Allergy and Clinical Immunology, University of Michigan, Ann Arbor, Michigan, USA

JONATHAN A. BERNSTEIN, MD
Department of Internal Medicine, Division of Immunology, Allergy Section, University of Cincinnati, Bernstein Allergy Group, Cincinnati, Ohio, USA

DEREK K. CHU, MD, PhD, FRCPC
Department of Medicine, McMaster University, Hamilton, Ontario, Canada

LINDA COX, MD
Associate Professor, Department of Medicine and Dermatology, Nova Southeastern University, Davie, Florida, USA; Department of Medicine, University of Miami, Coral Gables, Florida, USA

ANNE MARIE DITTO, MD, FAAAAI, FACAAI, FACP
US Medical Expert, Respiratory, US Medical Affairs, GlaxoSmithKline, Associate Professor of Medicine, Department of Medicine, Division of Allergy–Immunology, Northwestern Medicine, Northwestern University Feinberg School of Medicine, Chicago, Illinois, USA

MARK S. DYKEWICZ, MD
Raymond and Alberta Slavin Endowed Professor in Allergy & Immunology, Professor of Internal Medicine, Director, Allergy & Immunology Fellowship Program, Chief, Section of Allergy and Immunology, Division of Infectious Diseases, Allergy and Immunology, Department of Internal Medicine, Saint Louis University School of Medicine, St Louis, Missouri, USA

LUZ FONACIER, MD
Department of Internal Medicine, Section of Allergy and Immunology, NYU Winthrop University Hospital, Mineola, New York, USA

DAVID B.K. GOLDEN, MD
Department of Medicine, Johns Hopkins University School of Medicine, Baltimore, Maryland, USA

JUSTIN GREIWE, MD
Bernstein Allergy Group, Department of Internal Medicine, Division of Immunology, Allergy Section, University of Cincinnati, Cincinnati, Ohio, USA

DILAWAR KHOKHAR, MD
Allergy and Clinical Immunology Fellow, Department of Internal Medicine, Division of Allergy and Clinical Immunology, University of Michigan, Ann Arbor, Michigan, USA

FEI LI KUANG, MD, PhD
Human Eosinophil Section, Laboratory of Parasitic Diseases, National Institute of Allergy and Infectious Diseases, National Institutes of Health, Bethesda, Maryland, USA

JASON K. LAM, DO
Allergy and Immunology Fellow, Saint Louis University School of Medicine, St Louis, Missouri, USA

MAHBOOBEH MAHDAVINIA, MD, PhD
Assistant Professor, Division of Allergy and Immunology, Department of Internal Medicine, Rush University Medical Center, Chicago, Illinois, USA

DAVID J. McCULLAGH, MB BCh BAO, DTM&H, FRCPC
Department of Medicine, McMaster University, Hamilton, Ontario, Canada

ANIL NANDA, MD
Asthma and Allergy Center, Lewisville, Texas, USA; Asthma and Allergy Center, Flower Mound, Texas, USA; Division of Allergy and Immunology, University of Texas Southwestern Medical Center, Dallas, Texas, USA

STACY NASSAU, MD
Department of Internal Medicine, Section of Allergy and Immunology, NYU Winthrop University Hospital, Mineola, New York, USA

JONATHAN I. SILVERBERG, MD, PhD, MPH
Associate Professor, Northwestern University Feinberg School of Medicine, Director, Northwestern Medicine Multidisciplinary Eczema Center, Chicago, Illinois, USA

BAOTRAN B. TRAN, APRN
Nurse Practitioner, Division of Allergy-Immunology, Northwestern Medicine, Chicago, Illinois, USA

ANITA N. WASAN, MD
Allergy and Asthma Center, McLean, Virginia, USA

SUSAN WASERMAN, MD, MSc, FRCPC
Department of Medicine, McMaster University, Hamilton, Ontario, Canada

Contents

Approach to Patients with Eosinophilia 1

Fei Li Kuang

> Physicians may encounter blood or tissue eosinophilia through a routine complete blood count with differential or a tissue pathology report. In this article, the basic biology of eosinophils is reviewed and definitions of blood eosinophilia, as well as the challenges of defining tissue eosinophilia, are discussed. Conditions associated with eosinophilia are briefly discussed as well as a general approach to evaluating eosinophilia. Future challenges include determining which eosinophil-associated diseases benefit from eosinophil-targeted therapy and identifying biomarkers for disease activity and diagnosis.

Approach to the Patient with Hives 15

Justin Greiwe and Jonathan A. Bernstein

> Urticaria is a common presenting problem to the primary care provider. Acute urticaria lasting less than 6 weeks may be associated with a drug or food allergens. Chronic urticaria lasting more than 6 weeks is often associated without a known underlying cause. Inducible stimuli causing hives should be excluded using specific provocation testing. Treatment follows a standardized algorithmic approach as outlined by the Joint Task Force Practice Parameter and/or International Urticaria guidelines. Patients not responsive to steps 1 or 2 should be referred to an urticaria specialist for further evaluation and treatment. The prognosis and outcome of urticaria is generally very favorable for most patients.

Anaphylaxis for Internists: Definition, Evaluation, and Management, with a Focus on Commonly Encountered Problems 25

Derek K. Chu, David J. McCullagh, and Susan Waserman

> Anaphylaxis is an acute systemic allergic reaction that can be life threatening. In adults, the most common causes of anaphylaxis are foods, drugs, and insect stings. This article reviews the definition, classification, evaluation, differential diagnosis, prognosis, complications, and management of anaphylaxis. Tailored for internists, the article focuses on anaphylactic medication allergies. It provides a guide to optimally evaluate and manage patients with antibiotic allergy using a simple, rapid risk stratification technique, graded antibiotic challenge (test dose), and/or allergist-

guided drug desensitization. It also reviews other causes of anaphylaxis that internists are likely to encounter, and an approach to their management.

such as pulmonary function testing, can be used to aid in the diagnosis. There are multiple associated comorbidities with asthma, including rhinitis, sinusitis, gastroesophageal reflux disease, obstructive sleep apnea, and depression. There is often an allergic component of asthma, and patient education is vital.

Foreword

Overreactions

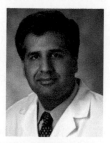

Bimal H. Ashar, MD, MBA, FACP
Consulting Editor

Charles Harrison Blackley was a mid-1800s English physician who was committed to finding out why he repeatedly suffered from "summer colds." Earlier theories had suggested the possibility that the trigger for such "colds" could be odors, dust, ozone, benzoic acid, or just the heat itself. Dr Blackley believed that pollens were the stimulant for these symptoms. In order to prove this, he applied serial dilutions of pollen to his own eyes and nose. He showed that just 2 µg of pollen could elicit symptoms of hay fever.[1] He went on to invent allergy skin testing, showing that the application of pollen to his skin could elicit a wheal reaction.

Over the last few decades, there has been a significant rise in numbers of people affected by allergies. It is estimated that allergies currently affect 30% of adults and 40% of children in the United States. It ranks as the sixth most common chronic disease in the United States, resulting in an estimated $18 billion cost to the health care system annually. In addition to allergic rhinitis, other categories of allergy, such as food, drug, insect, and skin, have caused significant morbidity in patients. The reason for the rise in body's overresponsiveness to allergens remains a mystery. Theories have suggested that increased use of antibiotics may play a role, but more support surrounds the "hygiene hypothesis." This theory suggests that the improvements in living conditions lead to a lack of exposure to germs, causing our immune system to overreact to potentially harmless irritants. Interestingly, Dr Blackley observed that farmers were less likely to come down with hay fever than those of higher socioeconomic classes.

In this issue of *Medical Clinics of North America*, Dr Ditto has assembled a team of experts to describe the triggers, presentations, and available treatments for the various

Med Clin N Am 104 (2020) xiii–xiv
https://doi.org/10.1016/j.mcna.2019.10.002
0025-7125/20/© 2019 Published by Elsevier Inc.

categories of allergy. In addition, a description of newly recognized symptoms associated with mast cell activation is provided.

Bimal H. Ashar, MD, MBA, FACP
Division of General Internal Medicine
Johns Hopkins University School of Medicine
601 North Caroline Street
#7143
Baltimore, MD 21287, USA

E-mail address:
Bashar1@jhmi.edu

REFERENCE

1. Crane J. Charles Harrison Blackley: The man who put the hay in hay fever. Hektoen International 2015. Available at: https://hekint.org/2017/01/28/charles-harrison-blackley-the-man-who-put-the-hay-in-hay-fever/. Accessed October 1, 2019.

Preface

Allergy: The "Whole" Story

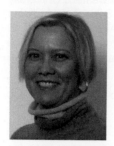

Anne Marie Ditto, MD
Editor

A subspecialist friend of mine once told me, in jest, "get an organ" as we were debating over which of us should manage a disease that overlapped in both of our specialties. However, to do so is impossible in the field of allergy. As allergist-immunologists, we quickly came to understand that allergic diseases are immunologic, and by definition, involve the entire body. It is true that many allergic diseases manifest predominantly in 1 organ, such as asthma involving the lung or atopic dermatitis involving the skin, yet all allergic diseases are systemic. This is why treating allergic rhinitis with antihistamines and topical steroids can improve asthma symptoms, and why immunotherapy can prevent further allergic sensitizations and even the development of asthma. It also explains why sinusitis can cause asthma exacerbations, and if left untreated, can be a cause of persistent asthma that is difficult to control. It explains why allergic drug reactions, which mainly manifest as skin rashes, can also cause fever, renal failure, and liver failure and why venom immunotherapy can markedly reduce the risk of anaphylaxis to stinging insects in high-risk patients.

Allergic diseases are on the rise, and allergic manifestations are ever changing. For example, de novo food allergy is presenting more commonly in adults, and gastrointestinal manifestations of food allergy, such as eosinophilic esophagitis and pollen-food allergy syndrome, are increasing in incidence. Atopic dermatitis, thought to be the first step in the "atopic march," is being recognized more commonly in adults with no previous history of childhood eczema. Asthma is increasing in epidemic proportions.

In our world of increasing specialization, it can be difficult to look beyond the target organ, yet this is oftentimes what is needed to provide the best patient care. My goal is that this issue will serve as a resource to you, the internist, to help shed light on allergic

Med Clin N Am 104 (2020) xv–xvi
https://doi.org/10.1016/j.mcna.2019.10.001
0025-7125/20/© 2019 Published by Elsevier Inc.

medical.theclinics.com

diseases, to assist in recognizing nuances in presentation, and to inform you of the most effective treatments.

Anne Marie Ditto, MD
Northwestern Medicine
Northwestern University
Feinberg School of Medicine
Division of Allergy–Immunology
211 East Ontario Suite 1000
Chicago, IL 60611, USA

E-mail address:
amditto@northwestern.edu

Dedication

I would like to dedicate this issue to my mother. Without her love, sacrifice, support, and encouragement, I would not have had the opportunity to specialize in Allergy-Immunology. Thank you, Mom!

In Loving Memory
Mary Elisa DiTullio Ditto
1932-2019

Med Clin N Am 104 (2020) xvii
https://doi.org/10.1016/j.mcna.2019.10.009
0025-7125/20/© 2019 Published by Elsevier Inc.

medical.theclinics.com

Approach to Patients with Eosinophilia

Fei Li Kuang, MD, PhD

KEYWORDS

- Eosinophil • IL-5 • Corticosteroids • Biologics • Hypereosinophilia
- Eosinophil granule proteins

KEY POINTS

- Peripheral blood eosinophilia is defined using absolute eosinophil count (AEC; cells/mm³). Eosinophil percentages can be misleading.
- Degree of eosinophilia is not always correlated with severity or seriousness of disease.
- Medications are the most common cause of eosinophilia in the developed world, whereas parasitic infections are the most common cause worldwide.
- Concomitant medications (eg, corticosteroids) and transient medical conditions (bacterial infection) can mask a greater degree of eosinophilia by temporarily suppressing the AEC.
- Sustained hypereosinophilia (AEC $\geq$1500 cells/mm³) without clear cause should prompt an evaluation for hypereosinophilic syndrome, especially if the patient is symptomatic.

INTRODUCTION

Physicians may encounter blood or tissue eosinophilia through a routine complete blood count (CBC) with differential or a tissue pathology report. In this article, the basic biology of eosinophils is reviewed and definitions of blood eosinophilia, as well as the challenges of defining tissue eosinophilia, are discussed. Conditions associated with eosinophilia are briefly discussed as well as a general approach to evaluating eosinophilia. Future challenges include determining which eosinophil-associated diseases benefit from eosinophil-targeted therapy and identifying biomarkers for disease activity and diagnosis.

EOSINOPHIL BIOLOGY

Eosinophils are myeloid cells that were first named by Paul Ehrlich in 1879 because of their bright red staining eosin-fast granules. These cells arise from the bone marrow

Disclosure: The author has nothing to disclose.
Funding: This research was supported by the Intramural Research Program of the NIH, NIAID, LPD.
Human Eosinophil Section, Laboratory of Parasitic Diseases, National Institute of Allergy and Infectious Disease, National Institutes of Health, 4 Memorial Drive, B1-27, Bethesda, MD 20892, USA
E-mail address: feili.kuang@nih.gov

Med Clin N Am 104 (2020) 1–14
https://doi.org/10.1016/j.mcna.2019.08.005
0025-7125/20/Published by Elsevier Inc.

and are released in mature form, circulate in the periphery, and become tissue-resident cells. Eosinophil development depends on several cytokines, including interleukin (IL)-5, IL-3, and granulocyte-macrophage colony-stimulating factor (GM-CSF). IL-5 is also critical for eosinophil activation and survival. Although eosinophils are found in the circulation, they are thought to be primarily tissue-dwelling cells, where they are 100-fold more abundant. In the blood, eosinophils have a half-life of 8 to 18 hours after departing the bone marrow. It is unclear how long they live in various tissues at homeostasis and it is possible their survival could be extended/sustained by exogenous factors such as IL-5.

Eosinophil Granules

Electron micrographs reveal that eosinophils contain multiple types of granules: primary granules, secondary (eosinophil-specific) granules, small granules, and microgranules (secretory vesicles). Primary granules are round and uniformly dense, and are composed of Charcot-Leyden crystal protein (galectin-10), which forms the well-known Charcot-Leyden crystals associated with the sputum of patients with asthma, described years before the discovery of eosinophils[1]. Despite this well-known association, it is now appreciated that these crystals are not pathognomonic for asthma but can form anywhere in which there is an excess of eosinophil turnover.

Eosinophil-specific or secondary granules have an electron-dense core and are surrounded by an electron-lucent matrix. These granules are composed of 4 granule proteins: major basic protein (MBP), which forms part of the core; eosinophil peroxidase (EPO); eosinophil-derived neurotoxin (EDN); and eosinophil cationic protein (ECP). Several preformed chemokines, growth factors, and cytokines are also found within eosinophil-specific granules, such as IL-4, IL-2, GM-CSF, IL-5, IL-13, CCL5/regulated on activation, normal T cell expressed and secreted (RANTES), and eotaxin.[2] Small granules contain acid phosphatase and arylsulfatase. In addition, secretory vesicles, also known as microgranules, are dumbbell-shaped and contain various receptors, adhesion molecules, and albumin.

Eosinophils also contain lipid bodies, which differ from granules because they are enclosed by a phospholipid monolayer. Lipid bodies are the sites of leukotriene synthesis and their formation is induced in a variety of experimental inflammatory conditions as well as in response to various stimuli.[3]

Eosinophils use a variety of degranulation processes to selectively or completely release their cellular contents. These processes include classic exocytosis (individual granules fuse with the plasma membrane and discharge its cargo), compound exocytosis (several granules fuse together and then fuse with the plasma membrane), piecemeal degranulation (small components of granules bleb off and fuse with the plasma membrane), and eosinophil cytolysis.[4] How these processes are regulated is still being understood. In addition, eosinophils also release DNA nets or traps with intact free granules and this is a regulated pathway of extracellular trap cell death mediated by eosinophils, known as ETosis. Recently, ETosis was directly associated with formation of Charcot-Leyden crystals.[5]

Role of Eosinophils

Eosinophils are thought to be effector cells in the body's defense against parasitic infections, and the mechanism of action may differ depending on the parasite. One proposed mechanism of action is the release of toxic eosinophil granule proteins via ETosis. Other mechanisms include antibody-dependent cytotoxic cell death performed by both eosinophils and neutrophils in schistosomiasis.[6,7] Eosinophils might use similar mechanisms to cause tissue damage and inflammation in eosinophil-associated diseases.

However, eosinophil-deficient mice can clear some parasitic infections, suggesting at least redundancy in the body's antiparasite defenses.[8] More recently, eosinophils have been ascribed roles in maintaining bone marrow plasma cells, vaccine recall responses, and modulating a variety of T cell–mediated responses, as well as roles in tissue repair, glucose and fat metabolism, and perhaps tumor surveillance (reviewed in Ref.[9]). Many of these studies have been in animal models and the extension to humans has yet to be made. Murine studies also suggest that eosinophils can be divided into inflammatory or homeostatic subsets and it is unclear whether these exist in humans.

Of relevance to this article is the role that eosinophils play in the pathogenesis of allergic disease. They are physically present in the airways of patients with eosinophilic asthma, within the polyps of those with chronic rhinosinusitis with polyps, and in the gastrointestinal (GI) tract of those with eosinophilic GI disease. They can also be present in the skin of those with drug-related skin eruptions.

DEFINITIONS OF EOSINOPHILIA
Blood Eosinophilia

In general, the degree of eosinophilia is defined using the absolute eosinophil count (AEC), which refers to the number of circulating eosinophils in peripheral blood. AEC can be ascertained by multiplying the total white blood cell count (WBC) by the percentage of eosinophils. The normal range of blood eosinophils is 0 to 500 cells/mm^3 and the typical percentage is less than 5% of WBC. However, the presence of eosinophilia cannot be determined by percentage alone because leukopenia would lead to a relative increase in eosinophil percentage, and vice versa.

Humans show diurnal variation in several hematologic parameters, including blood eosinophil counts, with a recent study showing a median within-subject variability of 40 cells/mm^3 or 20%, with the peak occurring at 1 AM and the maximum at noon in those with normal range eosinophil counts.[10,11] The within-subject change of eosinophil counts in 24 hours in those with increased eosinophil counts is unknown.

Eosinophilia is defined as greater than 500 eosinophils/mm^3. The degree of eosinophilia can be categorized as mild (500–1500 cells/mm^3), moderate (1500–5000 cells/mm^3), or severe (>5000 cells/mm^3). Hypereosinophilia is defined as moderate to severe eosinophilia ($\geq$1500 cells/mm^3). To meet the definition for hypereosinophilic syndromes requires evidence of end-organ damage as a result of hypereosinophilia.

The degree of blood eosinophilia is commonly thought to be correlated with the severity or seriousness of disease, but there is no evidence to support this except anecdotal experience in persons with severe eosinophilia and hypereosinophilic syndrome. End-organ damage can occur at moderate levels of eosinophilia. A recent study describes a rare group of people with asymptomatic hypereosinophilia and no evidence of end-organ damage despite exhaustive and regular evaluation for it.[12]

Concomitant medications (eg, corticosteroids) and transient medical conditions (bacterial infection) can also mask a greater degree of eosinophilia by temporarily suppressing the AEC. Thus, clinical evaluation and context are important.

Tissue Eosinophilia

During homeostatic conditions, most eosinophils reside in tissue, with most in the GI tract except for the esophagus. They are also found in the thymus, mammary glands, and uterus. Tissue residence is regulated by tissue expression of eosinophil-recruiting chemokines, such as eotaxin-1. In pathologic conditions, eosinophils are recruited to other anatomic sites, including the lung, skin, and esophagus, and they can be further increased in sites that normally contain eosinophils, such as the stomach. However, thresholds for what is considered a pathologic increase are not well defined.

The experience with esophageal eosinophilia shows how that could change. For the purposes of research and clinical care, a consensus standard was established by a multidisciplinary group of physicians interested in eosinophilic esophagitis in 2007.[13,14] With the appropriate clinical context and symptoms, and a lack of response to a trial of high-dose proton-pump inhibitors (to treat gastric reflux disease), esophageal tissue showing a peak eosinophil count greater than or equal to 15 eosinophils per high-power field (eos/hpf) was agreed on to be the minimum standard for diagnosis of eosinophilic esophagitis. This standard was often accompanied by other histologic features, such as basal zone hyperplasia, degranulated appearance of eosinophils, and presence of eosinophilic microabscesses.

Later studies revealed an entity described as proton-pump inhibitor–responsive esophageal eosinophilia (PPI-REE) and transcriptomic studies suggest that this entity is more like eosinophilic esophagitis than gastric reflux disease.[15] Thus, the most recent guidelines suggest that a trial of high-dose proton-pump inhibitor (PPI) is not required to establish a diagnosis of eosinophilic esophagitis if the right clinical context is present.[16] PPI might be considered as an initial treatment of eosinophilic esophagitis, although whether patients with PPI-REE would retain responsiveness to this treatment remains to be determined.

Beyond the esophagus, eosinophils are normally found in the GI tract and thus may play a role in maintaining homeostasis. There are few studies describing normal GI tissue eosinophil levels.[17,18] Debrosse and colleagues[17] performed a study in a pediatric population undergoing endoscopy with biopsies that were ultimately found to be normal. They proposed using 2 times the peak eosinophil counts in each GI segment as the threshold for tissue eosinophilia. This method results in different segments of the large bowel having different cutoffs, with the ascending colon having the highest threshold for diagnosis. At present, stomach eosinophilia is defined as having 30 eos/hpf in at least 5 high-power fields for the purposes of clinical and natural history study enrollment, with a similar threshold for the small bowel. More studies are needed to determine whether eosinophil number alone, and to what threshold, defines disease in each segment of the GI tract.[19]

Interpreting Eosinophilia

As with any laboratory value, clinical context is important. Is the abnormal value a new finding and is it persistent? What are the clinical symptoms and concomitant medications associated with the laboratory abnormality, and how does that change over the course of time and/or treatment? Thus, a thorough and detailed history and physical examination are critical in this setting. Mild eosinophilia in a patient taking high-dose corticosteroid while febrile would be interpreted differently than a patient with no symptoms but found to have a moderate eosinophilia. In addition, as discussed later, whether eosinophils are pathogenic and disease causing versus being part of the cellular milieu that are recruited to the site of disease remains an open question.

CONDITIONS ASSOCIATED WITH EOSINOPHILIA

Eosinophilia is associated with several medical conditions and disease states, including allergic diseases. This section will touch on general categories and a non-exhaustive list of specific conditions, from common ones, such as a drug reaction, to rare diseases of eosinophilia, such as hypereosinophilic syndromes.

Infections

Eosinophilia is classically associated with parasitic diseases, such as helminth infections. There are reviews devoted to this topic[20] and one approach is to consider the type of patient, previous travel, and exposure history to guide evaluation. If a patient is suspected of having a parasitic infection, referral to an infectious disease specialist may be warranted.

Human immunodeficiency virus (HIV) infection can be associated with eosinophilia,[21] although there are confounding factors, such as medication usage or concomitant opportunistic or parasitic infections. In a case-control study, approximately 10% of treatment-naive patients with HIV had associated blood eosinophilia and a slightly higher HIV RNA viral load, without differences in age, sex, race, or baseline cluster of differentiation CD4 counts, compared with a control group of treatment-naive patients with HIV without blood eosinophilia.[22] The presence of a rash, including but not exclusive to eosinophilic folliculitis, was more likely in patients with blood eosinophilia in that study (46% in cases vs 25% in controls). Both tuberculous[23–25] and nontuberculous mycobacterial infections[26] are associated with eosinophilia. It is noteworthy that bacterial infections are associated with **eosinopenia**.

Treatment is targeted at the underlying infection. Infection resolution is often associated with decrease or resolution of eosinophilia, although this might not occur immediately. For example, after single-dose diethylcarbamazine or ivermectin treatment of *Loa loa* infection, posttreatment-associated eosinophilia can be observed and may take days to weeks to resolve.[27] In a study of *Strongyloides stercoralis* infection in rural India, eosinophilia was decreased 6 months posttreatment, and, in some cases, not resolved.[28] Rarely, hypereosinophilic syndrome can occur as a result of active parasitic infection,[29,30] and treatment in those cases is still aimed at the underlying infection.

Medications

Medications are the most common cause of persistent eosinophilia in the developed world, but the laboratory finding is neither sensitive nor specific for a drug reaction. In a study of inpatient acute cutaneous drug reactions (n = 55), blood eosinophilia (defined as >700 cells/mm^3) was seen in only 18% and tissue eosinophils were seen in 24% of cases.[31] Furthermore, only half of those with biopsy-proven tissue eosinophils (ie, 12% of cases) had concurrent blood eosinophilia. Thus, lack of eosinophilia in blood or eosinophils detected on tissue biopsy should not be used to rule out allergic or eosinophilic drug reaction. In addition, there are many allergic drug reactions that are not thought to be mediated by or associated with eosinophils, including classic immunoglobulin (Ig) E–mediated type 1 hypersensitivity, delayed hypersensitivity (contact dermatitis), serum sickness, and toxic epidermal necrolysis/Stevens-Johnson syndrome (SJS).

Drug reactions associated with eosinophilia can range from benign, transient eosinophilia with or without skin eruption to more severe involvement of internal organs such as in drug reaction with eosinophilia and systemic symptoms (DRESS).[32] In a single-center prospective study to investigate inpatient eosinophilic drug reactions, the incidence of eosinophil-associated drug reactions was found to be 16.67 per 10,000 admissions, with 56% of those being asymptomatic, 13% with skin and soft tissue reactions, 7% with visceral involvement, and 23% with clinical presentation consistent with DRESS.[33]

DRESS is a potentially life-threatening disease and worth discussing in more detail. It presents in a delayed fashion (weeks) after drug initiation with symptoms that include fever (90%–100%), often high-grade, along with a morbilliform rash. There can also be facial swelling in the early phase. These symptoms can be followed or accompanied by visceral involvement with the most common 2 being hepatic and lymphadenopathy, but can include myocarditis, colitis, pneumonitis, and central nervous system involvement.

Drugs commonly associated with DRESS include allopurinol, sulfasalazine, antibiotics (β-lactam antibiotics, minocycline, dapsone, sulfamethoxazole, vancomycin), anticonvulsants (lamotrigine, valproic acid, carbamazepine, phenobarbital, phenytoin), antiretroviral agents (abacavir, nevirapine, raltegravir, efavirenz), and strontium ranelate.[32]

The cause of the disease is thought to be a combination of activated CD8+ T cells directed against the drug and viruses. Laboratory findings include eosinophilia, changes in T-helper cytokine milieu, and viral reactivation such as that detected with human herpesvirus (HHV) 6 polymerase chain reaction (PCR). Recent studies are beginning to parse out the factors that are associated with specific drugs or causes. Examples include correlation of increased serum thymus and activation regulated chemokine (TARC)/CCL17 levels in patients with DRESS with HHV6 reactivation[34] and clinical/laboratory differences between those with DRESS triggered by lamotrigine versus other drugs.[35] Although there have been studies that isolate drug-specific T cells from blood and skin of patients with DRESS, there currently is no validated testing to ascertain which drug is the culprit.

Diagnosis of DRESS can be difficult because of an incomplete clinical picture or an atypical presentation, and thus diagnostic scoring systems were instituted to simplify the approach, an example being the RegiSCAR scoring system, whose criteria are listed in **Table 1**.[36,37] Treatment of mild cases of DRESS includes drug withdrawal and supportive measures. Skin manifestations can be treated with topical corticosteroids, whereas, in patients with visceral organ involvement, high-dose corticosteroids are often used. Complete recovery after drug withdrawal can take weeks to months. Prior retrospective studies describe mortalities of 5% to 10%, whereas a recent prospective study reported 2 deaths out of 117 (1.7%) during the acute phase.[37–39]

Although any medication can result in a drug reaction, there are specific ones that are more well known for causing specific reactions, such as those delineated earlier for DRESS, and in some cases this is caused by genetic susceptibility. For example, severe cutaneous adverse reactions in response to abacavir, allopurinol, carbamazepine, and nevirapine are more likely to occur in people with specific human leukocyte antigen (HLA) alleles. HLA allele testing before initiation of carbamazepine and abacavir is now recommended.

It is also important to query the patient on use of supplements and over-the-counter medications. Eosinophil myalgia syndrome was described after exposure to a contaminant in the supplement L-tryptophan in the late 1980s, and resulted in skin thickening, myalgias, and other visceral organ involvement.[40] In addition, there are also allergic drug reactions that are neither associated with eosinophilia nor eosinophil mediated, such as SJS.

Malignancy

An occult neoplasm may be associated with blood eosinophilia and, in those patients with new-onset persistent eosinophilia without a clear cause, an age-appropriate evaluation for malignancy should be undertaken. A thorough history and physical examination might reveal symptoms and findings, such as fevers, chills,

Table 1
RegiSCAR scoring system for drug reaction with eosinophilia and systemic symptoms

	Details	Scoring
Fever ≥38.5°C	Absent/or present	−1 or 0
Enlarged lymph nodes	—	—
Eosinophilia	Absent or AEC 700–1499/μL or AEC ≥1500/μL	0 or 1 or 2
Atypical lymphocytes	Absent or present	0 or 1
Skin Findings		
Skin rash extent	Absent or ≥50%	0 or 1
Skin rash suggesting DRESS	Absent or uncertain or present	−1 or 0 or 1
Biopsy suggesting DRESS	Absent or present or uncertain	−1 or 0
Organ involvement[a] Liver, kidney, lung, muscle, heart, pancreas and others	Absent or present or >1 organ	0 or 1 or 2
Resolution >15 d	Absent or present	−1 or 0
Evaluation for other causes ANA Blood culture Serology HVA/HVB/HVC Chlamydia/Mycoplasma pneumoniae Other serology/PCR	>3 other causes evaluated and negative	1

Abbreviations: AEC, absolute eosinophil count; ANA, antinuclear antibody; HVA/HVB/HVC, hepatitis virus A/B/C.
[a] After exclusion of other explanations, points are tallied.
Final score: less than 2, no case; 2 to 3, possible case; 4 to 5, probable case; greater than 5, definite case.
Adapted from Kardaun SH, Sekula P, Valeyrie-Allanore L, et al. Drug reaction with eosinophilia and systemic symptoms (DRESS): an original multisystem adverse drug reaction. Results from the prospective RegiSCAR study. Br J Dermatol 2013;169(5):1074; with permission.

weight loss, lymphadenopathy, or splenomegaly, to direct specific evaluation. Laboratory evaluation might reveal alterations in other hematologic parameters (eg, cytopenias, dysplastic-appearing cells on smear). In such cases, a hematologic cause for eosinophilia should be pursued by referral to specialists. Various forms of mastocytosis are also associated with significant eosinophilia[41,42] but, in those cases, treatment is tailored toward the mastocytosis. In addition, after the malignancy is removed or treated, eosinophilia generally does resolve. In stem cell transplants for treatment of malignancy, posttransplant eosinophilia can be seen sometimes as part of graft-versus-host disease.[43,44]

Autoimmune Disorders/Immune Dysregulation

Several autoimmune disorders are associated with mild to moderate blood eosinophilia. In some cases, eosinophils are also found at the site of disease, such as in eosinophilic granulomatosis with polyangiitis (EGPA; formerly known as Churg-Straus). It is unclear whether eosinophils are causing direct damage, are attempting to resolve the inflammation, or are innocent bystanders. In general, treatments of autoimmune disease with or without blood eosinophilia are the same. A recent phase 3 trial of anti–IL-5 therapy to treat EGPA suggests that eosinophils themselves play some pathogenic role, because there was a significant decrease in disease flares in treated patients despite tapering of concomitant corticosteroid therapy, which would target cells beyond eosinophils.[45] Anti–IL-5 is now an approved therapy for EGPA. It remains to be seen whether eosinophil-targeted therapy would be helpful in other autoimmune diseases with associated blood eosinophilia.

Primary immunodeficiencies (PIDs) are associated with eosinophilia, and infrequently these can be more apparent in adulthood, with clinical presentation consisting of an array of autoimmune disorders.[46] One explanation for the correlation is that oligoclonal/restricted lymphocyte repertoires, such as those seen in several PIDs, lead to eosinophilia and this was experimentally shown in a murine model.[47] Again, definitive treatment targets the underlying PID.

Atopic Disorders

Mild to moderate eosinophilia can be associated with a wide variety of atopic disorders, including atopic dermatitis, allergic rhinitis, and asthma. Eosinophilic GI disease (EGID), such as eosinophilic esophagitis, is diagnosed by tissue eosinophilia along with clinical context. In eosinophilic esophagitis, very mild blood eosinophilia is often seen, whereas, in eosinophilic gastroenteritis (stomach or small bowel involvement), there is reportedly moderate to severe blood eosinophilia, but larger studies are needed to confirm this.

Many of these diseases are treated with corticosteroids (topical or systemic), which target both eosinophils and other immune cells such as lymphocytes that might be the inciting cell population. In the case of EGID, empiric food elimination diets have also been used, particularly in the pediatric population, and have a 70% to 80% efficacy in eosinophilic esophagitis.[48–50]

Most recently, treatment with eosinophil-targeted therapies in a subset of eosinophilic patients with asthma using anti–IL-5 or anti–IL-5R results in increased lung function and decrease diseases flares, and now both types of biologics have been approved for use as add-on to maintenance therapies in severe asthma with eosinophilic phenotype (moderate to severe for anti–IL-5R). This finding suggests that eosinophils play a direct pathogenic role at least in certain asthma endotypes. In contrast, treatment with anti–IL-4RA (blocking both IL-4 and IL-13 signaling) in all comers with moderate to severe asthma resulted in similar clinical improvement but was accompanied by transient increases in peripheral eosinophil counts as well as serum eosinophil granule protein levels.[51] With some individual exceptions (see supplemental appendix of Ref.[51]), the resultant eosinophilia did not seem to cause harm or affect efficacy, although a subgroup analysis stratifying patients with different degrees of peripheral blood eosinophil increase was not presented.

Other Conditions: Eosinophilia can be Associated with Cholesterol Embolization, Irradiation and Adrenal Insufficiency

Eosinophilia can be associated with cholesterol embolization, irradiation and adrenal insufficiency. Hypereosinophilic syndrome (HES) is a group of rare diseases defined as having a persistent blood eosinophilia count of greater than or equal to 1500 cells/mm^3 (for at least 4 weeks, unless imminent treatment was necessary[52]) and evidence of end-organ damage as a result of this eosinophilia. This definition has evolved over the years since Chusid first described the disease.[53] One way of subdividing this group can be into clinical subtypes. In myeloid HES, there is a genetic aberration in the eosinophil and/or myeloid lineage of cells, and this is accompanied by a dysplastic appearance of the eosinophils, increased serum vitamin B_{12} and tryptase levels, and clinical findings that could include splenomegaly. In lymphoid HES there is an aberrant T-cell clonal population (often CD3dimCD4 positive) that secretes high levels of IL-5, thus promoting eosinophilia. Occasionally, patients with single organ–restricted eosinophilic diseases such as EGID have peripheral blood eosinophilia that meet HES criteria and these patients are categorized as overlap HES. Associated HES is a category used for HES that develops in the presence of a malignancy or parasitic infection, or a drug reaction. Familial HES consists of rare families with autosomal dominant inheritance of blood eosinophilia, and often without many symptoms.[54,55]

A small group of patients show hypereosinophilia but do not have discernible symptoms or end-organ damage despite deliberate evaluation for them over several years.[12] These people are deemed to have hypereosinophilia of unknown significance and remain untreated but monitored over the years.

WORK-UP FOR EOSINOPHILIA

In addition to history and physical examination, it would be useful to obtain a repeat CBC with differential (to look for persistent eosinophilia), a basic metabolic panel and liver function test, and a peripheral blood smear to examine for dysplastic-looking cells. Depending on clinical context (and urgency) and likely causes, work-up for eosinophilia differs and sometimes subspecialist referral is warranted. It would be reasonable for older patients with lymphadenopathy, fevers, weight loss, and cytopenias to be referred to a hematologist/oncologist. Patients who have eosinophilia in association with a long history of GI symptoms, such as dysphagia, should be evaluated by both a gastroenterologist and an allergist/immunologist with experience in EGIDs. In addition, young men with new evidence of cardiac dysfunction in the setting of severe eosinophilia should be urgently evaluated for myeloid HES with bone marrow biopsy and testing for the causative genetic changes, including FIP1L1-PDGFRA translocation. Summary guidelines on evaluating for HES can found in Ref.[56] and include testing such as serum tryptase, vitamin B_{12}, serum IgE and flow cytometry for aberrant T cells, as well as imaging, cardiac, and pulmonary testing when indicated.

There are no validated tests to ascertain food triggers in EGID besides repeat invasive tissue sampling, and thus it is not helpful to measure for a panel of food-specific IgE or IgG4. Measuring serum IL-5 has not been useful thus far in determining the cause of eosinophilia, although it is a predictor of response to anti–IL-5 therapy in a subset of patients with HES.[57] Furthermore, limited data indicate that serum IL-5 level is affected by medications such as corticosteroids. Eosinophil granule proteins (MBP, EDN, EPO, ECP) can be measured in the blood and other body fluids and tissues, but the exact correlations with both diagnosis and disease activity have yet to be validated.

In addition, isolated, asymptomatic blood eosinophilia can be the earliest sign of HES.[58] Prospective multicenter studies are needed to better understand how many of such patients go on to develop hypereosinophilia or HES. Initial work-up for hypereosinophilic syndromes is separately described[53] but, in brief, should include evaluation for myeloid HES if AEC is markedly increased (>5000 cells/mm^3) with blood tests (tryptase, vitamin B_{12}), genetic testing for associated mutations such as FIP1L1/PDGFRA, and bone marrow evaluation. If the clinical scenario remains concerning (male patient with increased tryptase/B_{12} level, presence of splenomegaly, and dysplastic-appearing eosinophils) despite negative gene testing, it is worthwhile to refer to an HES specialist because false-negatives have been reported.[59]

Because symptoms can occur without warning, it is useful to periodically monitor an increased eosinophil count in the absence of symptoms or evidence of end-organ damage, with quarterly or annual history and physical examination, accompanied by targeted testing. There are no published consensus recommendations as to interval testing modalities because patients can have very different types of end-organ involvement. It is reasonable to perform yearly blood work, lung function tests, and echocardiography in those with hypereosinophilia, especially in the first 5 years.[12] In those with overlap HES (eg, EGID, EGPA), increases in eosinophil counts may precede or accompany a disease flare and those counts often return to the patient's baseline with treatment. If different or new symptoms accompany that disease flare, there should be targeted evaluation of those findings to elucidate whether they are caused by a new disease process or eosinophil related.

FUTURE DIRECTIONS: ROLE OF EOSINOPHIL-TARGETED THERAPY

In the past few years, eosinophil-targeted therapy has been shown to reduce disease flares and achieved US Food and Drug Administration approval in severe eosinophilic asthma (anti–IL-5, mepolizumab [100 mg subcutaneously] and reslizumab [weight based]; anti–IL-5R, benralizumab) and EGPA (mepolizumab 300 mg subcutaneously). In cases of life-threatening, treatment-refractory hypereosinophilic syndrome, high-dose mepolizumab (300 mg up to 700 mg) can be obtained through application to the compassionate use study (NCT00244686). A small phase 2 study of benralizumab (anti–IL-5R) therapy for patients with severe hypereosinophilic syndrome showed suppression of peripheral eosinophilia and symptomatic improvement over 48 weeks in 74% of patients.[60] Larger, phase 3, multicenter trials are still needed for both biologics in HES.

Drugs that target other eosinophil membrane receptors or have eosinophil count–reducing effects without a defined mechanism are being evaluated in a variety of eosinophil-associated conditions.[61–63]

Whether the IL-5/IL-5R biologics or other eosinophil-targeting therapies will be useful in other acute or chronic eosinophil-associated diseases remains an open question. For example, would they be useful in DRESS in the acute setting? Could they block posttreatment eosinophilia and reactions during treatment of certain helminth infections? These are unexplored questions.

There is more than a decade of safety data in using anti–IL-5 therapy for hypereosinophilic syndromes from a compassionate use study.[57,64] However, the effects of long-term eosinophil depletion with anti–IL-5R (benralizumab) therapy is unknown and may be different because this therapy seems to result in a more complete depletion of eosinophils, including tissue-resident ones. In addition, eosinophils might not be pathogenic in all conditions with which they are associated.[65] It is hoped that in the next decade, the use of these new eosinophil-targeted biologics will reveal in which diseases eosinophil level reduction is beneficial.

REFERENCES

1. Sakula A. Charcot-Leyden crystals and Curschmann spirals in asthmatic sputum. Thorax 1986;41(7):503–7.
2. Davoine F, Lacy P. Eosinophil cytokines, chemokines, and growth factors: emerging roles in immunity. Front Immunol 2014;5:570.
3. Melo RCN, Weller PF. Unraveling the complexity of lipid body organelles in human eosinophils. J Leukoc Biol 2014;96(5):703–12.
4. Spencer LA, Bonjour K, Melo RCN, et al. Eosinophil secretion of granule-derived cytokines. Front Immunol 2014;5:496.

5. Ueki S, Tokunaga T, Melo RCN, et al. Charcot-Leyden crystal formation is closely associated with eosinophil extracellular trap cell death. Blood 2018;132(20): 2183–7.
6. Sher A, Butterworth AE, Colley DG, et al. Immune responses during human schistosomiasis mansoni. II. Occurrence of eosinophil-dependent cytotoxic antibodies in relation to intensity and duration of infection. Am J Trop Med Hyg 1977;26(5 Pt 1):909–16.
7. Moser G, Sher A. Studies of the antibody-dependent killing of schistosomula of Schistosoma mansoni employing haptenic target antigens. II. In vitro killing of TNP-schistosomula by human eosinophils and neutrophils. J Immunol 1981; 126(3):1025–9.
8. Lee JJ, Rosenberg HF, editors. Eosinophils in health and disease. Elsevier; 2012.
9. Weller PF, Spencer LA. Functions of tissue-resident eosinophils. Nat Rev Immunol 2017;17(12):746–60.
10. Hilderink JM, Klinkenberg LJJ, Aakre KM, et al. Within-day biological variation and hour-to-hour reference change values for hematological parameters. Clin Chem Lab Med 2017;55(7):1013–24.
11. Sennels HP, Jørgensen HL, Hansen A-LS, et al. Diurnal variation of hematology parameters in healthy young males: the Bispebjerg study of diurnal variations. Scand J Clin Lab Invest 2011;71(7):532–41.
12. Chen Y-YK, Khoury P, Ware JM, et al. Marked and persistent eosinophilia in the absence of clinical manifestations. J Allergy Clin Immunol 2014;133(4):1195–202.
13. Furuta GT, Liacouras CA, Collins MH, et al. Eosinophilic esophagitis in children and adults: a systematic review and consensus recommendations for diagnosis and treatment. Gastroenterology 2007;133(4):1342–63.
14. Liacouras CA, Furuta GT, Hirano I, et al. Eosinophilic esophagitis: updated consensus recommendations for children and adults. J Allergy Clin Immunol 2011;128(1):3–20.e6 [quiz: 21].
15. Molina-Infante J, Bredenoord AJ, Cheng E, et al. Proton pump inhibitor-responsive oesophageal eosinophilia: an entity challenging current diagnostic criteria for eosinophilic oesophagitis. Gut 2016;65(3):524–31.
16. Dellon ES, Liacouras CA, Molina-Infante J, et al. Updated international consensus diagnostic criteria for eosinophilic esophagitis: proceedings of the AGREE conference. Gastroenterology 2018;155(4):1022–33.e10.
17. DeBrosse CW, Case JW, Putnam PE, et al. Quantity and distribution of eosinophils in the gastrointestinal tract of children. Pediatr Dev Pathol 2006;9(3):210–8.
18. Lwin T, Melton SD, Genta RM. Eosinophilic gastritis: histopathological characterization and quantification of the normal gastric eosinophil content. Mod Pathol 2011;24(4):556–63.
19. Khoury P, Akuthota P, Ackerman SJ, et al. Revisiting the NIH taskforce on the research needs of eosinophil-associated diseases (RE-TREAD). J Leukoc Biol 2018;104(1):69–83.
20. O'Connell EM, Nutman TB. Eosinophilia in infectious diseases. Immunol Allergy Clin North Am 2015;35(3):493–522.
21. Chou A, Serpa JA. Eosinophilia in patients infected with human immunodeficiency virus. Curr Hiv/AIDS Rep 2015;12(3):313–6.
22. Al Mohajer M, Villarreal-Williams E, Andrade RA, et al. Eosinophilia and associated factors in a large cohort of patients infected with human immunodeficiency virus. South Med J 2014;107(9):554–8.
23. Flores M, Merino-Angulo J, Tanago JG, et al. Late generalized tuberculosis and eosinophilia. Arch Intern Med 1983;143(1):182.

24. Vijayan VK, Reetha AM, Jawahar MS, et al. Pulmonary eosinophilia in pulmonary tuberculosis. Chest 1992;101(6):1708–9.
25. Driss V, Legrand F, Hermann E, et al. TLR2-dependent eosinophil interactions with mycobacteria: role of alpha-defensins. Blood 2009;113(14):3235–44.
26. Pfeffer PE, Hopkins S, Cropley I, et al. An association between pulmonary Mycobacterium avium-intracellulare complex infections and biomarkers of Th2-type inflammation. Respir Res 2017;18(1):93.
27. Herrick JA, Legrand F, Gounoue R, et al. Posttreatment reactions after single-dose diethylcarbamazine or ivermectin in subjects with loa loa infection. Clin Infect Dis 2017;64(8):1017–25.
28. Rajamanickam A, Munisankar S, Bhootra Y, et al. Elevated systemic levels of eosinophil, neutrophil, and mast cell granular proteins in strongyloides stercoralis infection that diminish following treatment. Front Immunol 2018;9:207.
29. Nutman TB, Miller KD, Mulligan M, et al. Loa loa infection in temporary residents of endemic regions: recognition of a hyperresponsive syndrome with characteristic clinical manifestations. J Infect Dis 1986;154(1):10–8.
30. Thaden J, Cassar A, Vaa B, et al. Eosinophilic endocarditis and Strongyloides stercoralis. Am J Cardiol 2013;112(3):461–2.
31. Romagosa R, Kapoor S, Sanders J, et al. Inpatient adverse cutaneous drug eruptions and eosinophilia. Arch Dermatol 2001;137(4):511–2.
32. Kuruvilla M, Khan DA. Eosinophilic drug allergy. Clin Rev Allergy Immunol 2016; 50(2):228–39.
33. Ramírez E, Medrano-Casique N, Tong HY, et al. Eosinophilic drug reactions detected by a prospective pharmacovigilance programme in a tertiary hospital. Br J Clin Pharmacol 2017;83(2):400–15.
34. Ogawa K, Morito H, Hasegawa A, et al. Elevated serum thymus and activation-regulated chemokine (TARC/CCL17) relates to reactivation of human herpesvirus 6 in drug reaction with eosinophilia and systemic symptoms (DRESS)/drug-induced hypersensitivity syndrome (DIHS). Br J Dermatol 2014;171(2):425–7.
35. Tashiro Y, Azukizawa H, Asada H, et al. Drug-induced hypersensitivity syndrome/drug reaction with eosinophilia and systemic symptoms due to lamotrigine differs from that due to other drugs. J Dermatol 2019;46(3):226–33.
36. Kardaun SH, Sidoroff A, Valeyrie-Allanore L, et al. Variability in the clinical pattern of cutaneous side-effects of drugs with systemic symptoms: does a DRESS syndrome really exist? Br J Dermatol 2007;156(3):609–11.
37. Kardaun SH, Sekula P, Valeyrie-Allanore L, et al. Drug reaction with eosinophilia and systemic symptoms (DRESS): an original multisystem adverse drug reaction. Results from the prospective RegiSCAR study. Br J Dermatol 2013;169(5): 1071–80.
38. Chen Y-C, Chiu H-C, Chu C-Y. Drug reaction with eosinophilia and systemic symptoms: a retrospective study of 60 cases. Arch Dermatol 2010;146(12): 1373–9.
39. Cacoub P, Musette P, Descamps V, et al. The DRESS syndrome: a literature review. Am J Med 2011;124(7):588–97.
40. Eosinophilia-myalgia syndrome—New Mexico. JAMA 1989;262(22):3116.
41. Böhm A, Födinger M, Wimazal F, et al. Eosinophilia in systemic mastocytosis: clinical and molecular correlates and prognostic significance. J Allergy Clin Immunol 2007;120(1):192–9.
42. Maric I, Robyn J, Metcalfe DD, et al. KIT D816V-associated systemic mastocytosis with eosinophilia and FIP1L1/PDGFRA-associated chronic eosinophilic leukemia are distinct entities. J Allergy Clin Immunol 2007;120(3):680–7.

43. Kalaycioglu ME, Bolwell BJ. Eosinophilia after allogeneic bone marrow transplantation using the busulfan and cyclophosphamide preparative regimen. Bone Marrow Transplant 1994;14(1):113–5.
44. Bush JW, Mohammad S, Melin-Aldana H, et al. Eosinophilic density in graft biopsies positive for rejection and blood eosinophil count can predict development of post-transplant digestive tract eosinophilia. Pediatr Transplant 2016;20(4):540–51.
45. Wechsler ME, Akuthota P, Jayne D, et al. Mepolizumab or placebo for eosinophilic granulomatosis with polyangiitis. N Engl J Med 2017;376(20):1921–32.
46. Williams KW, Milner JD, Freeman AF. Eosinophilia associated with disorders of immune deficiency or immune dysregulation. Immunol Allergy Clin North Am 2015;35(3):523–44.
47. Milner JD, Ward JM, Keane-Myers A, et al. Lymphopenic mice reconstituted with limited repertoire T cells develop severe, multiorgan, Th2-associated inflammatory disease. Proc Natl Acad Sci U S A 2007;104(2):576–81.
48. Lucendo AJ, Arias Á, González-Cervera J, et al. Empiric 6-food elimination diet induced and maintained prolonged remission in patients with adult eosinophilic esophagitis: a prospective study on the food cause of the disease. J Allergy Clin Immunol 2013;131(3):797–804.
49. Molina-Infante J, Arias Á, Alcedo J, et al. Step-up empiric elimination diet for pediatric and adult eosinophilic esophagitis: the 2-4-6 study. J Allergy Clin Immunol 2018;141(4):1365–72.
50. Kagalwalla AF, Sentongo TA, Ritz S, et al. Effect of six-food elimination diet on clinical and histologic outcomes in eosinophilic esophagitis. Clin Gastroenterol Hepatol 2006;4(9):1097–102.
51. Castro M, Corren J, Pavord ID, et al. Dupilumab efficacy and safety in moderate-to-severe uncontrolled asthma. N Engl J Med 2018;378(26):2486–96.
52. Valent P, Klion AD, Horny H-P, et al. Contemporary consensus proposal on criteria and classification of eosinophilic disorders and related syndromes. J Allergy Clin Immunol 2012;130(3):607–12.e9.
53. Chusid MJ, Dale DC, West BC, et al. The hypereosinophilic syndrome: analysis of fourteen cases with review of the literature. Medicine (Baltimore) 1975;54(1):1–27.
54. Prakash Babu S, Chen YYK, Bonne-Annee S, et al. Dysregulation of interleukin 5 expression in familial eosinophilia. Allergy 2017;72(9):1338–45.
55. Klion AD, Law MA, Riemenschneider W, et al. Familial eosinophilia: a benign disorder? Blood 2004;103(11):4050–5.
56. Klion AD. How I treat hypereosinophilic syndromes. Blood 2015;126(9):1069–77.
57. Kuang FL, Fay MP, Ware J, et al. Long-term clinical outcomes of high-dose mepolizumab treatment for hypereosinophilic syndrome. J Allergy Clin Immunol Pract 2018;6(5):1518–27.e5.
58. Ogbogu PU, Bochner BS, Butterfield JH, et al. Hypereosinophilic syndrome: a multicenter, retrospective analysis of clinical characteristics and response to therapy. J Allergy Clin Immunol 2009;124(6):1319–25.e3.
59. Pongdee T, Khoury P, Klion AD. Myeloproliferative hypereosinophilic syndrome: retrospective analysis of cytogenetic and molecular features. J Allergy Clin Immunol 2018;141(2):AB277.
60. Kuang FL, Legrand F, Makiya M, et al. Benralizumab for PDGFRA-negative hypereosinophilic syndrome. N Engl J Med 2019;380(14):1336–46.
61. Legrand F, Klion AD. Biologic therapies targeting eosinophils: current status and future prospects. J Allergy Clin Immunol Pract 2015;3(2):167–74.

62. Panch SR, Bozik ME, Brown T, et al. Dexpramipexole as an oral steroid-sparing agent in hypereosinophilic syndromes. Blood 2018;132(5):501–9.
63. Laidlaw TM, Prussin C, Panettieri RA, et al. Dexpramipexole depletes blood and tissue eosinophils in nasal polyps with no change in polyp size. Laryngoscope 2019;129(2):E61–6.
64. Roufosse FE, Kahn J-E, Gleich GJ, et al. Long-term safety of mepolizumab for the treatment of hypereosinophilic syndromes. J Allergy Clin Immunol 2013;131(2): 461–7.e1.
65. Lee JJ, Jacobsen EA, McGarry MP, et al. Eosinophils in health and disease: the LIAR hypothesis. Clin Exp Allergy 2010;40(4):563–75.

Approach to the Patient with Hives

Justin Greiwe, MD[a,b], Jonathan A. Bernstein, MD[a,b],*

KEYWORDS

- Chronic spontaneous urticaria • Inducible urticaria • Acute urticaria • Guidelines
- Treatment algorithm • Differential diagnosis

KEY POINTS

- Acute urticaria has been defined as lasting less than 6 weeks whereas chronic spontaneous urticaria persists more than 6 weeks.
- Chronic spontaneous urticaria is more common in women (2:1), typically begins in the third to fifth decades of life, and is a self-limited disorder in most patients, with the average duration of disease 1 to 5 years.
- Initial treatment includes a second-generation H1-receptor antagonist followed by incremental dose advancement up to 4 times the US Food and Drug Administration approved dose and/or adding an H2-antagonist or leukotriene receptor antagonist if therapy is ineffective.
- If hives are persistent then referral to an urticaria specialist is recommended for consideration of alternative therapies including omalizumab or cyclosporine.

INTRODUCTION

Urticaria is a common presenting clinical condition that the internist should be comfortable initially evaluating and treating but recognize that referral to a specialist is appropriate for further management when initial approaches are not effective or well tolerated by the patient. Urticaria episodes are usually of sudden onset, very pruritic, and evanescent meaning lesions come and go over 24 to 48 hours and reappear in different parts of the body. Acute urticaria has been defined as lasting less than 6 weeks whereas chronic spontaneous urticaria (CSU) persists for more than 6 weeks. CSU is more common in women (2:1) and typically begins in the third to fifth decades of life.[1–4] The economic burden of this condition is significant, with both direct and indirect

Disclosure Statement: J. Bernstein – PI, Consultant and Speaker for Novartis, Genentech, Sanofi-Regeneron, Astra Zeneca, Shire, CSL Behring, Pharming; PI and Consultant with Biocryst, Merck; Consultant and Speaker with Kalvista, Optinose.
^a University of Cincinnati Department of Internal Medicine, Division of Immunology, Allergy Section, University of Cincinnati, 231 Albert Sabin Way, ML#563, Cincinnati, OH 45267, USA;
^b Bernstein Allergy Group, 8444 Winton Road, Cincinnati, OH 45231, USA
* Corresponding author. 231 Albert Sabin Way, ML#563, Cincinnati, OH 45267.
E-mail address: jonathan.bernstein@uc.edu

Med Clin N Am 104 (2020) 15–24
https://doi.org/10.1016/j.mcna.2019.08.010
0025-7125/20/© 2019 Elsevier Inc. All rights reserved.
medical.theclinics.com

costs (ie, absenteeism defined as missed days from work and presenteeism defined as patients going to work but being less productive), although the absolute health care costs on our health care system are not known. One study from the UK estimated that the annual direct health care costs approximated a mean total cost of €2050 (US$2664).[5] This included medication use, outpatient office visits, emergency department/hospital costs, laboratory tests, and indirect costs including loss of earnings because of travel to outpatient visits and absenteeism from work A more recent European study found that costs seem to vary between countries from approximately €2400 in Italy (approximately US$2700) to almost €9000 (approximately US$10.121) in France based on purchasing power parity dollars.[6] From the patient's perspective, this condition can severely affect daily functioning and quality of life, with impairment comparable to other conditions such as ischemic heart disease and depression, with patients feeling a similar lack of energy, social isolation, and emotional distress.[7,8]

The 2 cases illustrated here are representative of common clinical presentations of patients with hives and should be reflected upon while reading this article.

CASE PRESENTATION I

A 32-year-old woman presents to the office with a history of sudden onset of hives that began after taking amoxicillin for a sinus infection. The hives began 2 days after completing a 10-day treatment course. The hives were irregularly shaped, polymorphic in size, raised, and extremely pruritic. They involved her face, neck, torso, arms, and upper legs. The hives would come and go over 24 hours and did not leave any scars. She noted some swelling of her lips and felt a constriction in her throat. She initially went to the emergency department, was treated with corticosteroids and antihistamines, and was told to follow up with her primary care physician. She was also given an epinephrine injector and told to avoid penicillin in the future. On presentation to her primary care provider, the hives had returned 1 day off corticosteroids, covered 50% of her, body and were very pruritic. She was miserable, and the hives were affecting both her work and sleep. She was unable to tolerate diphenhydramine owing to sedation. Her past medical history is remarkable for chronic rhinitis complicated by 3 to 4 sinus infections a year requiring frequent antibiotics. She has never had trouble taking penicillin or related derivatives. She is otherwise healthy without any known chronic medical problems.

CASE PRESENTATION II

A 62-year-old man with adult-onset diabetes mellitus presents with a history of hives for the past 2 years. The hives are persistent, evanescent, and aggravated by scratching. He is unable to relate the onset of the hives to medications or foods and denies any history of thyroid disease, autoimmune disorders, chronic infections, or malignancies. He has no associated lip, face, or tongue swelling. The hives respond to corticosteroids but he does not like taking them owing to his underlying diabetes. His medical history includes hypertension and hypercholesterolemia. His diabetes is controlled with oral medication and diet. He has dry skin and does not moisturize on a regular basis. He has tried daily antihistamines, which helps with the itch but does not prevent the hives from erupting.

TERMINOLOGY

The terminology related to urticaria is evolving. Chronic urticaria with no identified cause was referred to as idiopathic chronic urticaria. However, recent international guidelines endorsed by both the American Academy of Allergy, Asthma and Immunology and the American College of Allergy, Asthma and Immunology advocate using the term CSU with the terms intermittent or persistent to clinically describe this condition. The rationale for not using the term idiopathic is that it does not describe the clinical nature of the urticarial eruption, but rather refers to an unknown pathogenesis, which may or may not be the case when a patient presents to the clinic. Similarly, in discussing physical urticaria, consensus recommendations favor using the term chronic inducible urticaria, because many of the triggers identified to cause physical urticaria are not physical in nature but rather related to the autonomic nervous system such as cholinergic or adrenergic urticaria. It is also recommended to describe chronic urticaria as the presence of wheals, the presence of angioedema, or both because 40% of chronic urticaria presents with wheals alone, 40% with wheals and angioedema, and 20% with angioedema only.[9] **Fig. 1** summarizes the terminology recommended when discussing urticaria with patients or colleagues.[2]

PATHOGENESIS

There is still a poor understanding of the pathomechanisms related to CSU. Further research is needed to elucidate relevant biologic pathways and biomarkers that would predict responsiveness or unresponsiveness to conventional therapy with H1 antihistamines. It has been demonstrated that autoantibodies to the high-affinity IgE receptors on mast cells and basophils are prevalent in patients with CSU, but the clinical relevance of these antibodies remains unclear. Studies have been inconclusive as to whether certain therapies work better in patients with or without these antibodies.[10–12] However, with the advent of biologic therapies that target specific immune pathways for treatment of CSU, a better understanding of the relevance of IgE, effector cells such as mast cells, basophils and eosinophils, cytokines, cytokine receptors, and related biologic pathways is being increasingly recognized.

CLINICAL PRESENTATION

Urticaria is described as pruritic eruptions with serpiginous circumscribed borders that are usually raised, erythematous and blanching involving the superficial dermis. Lesions usually vary in size with each individual hive lasting minutes to hours (usually <24 hours). Approximately 20% of individuals experience acute spontaneous urticaria at some point in their life and up to 1% to 3% continue to have chronic spontaneous persistent or intermittent urticaria.[13] When urticaria occurs acutely, it is often difficult for clinicians to differentiate it from anaphylaxis because patients may report throat

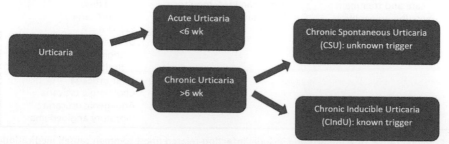

Fig. 1. Classification of urticaria based on the duration and the presence of triggering factors.

tightness and dyspnea. For this reason, in these situations, patients are often treated with oral corticosteroids, H1-antihistamines, and sometimes epinephrine. Furthermore, they may often be told empirically that medications (ie, nonsteroidal anti-inflammatory drugs [NSAIDs], aspirin, antibiotics, etc) or foods are responsible for the episode. Many times, these turn out to be associations versus cause and effect after a more thorough history and appropriate diagnostic testing excludes these suspected agents as triggers. It is important to recognize that complete avoidance of a suspected causative trigger should resolve the hives. If urticaria persists despite strict avoidance, it is possible that hives can persist for a short period of time before completely resolving; however, if they persist for a longer time period it is unlikely that the suspected agent is causative. It is crucial not to reinforce these associations because this further confuses the patient while increasing their anxiety and frustration, and often leads to a long list of erroneous drug and/or food allergies that can confound their general medical care and impact their quality of life. **Table 1** details the clinical approach to a patient who presents with urticaria as portrayed in the 2 case presentations, considering initial presentation, potential triggers, and duration of illness.

EVALUATION AND DIAGNOSIS

CSU is a clinical diagnosis based on the episodic and transient appearance of characteristic urticarial lesions with or without angioedema. A detailed history and physical examination are the cornerstones of the initial evaluation with a focus on the signs and symptoms associated with the lesions, duration of individual lesions, and accompanying angioedema. If symptoms and time course are consistent with CSU, then a more detailed clinical history focusing on identifying possible underlying causes and excluding a more serious systemic disease is indicated. Urticarial vasculitis is a rare form of chronic urticaria (0.1% of cases) confirmed by skin biopsy when patients have lesions that persist longer than 48 hours. However, a subsequent biopsy study

Table 1
Clinical approach to a patient presenting with urticaria

	Urticaria	
Anaphylaxis	**Acute (<6 weeks)**	**Chronic (>6 weeks)**
Urticaria and angioedema associated with signs/symptoms in organs other than the skin (pulmonary, cardiac, gastrointestinal) Appropriate emergency care and treatment Prescribe epinephrine autoinjector and refer to an allergist	Identifiable cause like a food or drug allergy[a] *Yes:* Avoid trigger, treat with antihistamines, refer to allergist *No:* Treat with antihistamines, monitor for resolution	*No obvious trigger:* CSU *Known physical trigger:* chronic inducible urticaria Dermatographism Heat urticaria (hot showers, extreme humidity) Cold urticaria Exercise Delayed-pressure urticaria/angioedema (tight clothing or straps) Solar urticaria Cholinergic urticaria Aquagenic urticaria Vibratory angioedema

[a] Common causes of acute urticaria include: infection-related (most common cause), medication-related, food-related, and contact-related. The majority of acute episodes do not go on to become a chronic issue.

found that even patients with traditional evanescent hives that dissipate over 24 to 48 hours can have a diagnosis of urticarial vasculitis. This caveat represents another reason to refer a patient refractory to treatment to an urticaria specialist for further evaluation and management. **Box 1** summarizes important components of a comprehensive clinical evaluation.[14]

A diagnostic algorithm for differentiating histaminergic and nonhistaminergic urticaria and/or angioedema is summarized in **Fig. 2**.[2,23]

TESTING

Routine laboratory tests for the evaluation of CSU is not recommended unless the clinical history suggests an underlying allergic etiology (ie, food or drug) or the presence of an underlying systemic disease such as thyroid disease, autoimmune diseases, chronic infections, and rarely malignancies. In general, broad panel serum specific-IgE or skin testing to foods or aeroallergens is not recommended.[1,23] In patients with a history of allergic rhinitis and testing is required to assess for allergen sensitization, serologic testing is recommended as skin testing can often be difficult to interpret correctly. If there is a concern about food allergy as a contributing cause, it is recommended that these patients be referred to an urticaria specialist for further evaluation before ordering extensive serologic food testing, which can lead to false-positive testing and obfuscate the patient's evaluation and management.

Box 1
Important components of a comprehensive clinical evaluation in a patient presenting with chronic urticarial lesions

Past medical history: recent foreign travel, infections, sexual history, and history of other atopic conditions.

Signs and symptoms of systemic disease: fever, weight loss, arthralgias, arthritis, cold or heat sensitivity, abdominal pain, or bone pain (autoimmune disorders including systemic lupus erythematosus, Sjogren syndrome, chronic urticarial vasculitis, dermatomyositis and polymyositis, and Still disease have been associated with CSU).

Possible triggers
- Inducible stimuli: exercise, heat, cold, and pressure.
- Newly administered drugs: antibiotics, NSAIDs, and hormonal therapies; NSAIDs worsen symptoms in 25% to 50% of patients with CSU.[15]
- Alcohol.
- Emotional stress and trauma: worsening hives often correlate with periods of physical or psychological stress.[16,17] Whether emotional stress is a cause or the result of hives is still debated however, rarely does treating underlying stress with nonhistaminic therapies resolve hives.[18]

Debate about diet: patients often identify foods as possible triggers for their symptoms and make dietary decisions without enough information. The interactions between diet and CSU is not fully understood and current guidelines do not advise dietary modifications to better control CSU owing to poor evidence in the medical literature and difficulty in adherence.[1]
- Pseudoallergen-free diet refers to avoidance of food additives like artificial preservatives, aromatic chemicals and dyes in processed foods and certain fruits, vegetables, seafood, spices, and a low histamine diet refers to avoiding foods high in vasoactive substances such as histamine have been advocated for initial treatment of patient by some investigators but the scientific data supporting these interventions is low.[19-21] Furthermore, while instituting dietary changes seems like a relatively benign recommendation, adhering to unnecessarily restrictive diets can potentially have a negative impact on the patient's quality of life and nutritional status.[22]

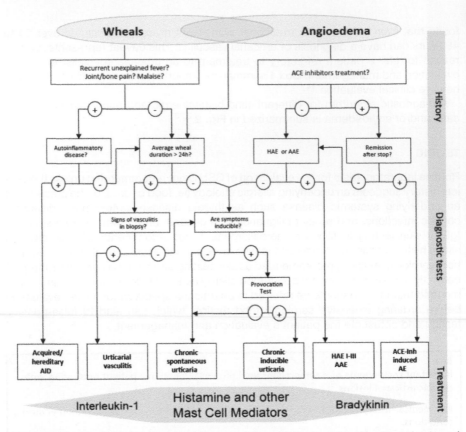

Fig. 2. Diagnostic algorithm for histaminergic and nonhistaminergic urticaria, urticaria and angioedema, or angioedema alone. AAE, acquired angioedema due to C1-inhibitor deficiency; AE, angioedema; ACE-Inh, angiotensin-converting enzyme inhibitor; AID, auto-inflammatory disease; HAE, hereditary angioedema. (*Adapted from* Zuberbier T, Aberer W, Asero R, et.al. The EAACI/GA^{2}LEN/EDF/WAO guideline for the definition, classification, diagnosis and management of urticaria. Allergy 2018;73(7):1400; with permission.)

ASSOCIATED CONDITIONS

There are several other clinical conditions, specifically autoimmune conditions, that have been associated with CSU. These disorders make up a small proportion of patients with chronic hives; therefore, screening tests to assess for autoimmune diseases and other rare conditions are not recommended during the initial evaluation unless there are clinical features or suspicions indicative of concurrent disease. A number of studies have associated thyroid autoantibodies, *Helicobacter pylori* infections, and celiac disease with CSU however, the quality of evidence supporting these relationships is weak.[1,23] Furthermore, clinical studies advocating treatment of these conditions, such as euthyroid patients with thyroid autoantibodies who are treated with thyroid supplementation, is considered highly controversial and not supported by the current medical literature.

TREATMENT

The most recent Joint Task Force (JTF) Practice Parameter for CSU recommends an algorithmic treatment approach detailed in **Box 2.**[1] Initial treatment includes a second-

---

Box 2
Updated step care approach to the management of chronic urticaria

Step 1: Monotherapy with second-generation antihistamine, avoidance of triggers (NSAIDs and relevant physical factors if present)

Step 2: Dose advancement of second-generation antihistamine used in step 1[a]
  Add another second-generation antihistamine
  Add an H2 antagonist
  Add a leukotriene receptor antagonist (montelukast [Singulair], zafirlukast)
  Add a first-generation antihistamine to be taken at bedtime[b]

Step 3: Dose advancement of potent antihistamines (eg, hydroxyzine or doxepin) as tolerated. Failure of steps 1 to 3: patients meet the definition of refractory CSU (not adequately controlled on maximal antihistamine therapy)

Step 4: Add an alternative agent
  Biologic (Omalizumab)
  Immunosuppressants (eg, cyclosporine)
  Other anti-inflammatory agents (eg, hydroxychloroquine, sulfasalazine, colchicine)
  Chronic, high-dose systemic corticosteroids should be avoided however short courses for 7 to 10 days are appropriate for severe hives

[a] Maximum dose of second-generation antihistamine, up to 4× the recommended US Food and Drug Administration dose.
[b] Patients with CSU and dermatographism had a 16 times higher odds of a favorable response to a first- or second-generation H1 antagonist[11,24]
Adapted from Bernstein JA, Lang DM, Khan DA, et al. The diagnosis and management of acute and chronic urticaria: 2014 update. J Allergy Clin Immunol 2014;133(5):1276; with permission.

---

generation H1-receptor antagonist followed by incremental dose advancements and/ or adding an H2-antagonist or leukotriene-modifying agent if therapy is ineffective.

The more recent International Urticaria Guidelines recommend a similar approach to steps 1 and 2 therapies, but do not advocate the use of H2 antagonists or a leukotriene-modifying agent owing to the low level of supporting clinical evidence.[23] **Fig. 3** compares the treatment recommendations advocated by the JTF Practice Parameters and the recently updated international chronic urticaria guidelines.

These treatment algorithms differ in many respects largely because the International Guidelines use GRADE methodology for determining evidence-based treatment recommendations, whereas the JTF guidelines used an evidence-based approach coupled with expert consensus to generate recommendations. The major differences between these guidelines, in addition to not advocating H2 antagonists and leukotriene-modifying agent, are that the international guidelines do not advocate first-generation or combination antihistamines, which cause significant sedation and can impact motor and cognitive skills, making it difficult for many patients to tolerate while working or at school. Furthermore, there is no difference between first and second generation antihistamines with respect to the antihistaminergic activity. If first-generation antihistamines such as doxepin and hydroxyzine are used to treat hives, they should be administered at bedtime at the lowest possible dose. Patients should be monitored regularly for side effects and once hives are well-controlled, stepping down on these agents is advisable. Caution should be exercised using these agents in older patients who are more susceptible to their anticholinergic side effects and the risk for cognitive decline. As with any medication, side effects should be discussed with the patient and whether or not to use them should be based on shared decision making that weigh benefits versus risks with patient preference. In addition, step 3

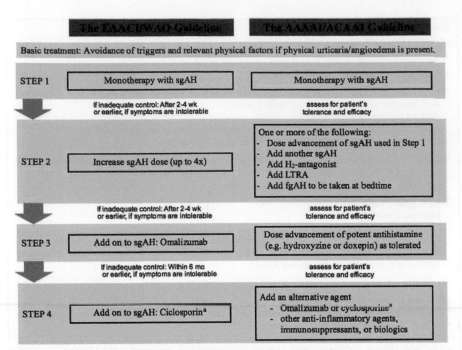

Fig. 3. Comparison of treatment algorithms between the international and American Academy of Allergy Asthma and Immunology (AAAAI)/American College of Allergy, Asthma & Immunology (ACAAI) guidelines. EAACI, European Academy of Allergology and Clinical Immunology; fgAH, first-generation antihistamine; LTRA, leukotriene receptor antagonist; sgAH, second-generation antihistamine; WAO, World Allergy Organization. [a] Different spellings as used in the respective guideline. Additional comments: EAACI/WAO: A short course of corticosteroids may be considered in case of severe exacerbation. AAAAI/ACAAI: Begin treatment at step appropriate for patient's level of severity and treatment history; step-down treatment is appropriate at any step, once consistent control of urticaria/angioedema is achieved. (*Adapted from* Zuberbier T, Bernstein JA. A Comparison of the United States and International Perspective on Chronic Urticaria Guidelines. J Allergy Clin Immunol Pract 2018;6(4):1148; with permission.)

treatment for the international guidelines advocates using omalizumab, an anti-IgE monoclonal antibody, approved for the treatment of CSU. Evidence supporting this treatment as first-line treatment of CSU after high-dose second-generation antihistamines was not available at the time of the publication of the JTF guideline. Finally, step 4 therapy for the international guideline advocates cyclosporin, whereas step 4 for the JTF guideline recommends a choice between omalizumab, cyclosporin, or other anti-inflammatory therapies such as hydroxychloroquine, dapsone, colchicine, or sulfasalazine to name a few.[23] Owing to the low quality of scientific evidence, these therapies have been recommended as alternative therapies by the international guidelines if steps 1 to 4 are not effective.[2,23] However, for the purpose of this review, discussion of treatment should focus on steps 1 and 2 only, as need for step 3 and 4 therapy should prompt referral to an urticaria allergy or dermatology specialist. It is important for the primary care physician to have a close working relationship with an urticarial specialist because only approximately 45% to 60% of patients achieve an adequate therapeutic response from steps 1 and 2.[25]

SUMMARY

Urticaria is a frequently encountered problem in the primary care setting in children and adults and therefore a better understanding of terminology and clinical course is important to provide optimal patient care. The evaluation of urticaria in the primary care setting can be complicated because patients present with an assortment of concerns for possible triggers and varied presentations. When obvious causes have been ruled out and symptoms persist despite maximizing step 1 and 2 therapy, referral to an urticaria specialist is indicated. With CSU affecting 1% to 3% of the general population, optimal care that completely controls the hives can significantly reduce the direct and indirect medical costs associated with this condition while improving patient quality of life.

REFERENCES

1. Bernstein JA, Lang DM, Khan DA, et al. The diagnosis and management of acute and chronic urticaria: 2014 update. J Allergy Clin Immunol 2014;133(5):1270–7.
2. Zuberbier T, Aberer W, Asero R, et al. The EAACI/GA²LEN/EDF/WAO guideline for the definition, classification, diagnosis and management of urticaria. Allergy 2018;73(7):1393–414.
3. Sanchez-Borges M, Asero R, Ansotegui IJ, et al. Diagnosis and treatment of urticaria and angioedema: a worldwide perspective. World Allergy Organ J 2012; 5:125–47.
4. Greaves M. Chronic urticaria. J Allergy Clin Immunol 2000;105:664–72.
5. O'Donnell BF. Urticaria: impact on quality of life and economic cost. Immunol Allergy Clin North Am 2014;34(1):89–104.
6. Maurer M, Abuzakouk M, Bérard F, et al. The burden of chronic spontaneous urticaria is substantial: real-world evidence from ASSURE-CSU. Allergy 2017; 72(12):2005–16.
7. O'Donnell BF, Lawlor F, Simpson J, et al. The impact of chronic urticaria on the quality of life. Br J Dermatol 1997;136:197–201.
8. Grob JJ, Gaudy-Marqueste C. Urticaria and quality of life. Clin Rev Allergy Immunol 2006;30:47–51.
9. Greiwe J, Bernstein JA. Therapy of antihistamine-resistant chronic spontaneous urticaria. Expert Rev Clin Immunol 2017;13(4):311–8.
10. Bagenstose SE, Levin L, Bernstein JA. The addition of zafirlukast to cetirizine improves the treatment of chronic urticaria in patients with positive autologous serum skin test results. J Allergy Clin Immunol 2004;113(1):134–40.
11. Amin P, Levin L, Holmes SJ, et al. Investigation of patient-specific characteristics associated with treatment outcomes for chronic urticaria. J Allergy Clin Immunol Pract 2015;3(3):400–7.
12. Metz M, Staubach P, Bauer A, et al. Clinical efficacy of omalizumab in chronic spontaneous urticaria is associated with a reduction of FcεRI-positive cells in the skin. Theranostics 2017;7(5):1266–76.
13. Kaplan AP. Urticaria and angioedema. In: Adkinson NF, Bochner BS, Busse WW, et al, editors. Middleton's allergy: principles and practice, 2, 7th edition. St Louis (MO): Mosby; 2009. p. 1063.
14. Saini S. Chronic spontaneous urticaria: clinical manifestations, diagnosis, pathogenesis, and natural history. Callen J, ed. UpToDate. Waltham (MA): UpToDate Inc. Available at: https://www.uptodate.com. Accessed March 07, 2019.
15. Grattan CE. Aspirin sensitivity and urticaria. Clin Exp Dermatol 2003;28(2):123–7.

16. Staubach P, Dechene M, Metz M, et al. High prevalence of mental disorders and emotional distress in patients with chronic spontaneous urticaria. Acta Derm Venereol 2011;91(5):557–61.
17. Ozkan M, Oflaz SB, Kocaman N, et al. Psychiatric morbidity and quality of life in patients with chronic idiopathic urticaria. Ann Allergy Asthma Immunol 2007; 99(1):29–33.
18. Ben-Shoshan B, Blinderman I, Raz A, et al. Psychosocial factors and chronic spontaneous urticaria: a systematic review. Allergy 2013;68(2):131–41.
19. Magerl M, Pisarevskaja D, Scheufele R, et al. Effects of a pseudoallergen-free diet on chronic spontaneous urticaria: a prospective trial. Allergy 2010;65(1): 78–83.
20. Siebenhaar F, Melde A, Magerl M, et al. Histamine intolerance in patients with chronic spontaneous urticaria. J Eur Acad Dermatol Venereol 2016;30:1774.
21. Wagner N, Dirk D, Peveling-Oberhag A, et al. A Popular myth - low-histamine diet improves chronic spontaneous urticaria - fact or fiction? J Eur Acad Dermatol Venereol 2017;31:650.
22. Yeung H, Swerlick RA. Evidence on pseudoallergen-free diet for chronic urticaria. J Am Acad Dermatol 2015;72(6):e181.
23. Zuberbier T, Bernstein JA. A comparison of the United States and international perspective on chronic urticaria guidelines. J Allergy Clin Immunol Pract 2018; 6(4):1144–51.
24. Kozel MM, Sabroe RA. Chronic urticaria: aetiology, management and current and future treatment options. Drugs 2004;64:2515–36.
25. Kaplan AP. Treatment of chronic spontaneous urticaria. Allergy Asthma Immunol Res 2012;4(6):326–31.

Anaphylaxis for Internists
Definition, Evaluation, and Management, with a Focus on Commonly Encountered Problems

Derek K. Chu, MD, PhD, FRCPC*,
David J. McCullagh, MB BCh, BAO, DTM&H, FRCPC,
Susan Waserman, MD, MSc, FRCPC*

KEYWORDS

- Anaphylaxis • Type I hypersensitivity (immediate hypersensitivity)
- Urticaria and pseudoallergy • Meta-analysis
- Antibiotic allergy (including penicillin and cephalosporin β-lactams)
- Graded challenge (test dose) • Desensitization • Epinephrine

KEY POINTS

- Anaphylaxis in adults is most commonly caused by medications, of which antibiotic allergy is the most commonly reported, but other causes of anaphylaxis in adults include immunoglobulin E–mediated allergy to food and insect stings.
- Mimickers of anaphylaxis include infectious, autoimmune, malignant, autoinflammatory, and pseudoallergic causes.
- The treatment of anaphylaxis involves the prompt administration of intramuscular epinephrine to the vastus lateralis (midouter thigh), with adjuncts of intravenous fluids, conservative supplemental oxygen, and H1 antihistamines. There may be a limited role for adjunctive corticosteroids for the low absolute risk for biphasic reactions (~4%).
- Penicillin allergy is often mislabeled out of fear of anaphylaxis, resulting in significant morbidity, increased hospital stays, medical costs, risk of hospital-acquired infections, and antibiotic-resistant infections.
- Internists can easily risk stratify patients labeled as antibiotic allergic. In urgent situations in which allergists are not available, internists should consider diagnostic graded challenge (test doses).

ANAPHYLAXIS: OVERVIEW FOR INTERNISTS

Defined by the National Institute of Allergy and Infectious Disease (NIAID)/Food Allergy and Anaphylaxis Network symposium 2005 to 2006 expert consensus criteria, anaphylaxis is a serious (systemic) allergic reaction that is rapid in onset and may

Disclosures: None.
Department of Medicine, McMaster University, 1200 Main Street West, HSC-3V49, Hamilton, Ontario L8N 3Z5, Canada
* Corresponding author.
E-mail addresses: chudk@mcmaster.ca (D.K.C.); waserman@mcmaster.ca (S.W.)

Med Clin N Am 104 (2020) 25–44
https://doi.org/10.1016/j.mcna.2019.08.007   medical.theclinics.com

cause death.[1,2] This article reviews the diagnosis and management of anaphylaxis, focusing on what may be most relevant for internists.

Classification

Diagnostic criteria for anaphylaxis are shown in **Table 1**. Although the NIAID and World Allergy Organization use the same definition for anaphylaxis, it is important to recognize that UK and Australian professional societies also consider isolated bronchospasm without typical skin features (urticaria, angioedema) as anaphylaxis.[3] Although it has been reported that up to 20% of anaphylaxis may present without cutaneous signs/symptoms,[1,2] our unpublished (Chu DK, et al. 2019) meta-analysis shows that 92% (95% confidence interval [CI], 89%–95%) of anaphylaxis presents with cutaneous signs (**Fig. 1**). Severity classification is complex, with more than 20 different scoring systems and no clear consensus on which has the best test characteristics.[4] Causes of anaphylaxis include immunoglobulin (Ig) E–mediated reactions to foods, drugs, insect stings, and latex. There are also non–IgE-mediated causes, such as to certain biologics, iron dextrans, radiocontrast media, and exercise. Previously these reactions were termed anaphylactoid reactions, but the term non–IgE-mediated anaphylaxis is instead now preferred.[2] As discussed later, non–IgE-mediated causes are amenable to pretreatment. Some food-related causes of exercise-induced anaphylaxis are managed as IgE-mediated anaphylaxis, with avoidance of the food before exercise. Spontaneous anaphylaxis can be idiopathic or can be caused by an underlying mast cell disorder such as systemic mastocytosis. About 80% of the latter cases involve multiple small yellow-tan to red-brown macules or slightly raised papules called urticaria pigmentosa (also known as maculopapular cutaneous mastocytosis) that urticate on being scratched, eponymously called Darier sign.

Table 1
Anaphylaxis is highly likely when any of these criteria are fulfilled

(1) Sudden onset of	(2) Two or More, After a Likely Allergen	(3) Hypotension After Exposure to a Known Allergen
Mucocutaneous manifestations (generalized hives, itching, flushing, angioedema)	Mucocutaneous manifestations (generalized hives, itching, flushing, angioedema)	SBP<90 mm Hg or >30% less than baseline
And either of:	Sudden (persistent) gastrointestinal symptoms (crampy abdominal pain, vomiting)	—
Sudden respiratory manifestations (dyspnea, wheeze, cough, stridor, hypoxemia)	Sudden respiratory manifestations (dyspnea, wheeze, cough, stridor, hypoxemia)	—
Hypotension or its consequences (hypotonia, incontinence)	Hypotension or its consequences (hypotonia, incontinence)	—

Abbreviation: SBP, systolic blood pressure.

Modified from Sampson HA, Muñoz-Furlong A, Campbell RL, et al. Second symposium on the definition and management of anaphylaxis: summary report–Second National Institute of Allergy and Infectious Disease/Food Allergy and Anaphylaxis Network symposium. J Allergy Clin Immunol 2006;117(2):393; with permission.

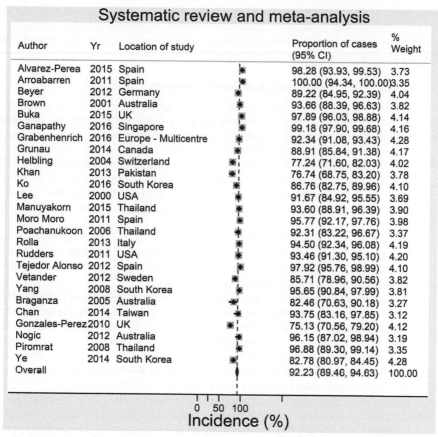

Systematic review and meta-analysis

Author	Yr	Location of study		Proportion of cases (95% CI)	% Weight
Alvarez-Perea	2015	Spain		98.28 (93.93, 99.53)	3.73
Arroabarren	2011	Spain		100.00 (94.34, 100.00)	3.35
Beyer	2012	Germany		89.22 (84.95, 92.39)	4.04
Brown	2001	Australia		93.66 (88.39, 96.63)	3.82
Buka	2015	UK		97.89 (96.03, 98.88)	4.14
Ganapathy	2016	Singapore		99.18 (97.90, 99.68)	4.16
Grabenhenrich	2016	Europe - Multicentre		92.34 (91.08, 93.43)	4.28
Grunau	2014	Canada		88.91 (85.84, 91.38)	4.17
Helbling	2004	Switzerland		77.24 (71.60, 82.03)	4.02
Khan	2013	Pakistan		76.74 (68.75, 83.20)	3.78
Ko	2016	South Korea		86.76 (82.75, 89.96)	4.10
Lee	2000	USA		91.67 (84.92, 95.55)	3.69
Manuyakorn	2015	Thailand		93.60 (88.91, 96.39)	3.90
Moro Moro	2011	Spain		95.77 (92.17, 97.76)	3.98
Poachanukoon	2006	Thailand		92.31 (83.22, 96.67)	3.37
Rolla	2013	Italy		94.50 (92.34, 96.08)	4.19
Rudders	2011	USA		93.46 (91.30, 95.10)	4.20
Tejedor Alonso	2012	Spain		97.92 (95.76, 98.99)	4.10
Vetander	2012	Sweden		85.71 (78.96, 90.56)	3.82
Yang	2008	South Korea		95.65 (90.84, 97.99)	3.81
Braganza	2005	Australia		82.46 (70.63, 90.18)	3.27
Chan	2014	Taiwan		93.75 (83.16, 97.85)	3.12
Gonzales-Perez	2010	UK		75.13 (70.56, 79.20)	4.12
Nogic	2012	Australia		96.15 (87.02, 98.94)	3.19
Piromrat	2008	Thailand		96.88 (89.30, 99.14)	3.35
Ye	2014	South Korea		82.78 (80.97, 84.45)	4.28
Overall				92.23 (89.46, 94.63)	100.00

0   50 100
Incidence (%)

Fig. 1. Proportion of anaphylaxis with cutaneous signs (Chu DK et al, unpublished).

Investigations and Differential Diagnosis

Anaphylaxis is a clinical diagnosis, although its pathophysiology is thought to be caused by systemic mast cell and basophil activation and resultant platelet-activating factor and histamine release.[5,6] Laboratory tests supportive of the diagnosis are time sensitive to obtain, of which the most widely available is measurement of serum or plasma tryptase level.[2] The latter must be drawn within 3 hours of a reaction and peaks after 30 to 90 minutes. Because the turnaround time of this test is in the order of days, it is most useful to retrospectively confirm whether or not a significant immediate hypersensitivity event mediated by mast cell activation occurred (significant increase defined as 1.2 × baseline serum tryptase level [ng/mL or μg/L] + 2).[7] This test is particularly useful when disorders mimicking anaphylaxis are present, such as asthma, vocal cord dysfunction, syncope, or flushing syndromes. Patients presenting with isolated angioedema (ie, without urticaria) should also be evaluated for bradykinin-mediated angioedema causes, such as angiotensin-converting enzyme (ACE) inhibitor or Dipeptidyl peptidase-4 (DPP4) inhibitor–induced angioedema, hereditary angioedema,[8] or acquired angioedema (most commonly associated with lymphoproliferative disease or monoclonal gammopathy of unknown significance).[9] A C4 level is the first-line screening test for investigation of suspected bradykinin-mediated angioedema. If it is low, C1-esterase inhibitor level and function should then be ordered to classify the type of bradykinin-mediated angioedema. Management is distinct from anaphylaxis in that bradykinin-mediated angioedema has little to no response to antihistamines and epinephrine.

Specific Mimickers of Anaphylaxis Relevant to Internists

Although the most common causes of anaphylaxis globally are foods, medications, and insect stings (**Fig. 2**), and it occurs primarily in a home setting (**Fig. 3**), internists are most likely to encounter drug-induced anaphylaxis in hospital. However, many drugs can be nonspecific mast cell activators, often causing acute-onset urticaria with or without associated angioedema and not mediated by any underlying allergy[10] (eg, specific IgE leading to anaphylactic mast cell degranulation). The 3 most common nonspecific mast cell activators that internists ae likely to face are opioids, vancomycin-induced red man syndrome, and nonsteroidal antiinflammatory drugs (NSAIDs).

Opioid-induced reactions are typically mild and only involve the skin (even if generalized; **Fig. 4**) and can be treated with nonsedating second-generation H1 antihistamines. Similarly, *Mycoplasma* and many viral infections can cause isolated mucocutaneous urticaria with or without angioedema.

Intravenous (IV) vancomycin's classic side effect, red man syndrome (upper body–erythema and pruritus), is a predictable pharmacologic side effect of nonspecific mast cell activation and histamine release that can be managed by slowing the infusion rate (eg, 10 mg/min or 1 g over 100 minutes) and treatment with second-generation nonsedating H1 antihistamines[10] (eg, cetirizine 10–20 mg, loratadine 5–10 mg, desloratidine 5–10 mg). It is not a true allergic response. If rapid vancomycin infusion is required (eg, 1 g in <60 minutes), premedication with oral or IV antihistamines 30 to 60 minutes before infusion has been shown in at least 3 randomized trials[11–13] to be effective in reducing the incidence of red man syndrome (random effects meta-analyzed risk ratio (RR) 0.57 [95% CI, 0.35–92]; **Fig. 5**). Vancomycin is a rare cause of immediate hypersensitivity; there are no large-scale epidemiologic analyses, but there are case reports.

NSAIDs are a common cause of both allergic and pseudoallergic reactions (**Table 2**), including urticaria and angioedema.[14] Although pseudoallergic reactions

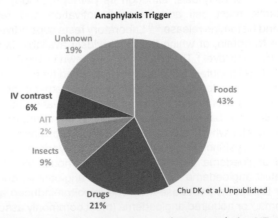

Fig. 2. Anaphylaxis triggers: systematic review and meta-analysis. AIT, allergen immunotherapy; IV, intravenous.

Location where anaphylaxis began

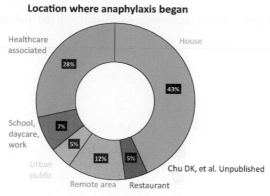

Healthcare associated 28%

House 43%

School, daycare, work 7%

Urban public 5%

Remote area 12%

Restaurant 5%

Chu DK, et al. Unpublished

Fig. 3. Anaphylaxis starting location: systematic review and meta-analysis.

are thought to be mediated by cyclooxygenase (COX) inhibition and the balance between prostaglandins and leukotrienes, allergic reactions are mediated by specific IgE. It follows that pseudoallergic reactions occur to any NSAID, often in a dose-dependent manner, whereas allergic reactions occur specifically to only 1 type of NSAID and are elicited even at small doses. Hence, NSAID-induced reactions can range from benign to life threatening and are best referred for evaluation by an allergist. It should be noted that acetylsalicylic acid (eg, aspirin) has been reported to cause only pseudoallergic reactions, not anaphylaxis. In many cases, selective COX-2 inhibitors (eg, celecoxib) can be used in place of nonselective NSAIDs.

Rare Syndromes with Urticaria that Might Lead to Hospital Admission

Urticaria with constitutional symptoms, fever, arthritis, or bruising (purpura or ecchymoses) might suggest an underlying autoinflammatory disease (including Schnitzler syndrome), urticarial vasculitis, or cryoglobulinemia, rather than recurrent anaphylaxis. A full discussion of these conditions is beyond the scope of this article.

Classic histamine-mediated urticaria is evanescent and migratory, with each lesion being pruritic and lasting less than 24 hours in any 1 location before the skin returns to

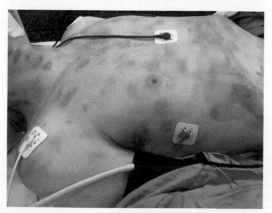

Fig. 4. Opioid-induced urticaria.

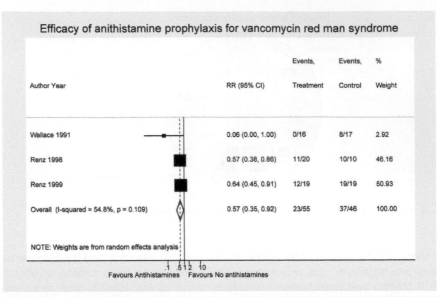

Fig. 5. Efficacy of antihistamine prophylaxis for red man syndrome, meta-analysis.

normal morphology. Urticaria that is atypical should prompt consideration of urticarial vasculitis, which may be classified as normocomplementemic or hypocomplementemic, with the latter having a more severe course. In contrast with histamine-mediated urticaria, urticarial vasculitis lesions are typically painful or burning in sensation, with each lesion lasting greater than 48 hours and healing with a bruise (**Table 3**).

Prognosis and Complications of Anaphylaxis

Prognostic factors for outcomes after anaphylaxis (**Table 4**) most consistently identify comorbid cardiac or pulmonary disease, especially asthma, as a risk factor for life-threatening or fatal reactions. Ensuring asthma control is therefore critical to

Table 2 Nonsteroidal antiinflammatory drug–induced allergic and pseudoallergic reactions classification	
Pseudoallergic: Reactions to any NSAID	**Allergic: Reactions to Only 1 Specific NSAID**
Type 1: AERD/Sampter triad (NSAID-induced naso-ocular and lower-respiratory responses)	Type 5: urticaria ± angioedema
Type 2: urticaria ± angioedema with a history of chronic urticaria	Type 6: anaphylaxis
Type 3: exacerbation of underlying urticaria ± angioedema without a history of chronic urticaria	—
Type 4: mixed respiratory and urticaria ± angioedema	—

Abbreviation: AERD, aspirin exacerbated respiratory disease.

Table 3
Features of classic urticaria versus urticarial vasculitis

	Classic (Histamine-mediated) Urticaria	Urticarial Vasculitis
Symptom/Sensation	Itch	Pain or burning
Duration of Each Lesion	<24 h (evanescent)	>48 h
Location of Each Lesion	Migratory	Fixed
Morphology at Resolution	Normal skin	Purpura/ecchymosis
Associations	Angioedema	Possible underlying CTD Arthritis/arthralgia, abdominal pain, and/or glomerulonephritis On skin biopsy: leukocytoclastic vasculitis

Abbreviation: CTD, connective tissue disease.
(*Modified from* Sampson HA, Muñoz-Furlong A, Campbell RL, et al. Second symposium on the definition and management of anaphylaxis: summary report–Second National Institute of Allergy and Infectious Disease/Food Allergy and Anaphylaxis Network symposium. J Allergy Clin Immunol 2006;117(2):393.)

the management of food allergy. Peanut and tree nuts are the most common cause of life-threatening and fatal reactions.[15,16] In contrast, it is commonly thought that the severity of previous reactions predicts the severity of future reactions, but in actuality the severity of one reaction compared with the next is unpredictable.[2] Several series

Table 4
Potential modifiable risk factors to reduce risk fatal anaphylaxis

Risk Factor	Possible Intervention
Before a Reaction	
Uncontrolled asthma	Optimize asthma control, frequent follow-up
Supported self-management in allergen avoidance	Discuss avoidance strategies. Referral to registered dietician and/or patient support groups
Not always carrying epinephrine on person	Stress importance of always carrying autoinjector
During a Reaction	
Delayed recognition of anaphylaxis	Reinforce anaphylaxis criteria, which might be facilitated by video and simulation sessions
Delayed or lack of epinephrine	Prompt epinephrine injection
Sitting or standing positioning	Keep supine ± legs raised
After a Reaction	
No referral to an allergist	Refer all patients with anaphylaxis
No prescription of autoinjector	Always prescribe an epinephrine autoinjector and educate on how and when to use it
Lack of education	Discuss strategies for allergen avoidance, cofactors, and asthma control

Data from Refs.[2,15,17,20]

have shown that most case mortality in food allergy is associated with a previous history of less severe reactions and therefore the thought that there was no need to carry an epinephrine autoinejctor.[15,17,18] Consistent with this is the observation that the delay or lack of prompt epinephrine autoinjector use after a reaction is associated with more severe outcomes, including mortality and biphasic reactions.[15,16,18] The association of β-blockers and ACE inhibitors with the severity and frequency of anaphylaxis, although potentially significant, is of very-low-quality (certainty) evidence.[19] Complications of anaphylaxis include repeat reactions typically within 4 to 8 hours (up to 72 hours) without additional allergen exposure, termed biphasic reactions, occur in about 4% of cases (3.65% [95% CI, 2.12–6.19]; **Fig. 6**), intensive care unit (ICU) admission in about 4% (4.41% [95% CI, 2.02–9.35], Chu DK, et al. 2019), and mortality in about 1% (1.04 [95% CI, 0.14–2.49], Chu DK, et al. 2019). Death is typically secondary to respiratory obstruction and/or shock and occurs within 60 minutes. Anaphylaxis may also result in coronary vasospasm with or without myocardial infarction, termed Kounis syndrome, but this entity is limited to case reports.

Treatment of Anaphylaxis in Hospital

Acute management is prompt administration of 0.3 to 0.5 mL of 1 mg/mL (previously known as 1:1000 concentration) epinephrine intramuscularly to the mid-outer thigh (vastus lateralis) and repeated every 3 to 5 minutes as needed.[2] This injection can be achieved by use of commercial autoinjectors or drawing up from a

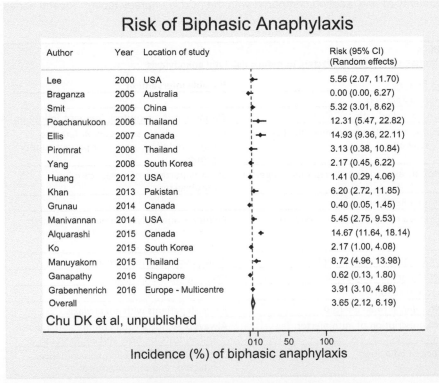

Risk of Biphasic Anaphylaxis

Author	Year	Location of study		Risk (95% CI) (Random effects)
Lee	2000	USA		5.56 (2.07, 11.70)
Braganza	2005	Australia		0.00 (0.00, 6.27)
Smit	2005	China		5.32 (3.01, 8.62)
Poachanukoon	2006	Thailand		12.31 (5.47, 22.82)
Ellis	2007	Canada		14.93 (9.36, 22.11)
Piromrat	2008	Thailand		3.13 (0.38, 10.84)
Yang	2008	South Korea		2.17 (0.45, 6.22)
Huang	2012	USA		1.41 (0.29, 4.06)
Khan	2013	Pakistan		6.20 (2.72, 11.85)
Grunau	2014	Canada		0.40 (0.05, 1.45)
Manivannan	2014	USA		5.45 (2.75, 9.53)
Alquarashi	2015	Canada		14.67 (11.64, 18.14)
Ko	2015	South Korea		2.17 (1.00, 4.08)
Manuyakorn	2015	Thailand		8.72 (4.96, 13.98)
Ganapathy	2016	Singapore		0.62 (0.13, 1.80)
Grabenhenrich	2016	Europe - Multicentre		3.91 (3.10, 4.86)
Overall				3.65 (2.12, 6.19)

Chu DK et al, unpublished

0 10   50   100

Incidence (%) of biphasic anaphylaxis

Fig. 6. Risk of biphasic anaphylaxis: systematic review and meta-analysis.

medication vial. Intramuscular epinephrine is preferred to bolus IV epinephrine as the initial treatment of anaphylaxis because the latter is associated with more complications (eg, arrhythmia) and dosing errors. There are no contraindications to epinephrine for anaphylaxis, including pregnancy, acute coronary syndrome, or co-morbid cardiovascular disease. Subsequent adjunctive treatment includes[2] supine positioning with legs raised[21] to encourage preload along with standard critical care management, including IV fluids with or without vasopressors for anaphylaxis-induced distributive and hypovolemic shock, conservative oxygen therapy to avoid hyperoxia-induced paradoxic tissue hypoxia,[22] early intubation if laryngeal edema is suspected (eg, stridor), and appropriate acuity monitoring (eg, Step-down unit or ICU). Upright posture during reactions is associated with fatal anaphylaxis,[15,21] thought to be caused by rapid vena cava emptying, loss of pre-load, and underfilled ventricles, a condition called empty heart syndrome.[21] Inhaled short-acting beta agonists (eg, salbutamol or albuterol) with or without short-acting antimuscarinics (eg, ipratropium) should also be considered for dyspnea, wheeze, or hypoxia. Additional adjuncts include H1 antihistamines (either second-generation nonsedating antihistamines or IV diphenhydramine) and H2-blockers (typically used for gastric acid suppression but may be helpful for allergic reactions) such as ranitidine.[1,2,23] Corticosteroids may have a modest relative effect on preventing biphasic reactions (**Fig. 7**), but whether this results in a clinically significant absolute risk reduction is less certain, because the risk of biphasic reactions is 3.65% without corticosteroids and 2.8% with corticosteroids, translating into a small absolute risk reduction of 0.85%. Risk factors for biphasic reactions are not clear.

Refractory anaphylaxis may require epinephrine infusion. Methylene blue may be helpful in severe refractory cases but supportive evidence is primarily from case reports and biological rationale of its effect on nitric oxide.[24] Glucagon (1 mg IV) may assist with inotropy and chronotropy in patients on β-blockers with refractory anaphylaxis.[25,26]

On discharge, all patients should be given an anaphylaxis action plan (eg, https://www.aaaai.org/Aaaai/media/MediaLibrary/PDF%20Documents/Libraries/Anaphylaxis-Emergency-Action-Plan.pdf or https://www.foodallergy.org/media/329), prescribed epinephrine autoinjectors (several different brands available in the United States), trained in its use, suggested a medical alert bracelet, and referred to an allergist for evaluation. Patients should be encouraged to always carry an autoinjector. Cost-savings programs are available to help ensure that all patients that require an autoinjector are able to access one (https://www.foodallergy.org/about-fare/blog/2018-patient-assistance-resources-for-epinephrine-auto-injectors). Further, the US Food and Drug Administration provides an updated site on any drug shortages (https://www.accessdata.fda.gov/scripts/drugshortages/dsp_ActiveIngredientDetails.cfm?AI=Epinephrine%20Injection,%20Auto-Injector&st=c).

These final steps at discharge are critical because many outpatient cases of fatal anaphylaxis occur in patients with a known history of food allergy, and are consistently associated with lack of or delayed use of epinephrine.[15,16,18,27,28] This problem is compounded by the fact that not all emergency medical technicians in the United States carry and/or are trained in the use of epinephrine for anaphylaxis.[29] Hence, patients should be informed that there can be a significant delay between onset of anaphylaxis as an outpatient and time to epinephrine administration. Prompt referral to an allergist helps to reinforce these points, and complete allergy testing can generate strategies for risk reduction (eg, allergen avoidance, venom immunotherapy, drug desensitization).

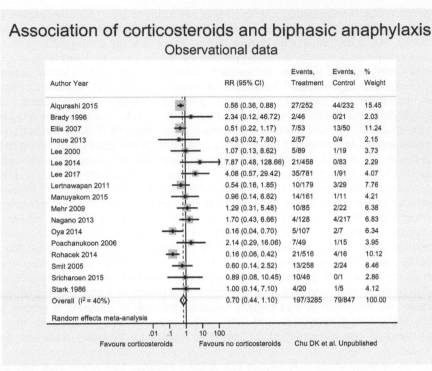

Association of corticosteroids and biphasic anaphylaxis
Observational data

Author Year	RR (95% CI)	RR (95% CI)	Events, Treatment	Events, Control	% Weight
Alqurashi 2015		0.56 (0.36, 0.88)	27/252	44/232	15.45
Brady 1996		2.34 (0.12, 46.72)	2/46	0/21	2.03
Ellis 2007		0.51 (0.22, 1.17)	7/53	13/50	11.24
Inoue 2013		0.43 (0.02, 7.80)	2/57	0/4	2.15
Lee 2000		1.07 (0.13, 8.62)	5/89	1/19	3.73
Lee 2014		7.87 (0.48, 128.66)	21/458	0/83	2.29
Lee 2017		4.08 (0.57, 29.42)	35/781	1/91	4.07
Lertnawapan 2011		0.54 (0.16, 1.85)	10/179	3/29	7.76
Manuyakorn 2015		0.96 (0.14, 6.62)	14/161	1/11	4.21
Mehr 2009		1.29 (0.31, 5.48)	10/85	2/22	6.38
Nagano 2013		1.70 (0.43, 6.66)	4/128	4/217	6.83
Oya 2014		0.16 (0.04, 0.70)	5/107	2/7	6.34
Poachanukoon 2006		2.14 (0.29, 16.06)	7/49	1/15	3.95
Rohacek 2014		0.16 (0.06, 0.42)	21/516	4/16	10.12
Smit 2005		0.60 (0.14, 2.52)	13/258	2/24	6.46
Sricharoen 2015		0.89 (0.08, 10.45)	10/46	0/1	2.86
Stark 1986		1.00 (0.14, 7.10)	4/20	1/5	4.12
Overall (I^2 = 40%)		0.70 (0.44, 1.10)	197/3285	79/847	100.00

Random effects meta-analysis

.01   .1   1   10 100

Favours corticosteroids   Favours no corticosteroids   Chu DK et al. Unpublished

Fig. 7. Corticosteroids for biphasic anaphylaxis: systematic review and meta-analysis (no available randomized controlled trials). M-H, Mantel-Haenszel.

WHY ANAPHYLAXIS TO ANTIBIOTICS IS PARAMOUNT TO INTERNISTS

Although there are many potential causes of anaphylaxis (**Table 5**), the most common cause in adults is drugs. Antibiotic allergies are the most common allergies reported by patients,[30] critically influencing everyday clinical decisions. The complications related to erroneous labeling of antibiotic allergy are mentioned earlier. Therefore, it is paramount for internists to have a core competency in antibiotic allergy, so that patients have access to appropriate first-line therapy. Next, this article provides a practical user's guide for internal medicine specialists (internists) to optimally evaluate and manage patients with presumed antibiotic allergy. This article builds on the recent summary of 5 critical points to know about penicillin allergy for patients and all health care providers.[31] There are also recent more general reviews on this topic,[14,32–35] regarding controversies and research priority setting.[36]

The largest and most commonly used antibiotic class used for inpatients are the β-lactams. This part of the article is therefore focused on the approach to patients with anaphylactic β-lactam allergy.

DEFINITIONS: IMMEDIATE VERSUS DELAYED HYPERSENSITIVITY; ALLERGY VERSUS SIDE EFFECT

Adverse reactions to drugs are classified into those that are known pharmacologic side effects and/or predictable/anticipated (eg, hypotension after taking an antihypertensive such as a dihydropyridine calcium channel blocker), that are unpredictable

Table 5
Causes of anaphylaxis most relevant to internists

Category of Cause	Specific Causes	Notes
Infectious	Hydatid	Risk with cyst aspiration or biopsy
Malignancy/ infiltrative[7]	Mast cell disorders	Comanagement with malignant hematology
Iatrogenic/ medications	Antibiotics NSAID (not ASA) Transfusion/blood product Radiocontrast Chlorhexidine NMBA NMBA reversal (Sugammadex) Total parental nutrition Latex Allergen immunotherapy	All cases of anaphylaxis: Trigger avoidance, prescribe epinephrine, refer to allergist Transfusion: Risk with complete selective IgA deficiency Radiocontrast: No diagnostic test. Shellfish allergy ≠ radiocontrast allergy
Idiopathic Food[38]	Exercise induced Seafood (fish, crustaceans, mollusks), peanut, tree nut most common and often lifelong in adults	Premedication protocols vary widely[37] Insects: Patient with systemic reactions are at high risk (50%) for
Insect stings[39]	Wasps (including yellow jacket), honeybees, fire ants	repeat reactions and venom immunotherapy is effective (RR ~0.2)

Abbreviations: ASA, acetylsalicylic acid; NMBA, neuromuscular blocking agent.

and idiosyncratic (eg, drug-induced lupus, DPP4 inhibitor–induced angioedema), and those that are predictably immune-mediated hypersensitivity responses (eg, penicillin-induced anaphylaxis). The focus here is on immediate hypersensitivity responses (eg, anaphylaxis, urticaria, bronchospasm). Severe delayed reactions are discussed in greater detail in other reviews.[32–34,40,41]

The term penicillin allergy can have different meanings among health care providers, patients, and researchers. Many use it to refer to immediate hypersensitivity to penicillins and cephalosporins, rather than solely either one, or the β-lactam class as a whole. This lack of specificity promotes misunderstanding and misnomers. For clarity, this article refers to penicillin allergy as solely to involving the subclass of β-lactams.

β-LACTAM ALLERGY
Penicillin Allergy

How common is penicillin allergy? What is the cost?
Penicillin allergy is the most common antibiotic allergy reported and its prevalence among inpatients can reach 15%.[30,41] However, studies evaluating penicillin allergy have shown that patients can tolerate a β-lactam more than 90% of the time.[42] The label of penicillin allergy has been shown to lead to increased health care costs. These costs occur for several reasons, including increased antibiotic costs from second-line therapies, increased length of stay, increased use of IV therapy, and higher readmission rates. Eight out of 10 patients with a penicillin allergy label that requires antibiotics receive inferior non–β-lactam antibiotics.[43] β-Lactam alternatives are broader spectrum and this leads to increases in antibiotic-resistant and hospital-acquired infections. Retrospective cohorts in the inpatient[44] and outpatient setting[45] have shown an increased risk of *Clostridioides difficile*, methicillin-resistant *Staphylococcus*

aureus, and vancomycin-resistant enterococcus in patients with the label of penicillin allergy. Meta-analyses show increased costs in the range of US$1125 to US$4254 per patient.[46] These estimates might underestimate the true cost of a penicillin allergy label, when the costs associated with resistant organisms are considered. Hence, the desire to avoid harm by commission may lead to harm by omission.

Is penicillin allergy a lifelong diagnosis?

IgE-mediated penicillin allergy wanes over time, likely because of weak IgE memory and short-lived IgE plasma cells.[47,48] Studies including prospective cohorts have shown that there is a significant reduction in the number of patients who are skin test positive for penicillin allergy over time. As an example, a study following patients who were skin test positive to benzylpenicillin, amoxicillin, or ampicillin were followed over the course of 5 years with repeated skin testing. After 5 years, 38 of 55 (69%) were no longer allergic by skin testing.[49] Approximately 80% of patients with true penicillin allergy are not allergic after 10 years.[41] Hence, there is a need to frequently reevaluate the diagnosis of penicillin allergy.

How to risk stratify, test for, and diagnose penicillin allergy

Like almost any other condition in medicine, diagnostic evaluation requires initial risk stratification by history. For β-lactam allergy, that means stratification into 1 of 3 categories:

1. Those who clearly are not allergic because the reaction was a known pharmacologic side effect (eg, antibiotic-induced isolated dyspepsia), or isolated family history of drug allergy without a personal history of penicillin allergy
2. Those in whom testing is contraindicated because of severe delayed drug reactions (eg, Steven-Johnson syndrome [SJS]/toxic epidermal necrolysis [TEN], drug reaction eosinophilia and systemic symptoms [DRESS])
3. Those appropriate for testing because of a possible history of immediate hypersensitivity (urticaria, angioedema, anaphylaxis) or delayed-onset nonspecific benign eruption

Although history alone does not always predict the outcome of skin testing,[50] pertinent information concerns the nature and course of the reported allergic reaction, when it occurred, its severity (eg, hospitalization, organ failure, skin desquamation, anaphylaxis), and whether or not the drug has been tolerated since.[33,41,51,52] Isolated family history is unimportant and nondiagnostic for immediate penicillin allergy, because it is not a strongly heritable trait.[41] The physical examination is, in general, not relevant to the diagnostic evaluation of a history of possible penicillin allergy.

Classically, skin testing is performed on all patients before challenge testing, but there is debate over whether and which patients can be challenged without skin testing, and what the optimal procedural technique is.[36,41] The classic rationale for sequential skin tests, including epicutaneous, intradermal, followed by challenge testing, is to minimize the risk of eliciting an iatrogenic anaphylactic response.

Interfering substances that lead to indeterminate allergy skin test results Skin testing relies on the patient to mount an urticarial (wheal and flare) response to a specific allergen, which is blocked by drugs with antihistaminic action. Common in-hospital drugs that can do this include H1-blocking antihistamines, diphenhydramine (Benadryl), dimenhydrinate (Gravol), tricyclic antidepressants, sleep aids/hypnotics (eg, zopiclone, benzodiazepines), and quetiapine. High-dose glucocorticoids might lead to false-negative skin responses, potentially through mast cell depletion over time.

What would allergists do? Challenge Negative skin tests are followed by administering a full, therapeutic dose of penicillin (eg, single-dose oral amoxicillin 250 or 500 mg, or the drug that caused the initial reaction if known) to prove tolerance.

Inpatient allergist evaluation with combined skin and challenge testing (including test dosing) of patients labeled as penicillin allergic has been shown to be rapid, safe, and cost-effective.[41–43,46]

Cross reactivity between and among (within) β-lactam antibiotics

The pathophysiologic basis of immediate penicillin hypersensitivity is thought to involve IgE antibodies specific to haptens formed from the breakdown of either the β-lactam core ring or chemical R-group side chains of β-lactams. The shared β-lactam core defining this family of antibiotics and shared or similar R side chains between specific β-lactams (eg, amino group, methoxyamino group) raises the possibility that allergy to 1 family member may imply allergy to other members, termed cross reactivity.[53]

Many internists face the situation in which the antibiotic of choice is a cephalosporin, but the patient reports a possible penicillin allergy, complicating therapeutic decision making. The authors and others[14,31,33,34,41,52] stress the importance of first clarifying whether the label of penicillin allergy is true or not. Internists can identify patients at very low risk of being truly allergic (such as nonsuggestive history; eg, isolated nausea with amoxicillin), and can easily offer a direct amoxicillin challenge (eg, 1 dose of 250 or 500 mg by mouth then observing for 30–60 minutes) to clarify the diagnosis.

There exists no published rigorous systematic review or guideline to inform evidence-based management of potential cross reactivity between β-lactams. However, for patients truly allergic to penicillin, our meta-analysis shows that rates of cross reactivity are ~1% with cephalosporins (0.72% [95% CI, 0%–2.24%]; **Fig. 8**). Rates of ~1% with carbapenems and 0% with monobactams (aztreonam) have been reported.[33,34,41,52,53] Historical reports quoting cross reactivity of 8% to 10%, which antibiotic package inserts reference, were erroneous owing to contamination of the cephalosporin test reagents with penicillin,[33,34,41,52,53] and this is supported by our meta-analysis. For penicillin-allergic patients, cross reactivity between other penicillins is thought to be high, but there are no rigorous analyses to support this.

Cephalosporin allergy

Cephalosporin allergy affects 2% of the population,[54] and is prevalent in the perioperative setting as a cause of anaphylaxis.[55] Although there are sparse data to robustly inform evidence-based decision making, increasingly frequent reports state that cephalosporin allergy is primarily specific to the R side group, which is variable between cephalosporins. Thus, the cross reactivity between most cephalosporins is thought to be low. Those with the highest potential to cross react are thought to be predictable by similarity in R side chains (**Table 6**). Consequently, guidance varies, with some clinicians recommending to use a cephalosporin with different side chains or alternative antibiotic (including penicillins), whereas others suggest test dosing for similar side chains and strictly avoiding identical side chains.[32–35,41,52,53]

β-Lactamase inhibitor allergy

Although a less frequent cause of allergic reactions, patients with a possible allergy to combination β-lactam/β-lactamase inhibitors (piperacillin-tazobactam, amoxicillin–

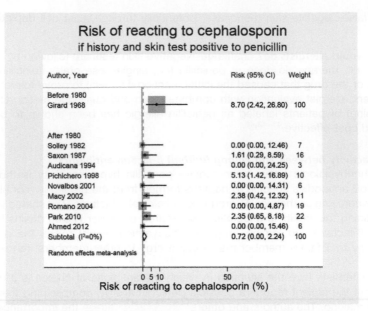

Fig. 8. Risk of cross reaction to cephalosporin in patients allergic to penicillin.

clavulanic acid, ticarcillin–clavulanic acid, ampicillin-sulbactam) could also be evaluated for allergy to the β-lactamase inhibitor component.

What should internists do in a pinch?

All patients identified carrying a label of penicillin allergy should be referred for outpatient allergy specialist evaluation to obtain diagnostic clarity. However, there are inevitably situations in which the internist has no immediate access to an allergy specialist. Here, the only rapid diagnostic tool is the history. As described earlier, the most informative pieces of information, even if collateral, for risk stratification are (1) whether the reaction was a known and predictable pharmacologic side effect; (2) whether the reaction was severe enough to cause hospitalization or had convincing features of anaphylaxis or severe delayed hypersensitivity reactions (SJS/TEN, DRESS, AIN); (3) when the reaction occurred, because more than 5 years ago, and especially more than 10 years ago, greatly decreases the risk of still having an immediate hypersensitivity; (4) whether the patient subsequently tolerated penicillins, because, if so, this strongly suggests the patient is not allergic.[14,31,33,34,41,52]

Using this approach, a substantial proportion of patients become eligible to receive penicillin. So long as there are no features of severe delayed hypersensitivity,

Table 6
Similar or identical side chains to consider when prescribing β-lactams for patients allergic to a different cephalosporin

Amino Group Shared	Methoxyamino Group Shared
Ampicillin: cephalexin, cefaclor	Cefuroxime, ceftriaxone, cefotaxime, cefepime
Amoxicillin: cefprozil, cefadroxil, cefratizine	—

penicillin-allergic patients have a ~1% chance of reacting to cephalosporins, and ~1% risk of reacting to carbapenems (see **Fig. 8**). Therefore, patients at intermediate risk of being truly penicillin allergic can undergo a graded challenge, also known as a test dose procedure.

Test dosing (graded challenge) For inpatients, in a monitored setting with anaphylaxis treatment medications and equipment at the bedside, the patient is administered either 1 in 100 (ie, 1%) or 1 in 10 (ie, 10%) of the intended full therapeutic dose (**Table 7**). After this, the infusion is paused and the patient monitored for 30 to 60 minutes for any allergic response. If there are no signs or symptoms of immediate hypersensitivity, the rest of the therapeutic dose is then infused and the patient monitored again for any signs of an allergic reaction. The same procedure can be done with oral antibiotics instead of IV. Although there are no rigorous analyses or evidence-based guidelines to determine contraindications to graded challenges, classic teaching is that uncontrolled cardiac or respiratory disease (primarily, asthma), or use of β-blockers may increase the risk of poor outcome if an allergic reaction did occur because of poor response to rescue epinephrine. A history of severe cutaneous adverse reaction (SCAR; eg, SJS/TEN, DRESS, acute generalized exanthematous pustulosis) is a contraindication to test dose.

Desensitization Desensitization is reserved for patients that definitely or likely have an immediate hypersensitivity to penicillin but must receive the penicillin to which they are allergic, and it is not possible to first test the patient by skin testing. Indications for this are typically those with an established long-term need for penicillins, such as syphilis (including in pregnancy), or possibly methicillin-sensitive staphylococcal bacteremia and/or its complications. Desensitization allows the patient to not react to the drug while they have routine (eg, daily) exposure to it. Without continual exposure, the allergy may regenerate in as little as 2 days if stopped. Allergist consultation is paramount to prepare for and guide management when allergic reactions during desensitization occur, which has been reported to occur in up to 20% of patients.[41,52,56]

NON–β-LACTAM ANTIBIOTICS

Skin testing to non–β-lactam antibiotics is not standardized and has uncertain diagnostic utility. Some non–β-lactams are notorious nonspecific mast cell activators that complicate evaluation because they result in presentations that appear like immediate hypersensitivity (eg, isolated urticaria), but are not truly allergy (ie, no underlying

Table 7
Graded challenge (test dose) and desensitization

	Graded Challenge (Test Dose)	Desensitization
Purpose	Diagnostic	Therapeutic
Result	Prove tolerance to a drug, if not remove allergy label	Allergy label must remain until it can be fully evaluated
β-Lactam Tolerance	Lifelong unless further event	Lasts only duration of desensitization procedure
Starting Dose	1 in 100 (ie, 1%) or 1 in 10 (ie, 10%) of therapeutic dose	1 in 1000 (ie, 0.1%) to 1 in 100 (ie, 1%) of therapeutic dose
Number of doses or steps	2–3	7–16

specific IgE response). Examples include vancomycin and fluoroquinolones. However, the principles for evaluation, graded challenge (test dose), and desensitization are similar for β-lactams and non–β-lactams.

Examples of Specific Scenarios Internists Might Encounter

No allergist and skin tests available

History of penicillin/amoxicillin allergy is low risk and needs a β-lactam: what do you do? A previously healthy 30-year-old woman is admitted to your rural community hospital at 10 PM with fevers, chills, and paronychia, with growth of methicillin-sensitive S aureus (MSSA) after 8 hours of blood culture. The overnight physician started empiric vancomycin because the patient reported a penicillin allergy. Her allergic reaction was not serious in that she was not hospitalized, and there was no organ failure (including jaundice suggestive of liver failure or hemolysis), mucocutaneous desquamation, or features of anaphylaxis. She was told that as a child she had a fever with possible middle ear infection for which she was given penicillin or amoxicillin; she is not sure which. Five days into the antibiotic course, she developed isolated macular erythema with urticaria over her torso. As a result, she was evaluated by a physician who told her mother that she was allergic to penicillin and to avoid all β-lactams forever. She has not been exposed to penicillin or related antibiotics since.

Knowing this is a low-risk history of true allergy because of its benign delayed features that could have been a manifestation of a viral infection, and lack of features of SCAR or anaphylaxis, and the history more than 10 years ago, you wish to remove the label of penicillin allergy, because penicillin and β-lactams are preferred for MSSA bacteremia and its complications.[57,58] If ordering a penicillin class antibiotic, you could choose to perform a supervised direct oral challenge to amoxicillin 250 mg and then monitor the patient for 30 to 60 minutes with medications to treat anaphylaxis at the bedside, because there is no available allergist in your community. If ordering a cephalosporin such as cefazolin, a direct oral challenge to amoxicillin 250 mg would still be a critical diagnostic procedure, because, if the label of penicillin allergy is removed, there is no specific concern for cross reactivity with cephalosporins. Should the patient be revealed to be allergic to amoxicillin after oral challenge, she would likely be able to tolerate a cephalosporin such as cefazolin because you know that cross reactivity with cephalosporins is ~1% (see **Fig. 8**), carbapenems ~1%, and aztreonam 0%.

History of penicillin/amoxicillin allergy is higher risk and needs a β-lactam: what do you do? If the scenario presented earlier was slightly different, with the patient reporting the allergic reaction as 1 year ago and immediate-onset urticaria and lip angioedema after the first dose, this would be an intermediate to high risk of true underlying allergy. Because of this, you consider alternative β-lactams, because this is preferable to vancomycin.[57,58] You recognize that the cross reactivity to cephalosporins in those allergic to penicillin is ~1% (see **Fig. 8**), with cross reactivity primarily being determined by shared R-group side chains (see **Table 6**). Therefore, you bring the patient to a monitored setting and do a test dose by administering 10% of a full therapeutic dose of cefazolin 2 g (ie, 200 mg) before pausing the infusion and monitoring the patient for 30 minutes with medications to treat anaphylaxis at the bedside. Because the patient did not react to this test dose, you then administer the remaining 90% of the cefazolin 2 g dose and again monitor for 30 minutes. If the patient reacts to this regimen, this would indicate allergy to cefazolin and you would then consider desensitization with expert allergist consultation (see **Table 7**), even if by remote telephone or electronic communication, or possibly patient transfer.

Allergist and skin tests available
History of immediate penicillin/amoxicillin allergy is any risk and needs a β-lactam: what do you do? If you had access to an allergist in either scenario discussed earlier, you would perform the initial risk stratification at the bedside in the same manner. With low-risk histories, you challenge the patient directly to oral amoxicillin 250 mg. With intermediate-risk or high-risk histories, you would refer for allergist evaluation and skin testing. Severe delayed hypersensitivity reactions (already defined) are contraindications to skin testing, challenge, or desensitization.

If the allergy skin testing to penicillin is positive, this would suggest the patient is likely allergic to penicillin and the allergist would help select an alternative antibiotic. Similarly, if the initial reaction was to a cephalosporin and the patient needs a different one, the allergist could help facilitate safe cephalosporin selection. In addition, all patients with a history of possible allergy should be referred to an allergist for evaluation because antibiotic allergy diagnoses are best clarified electively before urgent situations arise.

SUMMARY

This article reviews anaphylaxis, focusing on providing internists with a practical user's guide to its diagnosis, evaluation, and management, particularly to β-lactams. Internists also face patients who present with anaphylaxis to foods, insect stings, and non–antibiotic-related causes, such as NSAIDs. Less common causes are latex, radiocontrast, and exercise. Common scenarios that internists encounter are described earlier, along with considerations for their management. Being central to hospital and outpatient medicine, one of the most common problems encountered complicating therapeutic decision making is possible anaphylactic antibiotic allergies. The antibiotic allergy label is common and most patients thought to have antibiotic allergy are labeled as penicillin allergic. However, more than 9 out of 10 cases are mislabeled and can tolerate penicillin. New proactive efforts to reduce the label are needed, because they have been shown to be successful. Internists can routinely manage patients with the penicillin allergy label by risk stratifying and performing a graded challenge or referring for definitive testing and/or desensitization, depending on the acuity of the situation. Acute management of anaphylaxis entails prompt intramuscular epinephrine to the thigh, before moving on to several potential adjuncts.

ACKNOWLEDGMENTS

We thank the support of the Canadian Institutes of Health Research AllerGen NCE, Canadian Allergy, Asthma, and Immunology Foundation, Food Allergy Canada, Canadian Society of Allergy and Clinical Immunology, the Delaney family and the Walter and Maria Schroeder Foundation.

REFERENCES

1. Sampson HA, Munoz-Furlong A, Campbell RL, et al. Second symposium on the definition and management of anaphylaxis: summary report–second national institute of allergy and infectious disease/food allergy and anaphylaxis network symposium. J Allergy Clin Immunol 2006;117(2):391–7.

2. Simons FE, Ardusso LR, Bilo MB, et al. World allergy organization guidelines for the assessment and management of anaphylaxis. World Allergy Organ J 2011; 4(2):13–37.
3. ASCIA guidelines acute management anaphylaxis 2018. Available at: https://allergy.org.au/hp/papers/acute-management-of-anaphylaxis-guidelines/. Accessed May 1, 2019.
4. Eller E, Muraro A, Dahl R, et al. Assessing severity of anaphylaxis: a data-driven comparison of 23 instruments. Clin Transl Allergy 2018;8:29.
5. Arias K, Chu DK, Flader K, et al. Distinct immune effector pathways contribute to the full expression of peanut-induced anaphylactic reactions in mice. J Allergy Clin Immunol 2011;127(6):1552–61.e1.
6. Reber LL, Hernandez JD, Galli SJ. The pathophysiology of anaphylaxis. J Allergy Clin Immunol 2017;140(2):335–48.
7. Valent P, Akin C, Arock M, et al. Definitions, criteria and global classification of mast cell disorders with special reference to mast cell activation syndromes: a consensus proposal. Int Arch Allergy Immunol 2012;157(3):215–25.
8. Maurer M, Magerl M, Ansotegui I, et al. The international WAO/EAACI guideline for the management of hereditary angioedema-The 2017 revision and update. Allergy 2018;73(8):1575–96.
9. Zanichelli A, Azin GM, Wu MA, et al. Diagnosis, course, and management of angioedema in patients with acquired c1-inhibitor deficiency. J Allergy Clin Immunol Pract 2017;5(5):1307–13.
10. Zuberbier T, Aberer W, Asero R, et al. The EAACI/GA(2)LEN/EDF/WAO guideline for the definition, classification, diagnosis and management of urticaria. Allergy 2018;73(7):1393–414.
11. Renz CL, Thurn JD, Finn HA, et al. Antihistamine prophylaxis permits rapid vancomycin infusion. Crit Care Med 1999;27(9):1732–7.
12. Renz CL, Thurn JD, Finn HA, et al. Oral antihistamines reduce the side effects from rapid vancomycin infusion. Anesth Analg 1998;87(3):681–5.
13. Wallace MR, Mascola JR, Oldfield EC 3rd. Red man syndrome: incidence, etiology, and prophylaxis. J Infect Dis 1991;164(6):1180–5.
14. Demoly P, Adkinson NF, Brockow K, et al. International consensus on drug allergy. Allergy 2014;69(4):420–37.
15. Turner PJ, Jerschow E, Umasunthar T, et al. Fatal anaphylaxis: mortality rate and risk factors. J Allergy Clin Immunol Pract 2017;5(5):1169–78.
16. Sampson HA, Mendelson L, Rosen JP. Fatal and near-fatal anaphylactic reactions to food in children and adolescents. N Engl J Med 1992;327(6):380–4.
17. Pumphrey RS. Lessons for management of anaphylaxis from a study of fatal reactions. Clin Exp Allergy 2000;30(8):1144–50.
18. Pumphrey RS, Gowland MH. Further fatal allergic reactions to food in the United Kingdom, 1999-2006. J Allergy Clin Immunol 2007;119(4):1018–9.
19. Tejedor-Alonso MA, Farias-Aquino E, Perez-Fernandez E, et al. Relationship between anaphylaxis and use of beta-blockers and angiotensin-converting enzyme inhibitors: a systematic review and meta-analysis of observational studies. J Allergy Clin Immunol Pract 2019;7(3):879–97.e5.
20. Kastner M, Harada L, Waserman S. Gaps in anaphylaxis management at the level of physicians, patients, and the community: a systematic review of the literature. Allergy 2010;65(4):435–44.
21. Pumphrey RS. Fatal posture in anaphylactic shock. J Allergy Clin Immunol 2003; 112(2):451–2.

22. Chu DK, Kim LH, Young PJ, et al. Mortality and morbidity in acutely ill adults treated with liberal versus conservative oxygen therapy (IOTA): a systematic review and meta-analysis. Lancet 2018;391(10131):1693–705.

23. Lin RY, Curry A, Pesola GR, et al. Improved outcomes in patients with acute allergic syndromes who are treated with combined H1 and H2 antagonists. Ann Emerg Med 2000;36(5):462–8.

24. Evora PR, Simon MR. Role of nitric oxide production in anaphylaxis and its relevance for the treatment of anaphylactic hypotension with methylene blue. Ann Allergy Asthma Immunol 2007;99(4):306–13.

25. Zaloga GP, DeLacey W, Holmboe E, et al. Glucagon reversal of hypotension in a case of anaphylactoid shock. Ann Intern Med 1986;105(1):65–6.

26. Javeed N, Javeed H, Javeed S, et al. Refractory anaphylactoid shock potentiated by beta-blockers. Cathet Cardiovasc Diagn 1996;39(4):383–4.

27. Turner PJ, Gowland MH, Sharma V, et al. Increase in anaphylaxis-related hospitalizations but no increase in fatalities: an analysis of United Kingdom national anaphylaxis data, 1992-2012. J Allergy Clin Immunol 2015;135(4):956–63.e1.

28. Xu YS, Kastner M, Harada L, et al. Anaphylaxis-related deaths in Ontario: a retrospective review of cases from 1986 to 2011. Allergy Asthma Clin Immunol 2014; 10(1):38.

29. Brasted ID, Dailey MW. Basic life support access to injectable epinephrine across the United States. Prehosp Emerg Care 2017;21(4):442–7.

30. Lee CE, Zembower TR, Fotis MA, et al. The incidence of antimicrobial allergies in hospitalized patients: implications regarding prescribing patterns and emerging bacterial resistance. Arch Intern Med 2000;160(18):2819–22.

31. McCullagh DJ, Chu DK. Penicillin allergy. CMAJ 2019;191(8):E231.

32. Warrington R, Silviu-Dan F, Wong T. Drug allergy. Allergy Asthma Clin Immunol 2018;14(Suppl 2):60.

33. Shenoy ES, Macy E, Rowe T, et al. Evaluation and management of penicillin allergy: a review. JAMA 2019;321(2):188–99.

34. Blumenthal KG, Peter JG, Trubiano JA, et al. Antibiotic allergy. Lancet 2019; 393(10167):183–98.

35. Torres MJ, Celik GE, Whitaker P, et al. A EAACI drug allergy interest group survey on how European allergy specialists deal with beta-lactam allergy. Allergy 2019; 74(6):1052–62.

36. Schatz M, Fiocchi A, Jensen-Jarolim E, et al. Controversies in drug allergy: consensus documents from the world experts. World Allergy Organ J 2018; 11(1):41.

37. Lieberman P, Nicklas RA, Randolph C, et al. Anaphylaxis–a practice parameter update 2015. Ann Allergy Asthma Immunol 2015;115(5):341–84.

38. Sampson HA, Aceves S, Bock SA, et al. Food allergy: a practice parameter update-2014. J Allergy Clin Immunol 2014;134(5):1016–25.e3.

39. Golden DB, Demain J, Freeman T, et al. Stinging insect hypersensitivity: a practice parameter update 2016. Ann Allergy Asthma Immunol 2017;118(1):28–54.

40. Phillips EJ, Bigliardi P, Bircher AJ, et al. Controversies in drug allergy: testing for delayed reactions. J Allergy Clin Immunol 2019;143(1):66–73.

41. Joint Task Force on Practice Parameters; American Academy of Allergy, Asthma and Immunology; American College of Allergy, Asthma and Immunology; Joint Council of Allergy, Asthma and Immunology. Drug allergy: an updated practice parameter. Ann Allergy Asthma Immunol 2010;105(4):259–73.

42. Sacco KA, Bates A, Brigham TJ, et al. Clinical outcomes following inpatient penicillin allergy testing: a systematic review and meta-analysis. Allergy 2017;72(9): 1288–96.
43. King EA, Challa S, Curtin P, et al. Penicillin skin testing in hospitalized patients with beta-lactam allergies: effect on antibiotic selection and cost. Ann Allergy Asthma Immunol 2016;117(1):67–71.
44. Macy E, Contreras R. Health care use and serious infection prevalence associated with penicillin "allergy" in hospitalized patients: a cohort study. J Allergy Clin Immunol 2014;133(3):790–6.
45. Blumenthal KG, Lu N, Zhang Y, et al. Risk of meticillin resistant Staphylococcus aureus and Clostridium difficile in patients with a documented penicillin allergy: population based matched cohort study. BMJ 2018;361:k2400.
46. Mattingly TJ 2nd, Fulton A, Lumish RA, et al. The cost of self-reported penicillin allergy: a systematic review. J Allergy Clin Immunol Pract 2018;6(5):1649–54.e4.
47. Gould HJ, Ramadani F. IgE responses in mouse and man and the persistence of IgE memory. Trends Immunol 2015;36(1):40–8.
48. Jimenez-Saiz R, Chu DK, Mandur TS, et al. Lifelong memory responses perpetuate humoral TH2 immunity and anaphylaxis in food allergy. J Allergy Clin Immunol 2017;140(6):1604–15.e5.
49. Blanca M, Torres MJ, Garcia JJ, et al. Natural evolution of skin test sensitivity in patients allergic to beta-lactam antibiotics. J Allergy Clin Immunol 1999;103(5 Pt 1):918–24.
50. Wong BBL, Keith PK, Waserman S. Clinical history as a predictor of penicillin skin test outcome. Ann Allergy Asthma Immunol 2006;97(2):169–74.
51. Salkind AR, Cuddy PG, Foxworth JW. The rational clinical examination. Is this patient allergic to penicillin? An evidence-based analysis of the likelihood of penicillin allergy. JAMA 2001;285(19):2498–505.
52. Mirakian R, Leech SC, Krishna MT, et al. Management of allergy to penicillins and other beta-lactams. Clin Exp Allergy 2015;45(2):300–27.
53. Zagursky RJ, Pichichero ME. Cross-reactivity in beta-Lactam Allergy. J Allergy Clin Immunol Pract 2018;6(1):72–81.e1.
54. Macy E, Poon KYT. Self-reported antibiotic allergy incidence and prevalence: age and sex effects. Am J Med 2009;122(8):778.e1-7.
55. Cook T, Harper N. Anaesthesia, Surgery and Life-Threatening Allergic Reactions: Report and findings of the Royal College of Anaesthetists' 6th National Audit Project (NAP6)2018.
56. Castells M. Rapid desensitization for hypersensitivity reactions to medications. Immunol Allergy Clin North Am 2009;29(3):585–606.
57. Baddour LM, Wilson WR, Bayer AS, et al. Infective endocarditis in adults: diagnosis, antimicrobial therapy, and management of complications: a scientific statement for healthcare professionals from the American Heart Association. Circulation 2015;132(15):1435–86.
58. McDanel JS, Perencevich EN, Diekema DJ, et al. Comparative effectiveness of beta-lactams versus vancomycin for treatment of methicillin-susceptible Staphylococcus aureus bloodstream infections among 122 hospitals. Clin Infect Dis 2015;61(3):361–7.

Cough

A Practical and Multifaceted Approach to Diagnosis and Management

Baotran B. Tran, APRN[a,1], Anne Marie Ditto, MD[b],*

KEYWORDS

- Cough management • Approach to cough • Multifactorial cough • Cough reflex
- Causes of cough • Treatment of cough

KEY POINTS

- Cough is a common symptom often confronted in the clinical setting.
- The time and resources attributed to cough have been found to place an undue burden on patients and the health care system as a whole. One particular characteristic of cough that likely contributes to this is the multifactorial nature of cough, especially the lingering post-infectious cough.
- Physicians are trained to find a single diagnosis to explain symptoms. With cough, however, if all factors contributing are not identified and treated together, the cough often remains unresolved.

INTRODUCTION

Cough is a common symptom encountered in the clinical setting. It is the most prevalent complaint in the primary care setting and is present in 8% of primary care consultations.[1,2] In addition, approximately 40% of the population experiences a chronic cough in their lifetime.[3,4] The individual with cough often experiences embarrassment in social settings, hindered quality of life, and reduced work productivity.[4,5] An extensive evaluation and premature referral to secondary care are common reactions given the impact of cough on patients' lives. Premature referrals and an exhaustive work-up for cough, however, can be unnecessary and place an undue burden on patients and the health care system as a whole.[6] It has been shown that the majority of cough can be successfully managed with minimal investigation.[6,7]

Disclosure Statement: There are no relative conflicts of interest.
[a] Division of Allergy-Immunology, Northwestern Medicine, Chicago, IL, USA; [b] Division of Allergy-Immunology, Northwestern University Feinberg School of Medicine, 211 East Ontario Ste. 1000, Chicago, IL 60611, USA
[1] Present address: 211 East Ontario Street, 10th floor, Suite 1000, Chicago, IL 60611, USA.
* Corresponding author.
E-mail address: amditto@northwestern.edu

Med Clin N Am 104 (2020) 45–59
https://doi.org/10.1016/j.mcna.2019.08.011
0025-7125/20/© 2019 Elsevier Inc. All rights reserved.

medical.theclinics.com

In addition, there are often overlapping disorders that drive cough.[8–11] Successful management of cough requires the understanding of the interwoven nature of multiple conditions and their synergistic roles in driving cough. Sufficient treatment of cough involves consideration of not only the instigating cause but also the sequelae that potentiate the cough.[12,13] Multiple and concomitant management of all culprits of cough is often necessary for cough resolution.[7–10] This article discusses a practical and multifaceted approach to cough (**Fig. 1**).

PATHOPHYSIOLOGY OF COUGH

It is essential to understand the mechanism of the cough reflex in order to explore potential causes and appropriate management. Cough serves as a protective reflex to aid in the detection and clearance of debris and excess secretions from the respiratory tract.[3,12,14] The vagus nerve supplies a majority of cough receptors, which are found throughout both the upper and lower airways, spanning from the pharynx to the terminal bronchioles.[3,14]

Not only can cough arise from anywhere in the distribution of the vagus nerve but also the cough reflex has also been shown to have the ability of neuroplasticity. The formation of new neuronal connections and up-regulation of cough sensitivity can result from the behavior of cough itself.[15–19] The irritating nature of a repeated cough induces inflammation and tissue remodeling. An overly sensitive cough reflex is a consequence of these tissue changes.[19,20] In a sense, cough begets cough.

This positive feedback loop in which behavior reinforces cough in addition to the broad anatomic span of cough receptors are essential considerations in the management of cough because the etiology of cough tends to be multifactorial rather than a single source.[8–11] Treatment should encompass all contributors in order to sufficiently address the cough (**Fig. 2**).

THE ROLE OF HISTORY IN COUGH

A detailed history has not been shown to provide great benefit in the diagnosis and management of cough.[4,21,22] Some factors cannot be dismissed, however, when evaluating the risks for cough. These variables include duration of cough, medications taken by the patient with cough, a patient's response to them or lack thereof, and the milieu in which the cough occurs.[13]

Duration

Cough is categorized as acute (lasting <3 weeks), subacute (3–8 weeks), and chronic (>8 weeks).[10] Recognition of the subtyping of cough relative to duration narrows the list of potential differential diagnoses.[8] An exception to the significance of cough duration is tuberculosis (TB). A diagnosis of TB should be considered regardless of duration if a patient is at high risk for TB, including living in endemic areas or exposure to high-risk populations.[8]

Medications

A practical approach to evaluation of cough begins by assessing for pharmacologic causes. Angiotensin-converting enzyme inhibitors (ACEIs) are well recognized for their role in cough. There is evidence that up to 35% of patients on an ACEI experience a dry, persistent cough.[2,23] A simple approach to a hypertensive patient with cough on an ACEI is to stop the ACEI. Cessation of the ACEI should be trialed regardless of when the cough began in relation to initiation of the ACEI because cough can present

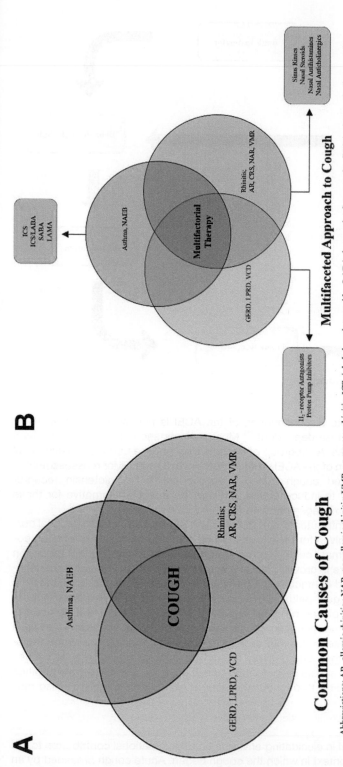

Common Causes of Cough

Multifaceted Approach to Cough

Abbreviations: AR, allergic rhinitis ; NAR, non allergic rhinitis; ICS, inhaled corticosteroid; LABA, long acting beta agonist; SABA, short acting beta agonist.

Fig. 1. (A) Common causes of cough and (B) multifaceted approach to treatment. AR, allergic rhinitis; CRS, chronic rhinosinusitis; GERD, gastroesophageal reflux disease; ICS, inhaled corticosteroid; NAR, non allergic rhinitis; LABA, long acting beta agonist; SABA, short acting beta agonist; VMR, vasomotor rhinitis.

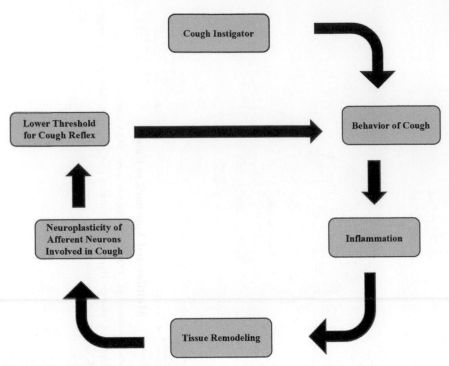

Fig. 2. Cyclical nature of cough.

sporadically.[24] Complete discontinuation of the ACEI is necessary because ACEI-induced cough is not dose dependent.[23] Most patients see improvement of cough within 1 week to 4 weeks. A subgroup of patients may not see benefit, however, until 3 months after cessation of the ACEI. Thus, follow-up at 3 months for reassessment of suspected ACEI-induced cough may be appropriate.[23,24] Angiotensin receptor blockers are less likely to induce cough and may be a viable alternative for those requiring hypertension management with ACEI-induced cough.[25]

A counterintuitive contributor of cough is the use of oral corticosteroids. Oral corticosteroids are often given for the purpose of relieving cough via its effects on eosinophils, neutrophils, mast cells, macrophage function, and consequent reduction of inflammation.[26] There is growing evidence, however, that oral corticosteroids increase esophageal acid contact. A link between higher doses of oral corticosteroid use and gastroesophageal reflux (GER) has been shown.[27] As discussed subsequently, GER is a key player in myriad potential causes of cough.[28] If corticosteroids are indicated in the management of cough and there is suspicion that GER may be contributing, alternative methods of delivery, such as inhaled or intramuscular injection, rather than oral delivery should be considered in order to reduce potential for acid reflux and its perpetuating role in cough.[27] The temporary addition of a proton pump inhibitor throughout the course of oral corticosteroids also may provide benefit.

Environment

A history can be helpful in elucidating environmental or situational contributors to the cough. Consider the context in which the cough began. Acute cough preceded by an upper respiratory tract infection is suggestive of a postinfectious cough and support-ive therapy is indicated. Questions regarding formal diagnoses of chronic rhinosinusi-tis (CRS) and GER, or symptoms suggestive of these disease processes, are imperative when collecting patients' history because sinusitis and GER are common contributors of a persistent cough.[2,8,15] Inquiries should include subtle symptoms or less recognized symptoms of either sinusitis or GER or both. These may include facial pressure (not pain), change in sense of smell, increased postnasal drip (PND) and/or intermittent drainage for sinusitis and throat clearing, cough when eating or lying down, and intermittent hoarseness for GER disease (GERD).

Those with cough living in an overcrowded urbanized or poverty-stricken environ-ment should be assessed for risk of TB.[13,29] Individuals with insidious, progressive dry cough and shortness of breath in the setting of high-risk sexual behaviors should be evaluated for immunosuppression associated with human immunodeficiency syn-drome (HIV) or AIDS.[30,31] A history that includes recent prolonged travel and sedentary state in an obese patient or risk factors for venous thrombosis and pulmonary embo-lism may warrant an investigation to assess for these processes.[32,33] It would be remiss not to consider the milieu and risk factors that precede the cough.

Another consideration for cough is potential irritants in the home or work setting. Smoking is a well-recognized risk factor for lung cancer and chronic cough.[34,35] Occu-pational risks for cough include acute or chronic exposures to irritating inhalants.[36] Avoidance measures from environmental irritants that may trigger cough is a practical, cost-effective, and safe approach that should not be disregarded when considering methods of cough management.

COMMON CULPRITS OF COUGH

If a basic history provides little insight to the etiology of cough, a practical approach is to then assess for the most common culprits. As delineated by the 2006 *CHEST* Guideline and Expert Panel Report, the most common causes of cough include upper airway cough syndrome (UACS), GER, asthma, nonasthmatic eosinophilic bronchitis (NAEB), or a combination of these 4 conditions.[8,37,38] A patient with chronic cough may not show improvement until all contributing factors are treated. In a patient with longstanding cough, initiating simultaneous treatment of UACS, infection, GER/LPRD, and NAEB/cough equivalent asthma (CEA) should be considered. If a more conservative approach is desired, the condition that seems to contribute greatest to the cough should be treated. Then, therapy should be sequentially escalated by add-ing on to the treatment rather than discontinuing and starting an alternative monother-apy. Cough in a nonhypertensive, nonsmoking patient with a history lacking in evidence of environmental irritants should be evaluated for these potential causes of cough.

Upper Airway Cough Syndrome

UACS, also known as PND syndrome, is a common precipitate for cough. Previous studies show that UACS can be implicated in up to 87% of patients with cough.[8,10,15,39] Rhinitis plays a provocative role in PND via inflammation and excess secretions resulting in induction of the cough reflex.[9,12,40]

Laryngopharyngeal Reflux Disorder, Gastroesophageal Reflux, and Vocal Cord Dysfunction

In a similar fashion, PND can be driven by laryngopharyngeal reflux disorder (LPRD), GER, or vocal cord dysfunction (VCD) through chronic irritation from gastric fluids and frequent throat clearing. It has been shown that up to 75% of patients presenting with chronic cough have LPRD.[28]

Empiric treatment of UACS has high yield for success with minimal risks.[8,41] Generally, the risks of short-term comprehensive therapy (LPRD, GER, and CRS) for UACS poses minimal adverse outcomes and the high yield for treatment of UACS is worth exploring before an extensive work-up is initiated.[8,41] For example, initiating a trial of simultaneous therapy for LPRD with antireflux therapy and nasal steroids for rhinitis generally poses minimal risk when used appropriately. These therapies usually are inexpensive and found over the counter, and their combined use often results in an improvement if not resolution of the bothersome cough.

In addition to UACS, asthma and NAEB are common culprits of cough that benefit from an inexpensive work-up and relatively low-risk therapies while often producing favorable outcomes.[8–10,42]

Asthma

Asthma can present with an array of symptoms, including cough, shortness of breath, chest tightness, or wheezing. Complicating the diagnosis of asthma is its expansive continuum in clinical presentation. Asthma may present as several congruent symptoms or as just a single symptom.[43] It has been shown that a substantial subset of asthmatics present with the sole symptom of cough via CEA.[44] This is not uncommon with early-onset allergic asthma, especially with children but also can be seen after an infection at any age.[43,45] Not only can a trial of asthma management provide timely and safe treatment of cough but also it may also prevent CEA from progressing into classic asthma when found in its early stages.[12,43]

Nonasthmatic Eosinophilic Bronchitis

NAEB accounts for up to 13% to 30% of cough cases referred to a specialist despite its prevalence and simple management.[10,42] Eosinophilic airway inflammation, as seen in NAEB, has been found to play a prevalent role in cough especially after an acute upper respiratory tract infection.[46] Asthma (in particular, eosinophilic asthma) and NAEB may present similarly because they both usually involve eosinophilic inflammation of the airways. Reversibility of airway obstruction, however, which is commonly seen in asthma (but not diagnostic of asthma), is not seen with NAEB.[9] In addition, bronchoprovocation tests (ie, methacholine challenge) usually show differing results in classic asthma and CEA compared with NAEB, where methacholine challenge is negative in NAEB and is positive in classic asthma and CEA.[47] Regardless, patients with CEA, NAEB, or asthma should all show benefit from a trial of systemic or inhaled corticosteroids. Lack of response to corticosteroids should prompt reconsideration of the diagnosis.[9,10,42] An improvement in cough for patients with asthma or NAEB-related cough should see improvement within approximately 4 weeks.[42]

In addition to distinguishing the role of asthma and NAEB in cough, spirometry can provide insight into chronic obstructive pulmonary disease (COPD) as a component of the cough.[48,49] Although less commonly a culprit compared with asthma and NAEB, COPD is a known precipitate of cough and formal pulmonary function tests (eg, low diffusing capacity of the lungs for carbon monoxide) can help identify or strengthen the argument for COPD targeted management. Long-acting β-agonists with or without inhaled corticosteroids and inhaled long-acting muscarinic antagonists (LAMAs) for treatment of COPD are generally well tolerated.[13,50]

It is also important to understand the cough in the context in which it first occurred, the nature of the cough, and its exacerbating factors. For example, if it is postinfectious, continued infection, such as subacute sinusitis, is likely to continue to cause cough. Coughing fits/spasms or coughing during the night, with exercise, or with a deep breath are symptoms consistent with airway hyper-reactivity whereas cough with eating or lying down may indicate a GERD component. Often, the cough is multifactorial and treatment of all causes and exacerbating factors is needed to fully resolve the cough, after which medication often is no longer needed.

LESS COMMON CAUSES OF COUGH

If the cough remains recalcitrant despite exploration of the most common causes, less frequent causes of cough should be considered.

Pneumonia

Pneumonia, whether viral or bacterial, is a diagnosis that should not be neglected in the evaluation of cough. A patient presenting with cough accompanied by fever, tachypnea, and pain with inspiration should be considered for work-up and treatment of pneumonia. Health care providers should consider atypical presentations of pneumonia in those who are older or immunosuppressed.[1] Patients with a confirmed diagnosis of pneumonia should be prepared for the potential for a postinfectious cough and to address any instigating factors that may contribute to the cough, such as LPRD/GER, and sinusitis.[2,8] Anticipating the likelihood of a postinfectious cough can help direct management and also provide reassurance to patients.

Aspiration and Dysphagia

Unlike viral and bacterial pneumonias, aspiration pneumonia results from the misdirection of materials into the airway rather than the esophagus. Cough can be a consequence of the proximity of the airway and the esophagus and can present in patients with an underlying disorder that results in food retention in the esophagus (eg, achalasia and eosinophilic esophagitis).[13] Treatment of the underlying cause(s) for dysphagia may improve the cough.

Cardiovascular Disease, Congestive Heart Failure

Similar to the retention of materials in the gastrointestinal system, fluid congestion secondary to cardiovascular dysfunction can trigger the cough reflex. Shortness of breath and cough are common presentations in the patient with uncontrolled congestive heart failure. An imbalance in fluid distribution from the cardiovascular system into the pulmonary system leads to fluid congestion in the lungs resulting in shortness of breath and cough. Measures to correct the fluid distribution in congestive heart failure (CHF) often result in improvement of the presenting cough.[51]

Bronchiectasis

Another disease process that commonly presents with cough is bronchiectasis. Bronchiectasis is the permanent damage and widening of the bronchi usually as a result of recurrent infections and the repeated inflammation that ensues.[52] Therefore, disorders that predispose the airways to recurrent infections or inflammation (eg, allergic bronchopulmonary aspergillosis, cystic fibrosis, common variable immunodeficiency, and specific antibody deficiency) often are associated with bronchiectasis. Bronchiectasis can self-perpetuate the cough reflex by impairing muco-ciliary clearance via chronic inflammation, predisposing the patient to more infections.[52]

Tracheobronchomalacia

Tracheobronchomalacia (TBM) also entails a mechanistic impairment in the airway that can result in cough. TBM involves the softening of the trachea and bronchial cartilage, resulting in a narrowed airway lumen. The literature describes an excessive dynamic airway collapse that often presents with a dry, barking cough stubborn to pharmacologic treatment.[53] Complicating the treatment of cough in TMB is the proclivity of the disorder to be associated with other pulmonary comorbidities, such as asthma or COPD.

Neurogenic Cough

When discrete sources for the cough elude these treatments and the cough remains refractory, the neurogenic cough should be considered. Appreciation for the physical and mechanistic consequences of cough is essential in understanding the neurogenic cough.[54] The instigating cause of cough (eg, respiratory infection, environmental irritant, and GER) may be controlled. The physiologic changes that ensue, however, despite removing the initial cause(s) may continue to potentiate the cough. These changes lower the threshold for physical and chemical stimuli to induce cough and result in an easily provoked cough reflex.[55] The treatment of neuropathic pain in the setting of cough has shown success for a subgroup of patients and gives greater clout to the influence of the nervous system on cough.[54]

WORK-UP

If a cough remains stubborn to a trial treatment of the leading diagnoses for cough, a work-up is indicated.[17,18] Objective findings from a work-up can strengthen the argument for a specific treatment approach or help providers reconsider other differentials. The work-up should be focused and should heed patient risk factors and previously failed or beneficial therapies.

Although not traditionally considered part of a work-up, vital signs provide convenient and safe objective data in assessing a patient who presents with cough. An elevated temperature may direct care toward an infectious etiology. Pulse oximetry assesses oxygenation whereas a review of the heart rate and respiration rate may reveal compensatory mechanisms for suboptimal oxygenation, such as CHF or PE. For those with a history of cardiovascular disease, blood pressure is an important consideration, especially in those who might be in acute CHF. These data are generally easily accessible in most clinical settings.

The physical examination can help elucidate characteristics of the cough. Patients who cough with deep inspiration for the lung examination may have a component of bronchial hyperreactivity that is seen in asthma and the postinfectious cough. Erythematous nasal mucosa with purulent drainage suggests sinusitis may be contributing whereas pale, edematous turbinates may point to an allergic component. Presence of nasal polyps should increase suspicion of CRS. Often with CRS, drainage is intermittent and not seen on examination, and sometimes a CT of the sinuses is needed because one of the only symptoms of CRS may be cough.

Assessment of Lung Function

As discussed previously, spirometry is a simple tool that can elucidate several common causes of cough. The negative predictive value for a negative result is reliable and approaches 100%.[37,38] Despite being the gold standard for diagnosis of obstructive airway diseases, spirometry is underutilized.[56] It has been shown that approximately 45% of patients referred to a specialty for cough had not obtained a prior spirometry.[6] Although there is debate as to whether or not ubiquitous use of spirometry would specifically improve COPD detection and treatment, it is questionable to say that spirometry is not a valuable and safe tool in detecting many contributors of cough. In addition to the ability to help identify obstructive airway diseases, spirometry provides a visual of the inspiratory loop and the ratio of forced expiratory flow over forced inspiratory flow to help identify the presence of variable extrathoracic obstruction often seen in VCD, LPR, or GER. Spirometry also allows for the assessment of forced vital capacity and may help identify restrictive disorders contributing to cough, such as fibrotic disease. Similar to that of cough with deep inspiration on lung examination, cough can be induced by performing spirometry and can be indicative of bronchial hyperreactivity, as seen in asthma and a postinfectious cough. If interpretation for point of care spirometry is indeterminate or difficult, a formal pulmonary function test with or without a bronchoprovocation can provide a more conducive environment to obtain results.[48,49,56] Bronchoprovocation often is not necessary because it usually does not change management and may be misleading in cases of NAEB in which bronchoprovocation testing is negative but the treatment is the same as of asthma/CEA.

Assessment of Anatomic Abnormalities in Cough

A chest radiograph (CXR) is another valuable tool in elucidating several causes of cough. Despite being widely available and generally inexpensive, it has been found that fewer than 75% of patients had obtained a CXR prior to referral to a specialist.[6] A CXR may not be indicated for an acute or subacute cough (eg, postinfectious cough). A CXR should be obtained, however, if the cough is not responding to treatment and prior to referral to a specialist. A CXR can direct the need for further work-up, such as a chest CT or bronchoscopy.[57]

Assessment of Cardiovascular Disease in Setting of Cough

If a cardiovascular etiology is suspected, an electrocardiogram or echocardiogram in addition to trending blood pressures can provide a noninvasive assessment of cardiovascular function.[51]

Assessment of Blood Work in Cough

In addition to imaging, review or obtaining blood work can provide insight on several causes of cough. See **Table 1** for specific laboratory tests that may provide insight into etiology of the cough.

MANAGEMENT

Management of cough should involve a multipronged approach. In addition to pharmacologic therapies (**Tables 2** and **3**), addressing environmental exposures and patient behaviors that potentiate the cough reflex is essential to symptomatic improvement:

- Cessation of exposure to offending agents, whether environmental irritants or medications (eg, ACEI), is a practical first step in treating cough.[2,23,34–36] Further work-up may be indicated, such as allergy testing to aeroallergens.

Table 1
Differential diagnoses for cough and indicated work-up

Suspected Cause	Indicated Work-up
Asthma	Spirometry, PFT with bronchoprovocation
Bronchiectasis	Chest CT
CHF	BNP, ECHO
CRS	Sinus CT
HIV/AIDS	HIV antigen/antibody
Lung mass	CXR, chest CT
NAEB	Sputum culture
Pneumonia	CXR, procalcitonin
Pulmonary embolism	D dimer, chest CT with angiogram
TBM	Chest CT
TB	CXR
VD	Spirometry, PFT

Abbreviations: BNP, B-type natriuretic peptide; CT, computerized tomography scan; ECHO, echocardiogram; PFT, pulmonary function test.

- Behavioral changes, such as limiting throat clearing in VCD or dietary and lifestyle modifications in LPRD/GER.[8,15,18,28]
- Reiterating role of cough in perpetuating inflammation can help address behaviors that lower the threshold to induce cough.[19,20,54]

INDICATIONS FOR REFERRAL

If the cough persists despite these considerations and efforts, referral to a specialist may be warranted. This may be necessary for collaboration and second opinion. Referral to a specialist also may be beneficial even if the cause of cough has been identified but better treatment resources are necessary for complete

Table 2
Specified therapies for cough management

Category	Specified Therapies
Airway clearance	Positive expiratory pressure device, airway clearance vest, chest percussions
Antireflux Tx	H_2-receptor antagonists, proton pump inhibitors
Avoidance measures	Avoidance of culprits (eg, allergens, environmental/occupational triggers, irritants, ACEIs)
Behavioral changes	Dietary and lifestyle modifications, behavioral exercises (eg, voice therapy)
Nasal sprays	Saline sinus rinses, corticosteroids sinus rinses, nasal steroids, nasal antihistamines, anticholinergics
Neuropathic Tx	Antineuralgic medications (eg, amitriptyline)
Respiratory inhalers	ICS, combination ICS/LABA, LAMA, SABA
Systemic Tx	Systemic corticosteroids (PO/IM), antibiotics

Abbreviations: ICS, inhaled corticosteroid; LABA, long acting beta agonist; SABA, short acting beta agonist; Tx, treatment.

Table 3
Treatment of cough

	Airway Clearance	Antireflux Therapy	Avoidance Measures	Behavioral Changes	Nasal Sprays	Neuropathic Therapy	Respiratory Inhalers	Systemic Therapy
AR			●		●			
NAR			●		●			
VMR			●		●			
CRS					●			●
Dysphagia		●		●	●			
GERD		●	●	●				
LPRD		●	●	●				
VCD		●	●	●				
Aspiration		●	●	●				
Asthma							●	
COPD	●			●			●	
NAEB							●	
Bronchiectasis	●						●	●
TBM				●				●
Pneumonia							●	●
TB			●					●
CVD			●					
Neurogenic				●		●		

Abbreviations: AR, allergic rhinitis; CVD, cardiovascular disease; NAR, non allergic rhinitis; VMR, vasomotor rhinitis.

resolution of cough. For example, referral to ear, nose, and throat specialist can provide resources for voice therapy in VCD or evaluation of surgical intervention in the setting of uncontrolled CRS. As discussed previously, cough often is multifactorial. As a result, a multifaceted approach is necessary and may require a multidisciplinary approach (**Fig. 3**).

UC AR, UC NAR, Recurrent Infections, SAD, CVID, Spirometry	➡ **Allergy/Immunology**
Antihypertensive management, CHF management	➡ **Cardiology**
UC LPRD, UC CRS, VCD, Voice therapy	➡ **Ear, Nose, Throat**
UC GER, Achalasia, Dysphagia, EOE	➡ **Gastroenterology**
Abnormal Chest CT, Bronchiectasis, HP, PFT, TBM	➡ **Pulmonary**

Fig. 3. Referral considerations for cough. AR, allergic rhinitis; CT, computerized tomography scan; CVID, common variable immunodeficiency; EoE, eosinophilic esophagitis; HP, hypersensitivity pneumonitis; NAR, non allergic rhinitis; SAD, specific antibody deficiency; UC, uncontrolled.

SUMMARY

Cough is a prevalent symptom that can be difficult to treat. Addressing the many layers of cough is essential to providing sufficient relief for the coughing patient. Often, new-onset cough, such as the postinfectious cough, can be multifactorial, involving both the upper and lower airways. It is not uncommon for GERD to contribute to cough regardless of the initial cause, with cough and possibly throat clearing being the only symptoms making the role of GERD more difficult to appreciate. If all contributing factors are not recognized, addressed, and treated, resolution may be difficult to achieve, with the cough lasting months or even years. Although the cause of cough often can be diagnosed with minimal work-up and treatment is usually inexpensive and accessible, a recalcitrant cough may require referral to a specialist for a more thorough work-up or to provide additional treatment resources.

REFERENCES

1. Holzinger F, Beck S, Dini L, et al. The diagnosis and treatment of acute cough in adults. Dtsch Arztebl Int 2014;111(20):356–63.
2. Yu ML, Ryu JH. Assessment of the patient with chronic cough. Mayo Clin Proc 1997;72(10):957–9.
3. Nasra J, Belvisi MG. Modulation of sensory nerve function and the cough reflex: understanding disease pathogenesis. Pharmacol Ther 2009;124(3):354–75.
4. Andersson C, Bonvini SJ, Horvath P, et al. Research highlights from the 2017 ERS International Congress: airway diseases in focus. ERJ Open Res 2018;4(1) [pii: 00163-2017].
5. Dicpinigaitis PV, Eccles R, Blaiss MS, et al. Impact of cough and common cold on productivity, absenteeism, and daily life in the United States: ACHOO Survey. Curr Med Res Opin 2015;31(8):1519–25.
6. Turner RD, Bothamley GH. Chronic cough and a normal chest X-ray - a simple systematic approach to exclude common causes before referral to secondary care: a retrospective cohort study. NPJ Prim Care Respir Med 2016;26:15081.
7. Ojoo JC, Everett CF, Mulrennan SA, et al. Management of patients with chronic cough using a clinical protocol: a prospective observational study. Cough 2013;9(1):2.
8. Irwin RS, French CL, Chang AB, et al. Classification of Cough as a Symptom in Adults and Management Algorithms: CHEST Guideline and Expert Panel Report. Chest 2018;153(1):196–209.
9. Mahashur A. Chronic dry cough: Diagnostic and management approaches. Lung India 2015;32(1):44–9.
10. Pratter MR. Overview of common causes of chronic cough: ACCP evidence-based clinical practice guidelines. Chest 2006;129(1 Suppl):59S–62S.
11. Irwin RS, Corrao WM, Pratter MR. Chronic persistent cough in the adult: the spectrum and frequency of causes and successful outcome of specific therapy. Am Rev Respir Dis 1981;123(4 Pt 1):413–7.
12. Lalloo UG, Barnes PJ, Chung KF. Pathophysiology and clinical presentations of cough. J Allergy Clin Immunol 1996;98(5 Pt 2):S91–6 [discussion: S96–97].
13. Irwin RS, Baumann MH, Bolser DC, et al. Diagnosis and management of cough executive summary: ACCP evidence-based clinical practice guidelines. Chest 2006;129(1 Suppl):1S–23S.
14. Simpson CB, Amin MR. Chronic cough: state-of-the-art review. Otolaryngol Head Neck Surg 2006;134(4):693–700.

15. Chung KF, Pavord ID. Prevalence, pathogenesis, and causes of chronic cough. Lancet 2008;371(9621):1364–74.
16. Chung KF. Chronic cough: future directions in chronic cough: mechanisms and antitussives. Chron Respir Dis 2007;4(3):159–65.
17. Birring SS. New concepts in the management of chronic cough. Pulm Pharmacol Ther 2011;24(3):334–8.
18. Birring SS. Controversies in the evaluation and management of chronic cough. Am J Respir Crit Care Med 2011;183(6):708–15.
19. Chung KF, McGarvey L, Mazzone S. Chronic cough and cough hypersensitivity syndrome. Lancet Respir Med 2016;4(12):934–5.
20. Dicpinigaitis PV, Kantar A, Enilari O, et al. Prevalence of arnold nerve reflex in adults and children with chronic cough. Chest 2018;153(3):675–9.
21. Mello CJ, Irwin RS, Curley FJ. Predictive values of the character, timing, and complications of chronic cough in diagnosing its cause. Arch Intern Med 1996;156(9):997–1003.
22. Smyrnios NA, Irwin RS, Curley FJ. Chronic cough with a history of excessive sputum production. The spectrum and frequency of causes, key components of the diagnostic evaluation, and outcome of specific therapy. Chest 1995;108(4):991–7.
23. Dicpinigaitis PV. Angiotensin-converting enzyme inhibitor-induced cough: ACCP evidence-based clinical practice guidelines. Chest 2006;129(1 Suppl):169S–73S.
24. Israili ZH, Hall WD. Cough and angioneurotic edema associated with angiotensin-converting enzyme inhibitor therapy. A review of the literature and pathophysiology. Ann Intern Med 1992;117(3):234–42.
25. Caldeira D, David C, Sampaio C. Tolerability of angiotensin-receptor blockers in patients with intolerance to angiotensin-converting enzyme inhibitors: a systematic review and meta-analysis. Am J Cardiovasc Drugs 2012;12(4):263–77.
26. Belvisi MG. Regulation of inflammatory cell function by corticosteroids. Proc Am Thorac Soc 2004;1(3):207–14.
27. Lazenby JP, Guzzo MR, Harding SM, et al. Oral corticosteroids increase esophageal acid contact times in patients with stable asthma. Chest 2002;121(2):625–34.
28. Irwin RS. Chronic cough due to gastroesophageal reflux disease: ACCP evidence-based clinical practice guidelines. Chest 2006;129(1 Suppl):80S–94S.
29. Schmidt CW. Linking TB and the environment: an overlooked mitigation strategy. Environ Health Perspect 2008;116(11):A478–85.
30. Pinheiro MVC, Ho YL, Nicodemo AC, et al. The diagnosis of multiple opportunistic infections in advanced stage AIDS: when Ockham's Razor doesn't cut it. Autops Case Rep 2018;8(2):e2018028.
31. Tchatchouang S, Nzouankeu A, Donkeng V, et al. Prevalence of opportunistic pathogens Pneumocystis jiroveci and tubercle bacilli in HIV-infected patients with respiratory infections in Yaounde, Cameroon. AIDS Res Hum Retroviruses 2019;35(5):428–9.
32. Ji QY, Wang MF, Su CM, et al. Clinical symptoms and related risk factors in pulmonary embolism patients and cluster analysis based on these symptoms. Sci Rep 2017;7(1):14887.
33. Kline JA. Diagnosis and exclusion of pulmonary embolism. Thromb Res 2018;163:207–20.
34. Dicpinigaitis PV. Effect of tobacco and electronic cigarette use on cough reflex sensitivity. Pulm Pharmacol Ther 2017;47:45–8.

35. Dicpinigaitis PV, Sitkauskiene B, Stravinskaite K, et al. Effect of smoking cessation on cough reflex sensitivity. Eur Respir J 2006;28(4):786–90.

36. Katoto PDMC, Murhula A, Kayembe-Kitenge T, et al. Household air pollution is associated with chronic cough but not hemoptysis after completion of pulmonary tuberculosis treatment in adults, rural eastern democratic republic of congo. Int J Environ Res Public Health 2018;15(11) [pii:E2563].

37. Lin L, Poh KL, Lim TK. Empirical treatment of chronic cough–a cost-effectiveness analysis. Proc AMIA Symp 2001;383–7.

38. Irwin RS, Madison JM. The diagnosis and treatment of cough. N Engl J Med 2000;343(23):1715–21.

39. Pavord ID, Chung KF. Management of chronic cough. Lancet 2008;371(9621): 1375–84.

40. Cruz AA. The 'united airways' require an holistic approach to management. Allergy 2005;60(7):871–4.

41. Pratter MR, Bartter T, Akers S, et al. An algorithmic approach to chronic cough. Ann Intern Med 1993;119(10):977–83.

42. Brightling CE. Chronic cough due to nonasthmatic eosinophilic bronchitis: ACCP evidence-based clinical practice guidelines. Chest 2006;129(1 Suppl): 116S–21S.

43. Niimi A. Cough and Asthma. Curr Respir Med Rev 2011;7(1):47–54.

44. Niimi A, Ohbayashi H, Sagara H, et al. Cough variant and cough-predominant asthma are major causes of persistent cough: a multicenter study in Japan. J Asthma 2013;50(9):932–7.

45. Goldsobel AB, Chipps BE. Cough in the pediatric population. J Pediatr 2010; 156(3):352–8.

46. Lai K, Lin L, Liu B, et al. Eosinophilic airway inflammation is common in subacute cough following acute upper respiratory tract infection. Respirology 2016;21(4): 683–8.

47. Dicpinigaitis PV. Chronic cough due to asthma: ACCP evidence-based clinical practice guidelines. Chest 2006;129(1 Suppl):75S–9S.

48. Bouharaoua S, Combe-Cayla P, Rakotonirina S, et al. Spirometry in primary care to screen for COPD: Feedback from a feasibility study in a semi-rural area. Rev Mal Respir 2017;34(9):1037–9 [in French].

49. Ferguson GT, Enright PL, Buist AS, et al. Office spirometry for lung health assessment in adults: a consensus statement from the National Lung Health Education Program. Respir Care 2000;45(5):513–30.

50. Pires N, Pinto P, Marçal N, et al, GI DPOC Interest Group on Chronic Obstructive Pulmonary Disease. Pharmacological treatment of COPD - New evidence. Pulmonology 2019;25(2):90–6.

51. Currens JH, White PD. Cough as a symptom of cardiovascular disease. Ann Intern Med 1949;30(3):528–43.

52. King PT. The pathophysiology of bronchiectasis. Int J Chron Obstruct Pulmon Dis 2009;4:411–9.

53. Dal Negro RW, Tognella S, Guerriero M, et al. Prevalence of tracheobronchomalacia and excessive dynamic airway collapse in bronchial asthma of different severity. Multidiscip Respir Med 2013;8(1):32.

54. Chung KF. Approach to chronic cough: the neuropathic basis for cough hypersensitivity syndrome. J Thorac Dis 2014;6(Suppl 7):S699–707.

55. Lim K. Neurogenic cough. J Allergy Clin Immunol 2014;133(6). 1779-.e3.

56. Vanjare N, Chhowala S, Madas S, et al. Use of spirometry among chest physicians and primary care physicians in India. NPJ Prim Care Respir Med 2016; 26:16036.
57. Speets AM, van der Graaf Y, Hoes AW, et al. Chest radiography in general practice: indications, diagnostic yield and consequences for patient management. Br J Gen Pract 2006;56(529):574–8.

Allergic Contact Dermatitis

Stacy Nassau, MD*, Luz Fonacier, MD

KEYWORDS

- Contact dermatitis • Allergic contact dermatitis • Irritant contact dermatitis
- Systemic contact dermatitis • Eczema • Nickel allergy

KEY POINTS

- Allergic contact dermatitis is a common skin disorder affecting millions of Americans.
- Common allergens are seemingly ubiquitous and are found in daily products, at work, and even in foods.
- Allergic contact dermatitis can present as an acute, subacute, or chronic dermatitis.
- Diagnosis of allergic contact dermatitis is based on a thorough history, physical examination, and patch testing.
- Once the allergen is identified, the mainstay of treatment is avoidance.

INTRODUCTION

Contact dermatitis is a common inflammatory skin disorder affecting millions of Americans and is the chief complaint for thousands of clinic visits to the internist every year. The disorder is characterized by pruritus, erythema, vesicles and scaling of the skin. Contact dermatitis can be further divided into allergic contact dermatitis (ACD) and irritant contact dermatitis (ICD), with ICD being more common (~80% of contact dermatitis)[1] ACD is a type IV-mediated hypersensitivity to a specific allergen, resulting in an inflammatory response with exposure. ICD is a nonimmunologically driven, inflammatory reaction to an irritating substance. These 2 types of dermatitis are often indistinguishable clinically.

PATHOPHYSIOLOGY

ACD is a type IV delayed-type hypersensitivity reaction resulting from the activation of allergen-specific T cells. The first phase is sensitization, when a person is first exposed to an allergen. The allergen is a hapten, which is defined as a low-molecular-weight antigen that, when bound to a larger carrier, can elicit an immune response. Initially, the hapten is engulfed by Langerhans cells or dermal dendritic cells. The hapten–peptide

Disclosure Statement: The authors have nothing to disclose.
Department of Internal Medicine, Section of Allergy and Immunology, NYU Winthrop University Hospital, 120 Mineola Boulevard, Suite 410, Mineola, NY 11501, USA
* Corresponding author.
E-mail address: Stacy.Nassau@nyulangone.org

Med Clin N Am 104 (2020) 61–76
https://doi.org/10.1016/j.mcna.2019.08.012

medical.theclinics.com

complexes migrate to regional lymph nodes of the skin, where they prime hapten-specific T cells (Th1, Th2, Th17, and T regulatory cells) that proliferate and circulate in the blood. The naïve T cells that specifically recognize allergen–major histocompatibility complex molecule complexes expand and create effector and memory T cells. The next phase is elicitation, where reexposure to the allergen results in recognition by the now-sensitized, hapten-specific T cells, causing an inflammatory cascade of cytokines and cellular infiltrates producing the clinical symptoms of ACD.[2]

EPIDEMIOLOGY

ACD is common, with some studies demonstrating prevalence rates as high as 20% of the general population.[3] Certain groups are at higher risk of developing ACD, which seems to be a result of both genetic tendencies and environmental exposures. Not all people exposed to a particular allergen become sensitized. Individuals sensitized to 1 allergen are more susceptible to sensitization with another.[4] Family members have been shown to have an increased rate of developing ACD, suggesting a genetic predisposition; however, a confounding factor is the shared environment.[4] Studies further evaluating genetic contributions to ACD are vast and ongoing. Patients with a history of atopic dermatitis have higher susceptibility in developing ICD, which is likely related to disruptions in the skin barrier and a greater inflammatory response.[2]

Contact dermatitis, both allergic and irritant, accounts for the vast majority of occupational skin disorders in the Western world.[5] Hairdressers, health care workers, food handlers, building and construction workers, and metal workers have high rates of developing ACD based on their close and repeated contact with common allergens.[6] ACD can have a significant negative impact on workplace productivity and expenses.[7] Many workers with significant disease require prolonged absences from work, need to alter practices at work, or may even change to another line of work based on the severity of their disease.[8]

Women seem to be at higher risk of developing ACD. This difference is thought to be a result of exposures as opposed to inherent to sex; for example, women have higher rates of nickel allergy potentially owing to the increased frequency of wearing jewelry.[9]

DIFFERENTIAL DIAGNOSIS

It can be difficult to distinguish ACD from other forms of dermatitis. A wide range of disorders, from common entities such as ICD, atopic dermatitis, seborrheic dermatitis, psoriasis and tinea, to the less common, mycosis fungoides, are all part of the differential diagnosis.[1] Importantly, these various disorders may coexist in the same patient.[1] History, patch testing, and other forms of testing (ie, biopsy, potassium hydroxide scraping) may help to clarify the diagnosis.

DIAGNOSIS

A thorough history is central to making the diagnosis of ACD. It is important to elucidate when the lesions developed, how they have evolved over time, and any suspected agents. Suspicious agents may be difficult to identify, because the reaction to the allergen is not always immediate. This delay in reaction, which can be up to 72 hours, can make identifying exposures difficult for both the patient and health care providers. The location and distribution of the lesions can aid in the diagnosis. Often it is difficult to identify any suspect agents at all, especially when the dermatitis has been longstanding. Thorough questioning of occupation, hobbies, and any changes in personal products or clothing is helpful.[10] When asking about work, questions should include the type of work performed, potential allergens or irritants the patient is in contact with, duration of exposure, and any improving or aggravating factors. In particular, skin improvement during vacation or sick leave can be an important clue.[11] Previous treatments, both prescription and over the counter, and the response to such treatment are important. If previous treatment resulted in worsening of the lesions, suspect a contact dermatitis to those agents.[12] A history of atopy, especially atopic dermatitis, may be a contributing factor in the development of ACD. A family history of psoriasis or other skin diseases is also important, because these entities may be confused for ACD.[4]

ACD may present as acute, subacute, or chronic dermatitis. Acute ACD is most often characterized by erythematous papules and vesicles. Severe cases may present with bullae. Chronic ACD tends to present as erythematous and pruritic lesions that may display the stigmata of more long-standing inflammation, such as lichenification, scaling, and fissuring. With disruption of the epidermal barrier, as can been seen in chronic ACD, superinfection can result. Subacute ACD is more difficult to characterize and can display a mixture of features.

Distribution is helpful in the diagnosis of ACD. Certain distributions, such as on the eyelid, lateral face, central face, neck, or hands, should trigger the consideration of ACD to cosmetics and personal products. **Table 1** lists the top 10 primary sites of ACD. The most common sites are the hands, a scattered or generalized pattern, and the face.[13]

Hands

The hands are the most common primary body site involved in contact dermatitis.[13] The majority of hand dermatitis is due to ICD. Classically, lesions of irritant hand dermatitis involve the palms, dorsal hand, and distal dorsal digits, but may also involve the interdigital web spaces where irritants get caught. In contrast, ACD of the hand usually presents as well-demarcated plaques and vesicles involving the dorsal hands, fingers, and wrists. Common allergens include preservatives, fragrances, metals, rubber, and topical antibiotics.[14]

Vesicular hand dermatitis can be a manifestation of systemic contact dermatitis (SCD), such as after the ingestion of nickel-containing foods by patients sensitized

Table 1	
Body sites of dermatitis as the primary involvement	
Dermatitis Site	**N (%)**
Hand	1230 (22.0)
Scattered generalized	995 (17.8)
Face	946 (16.9)
Eyelids	535 (9.6)
Trunk	307 (5.5)
Lips	274 (4.9)
Arm	230 (4.1)
Scalp	225 (4.0)
Leg	207 (3.7)
Foot	120 (2.1)
Total n	5591

Adapted from DeKoven JG, Warshaw EM, Zug KA, et al. North American Contact Dermatitis Group Patch Test Results: 2015-2016. Dermatitis 2018:29(6):297-309; with permission.

to nickel. Other causes of hand dermatitis are atopic dermatitis (more common in adults)[15] as well as dyshidrotic hand eczema, which presents as intensely pruritic, deep-seated vesicles appearing in clusters on the palms (most commonly on the thenar eminence), dorsal hands, and sides of the fingers. The feet can also be affected by dyshidrotic eczema in the same distribution.

Face

The following are general patterns of facial contact dermatitis.

1. Central face
   - Dermatitis involving the central face (cheeks, nose, chin, and forehead) may be due to ACD to gold (released from gold jewelry and contaminating titanium-containing foundation), make-up, moisturizers, wrinkle creams, and topical medications.
2. Lateral face
   - Dermatitis involving the lateral face (preauricular areas, postauricular area, jaw lines, and/or lateral neck) is most commonly due to shampoo and/or conditioner dripping down over these areas (**Fig. 1**).
3. Full face
   - Full facial dermatitis may be due to make-up foundation, facial cleansers, moisturizers, or airborne contactants.
4. Unilateral predominance
   - Unilateral facial dermatitis may be due to an ectopic transfer from the hands of contact allergens in nail products, fragrances, and topical medication. Connubial or consort contact dermatitis to products used by the partner or parent may also be transferred predominantly to 1 side of the face.[16]

Eyelids

The eyelids are one of the most sensitive areas of skin, and thus are susceptible to irritants and allergens. ACD of the lids and periorbital area is primarily caused by cosmetics applied to the hair, face, or fingernails, and include shampoo, conditioner, facial cleansers, make-up remover, mascara, nail polish, acrylic nails, make-up

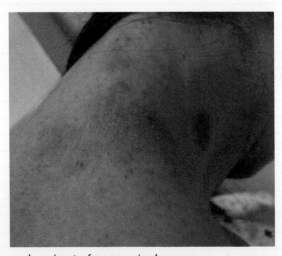

Fig. 1. ACD of the neck owing to fragrance in shampoo.

sponges, eyelash curlers, and allergens transferred from the hands. Marked edema of the eyelids is often a feature of poison ivy or hair dye dermatitis. Airborne pollen, dust and all types of volatile agents may affect the eyelids, and manifest as a type 4 cell-mediated hypersensitivity reaction. This entity should be distinguished from a type 1 IgE-mediated allergic conjunctivitis.

Other common allergens associated with eyelid dermatitis include gold, fragrances, formaldehyde-related preservatives, methylisothiazolinone (MI; a preservative in both industrial and consumer products), and cocamidopropyl betaine (a surfactant in shampoos and soaps).[17] Shellac and pigments in mascara can also cause ACD of the eyelids.[18–20] Shampoos and conditioners are probably the most common causes of isolated ACD of the eyelids.[21] Other hair products such as dyes, bleaching agents, setting lotions, sprays, gels, and mousses are more likely to involve the scalp or forehead in addition to the eyelid. Facial cleansers may cause dermatitis of the eyelid and the face. Ectopic dermatitis from nail polish and acrylic nail dermatitis more commonly affects some combination of the eyelids, face, and neck rather than an isolated eyelid dermatitis.[16] Eyelid dermatitis may also be due to seborrheic dermatitis, atopic dermatitis, or ICD.[22]

OTHER MANIFESTATIONS OF ALLERGIC CONTACT DERMATITIS
Occupational Allergic Contact Dermatitis

The hand is commonly involved in occupational contact dermatitis. The following is a list of some of the more common allergens responsible for ACD in the occupational setting: rubber accelerators, carbamates and thiurams (**Fig. 2**) are used in rubber processing (vulcanization) to speed up the reaction. They are found in the elastic that is commonly used in undergarments, socks, waistbands, surgical bonnets, wrists of surgical gowns, hair ornaments, shoe covers, and shoes. In the workplace, they can also be found in both latex and latex-free gloves.

Epoxy resin exposure can be found in the maritime industry, the electronics industry, dentistry, flooring industry, and industries working with epoxy glues. Epoxy resin is a frequent occupational allergen.[23]

Formaldehyde is a common occupational allergen used in many fields, such as in anatomic pathology laboratories (where it is used to preserve the bodies), farming, furniture making, wood manufacturing, laboratory work, pest control, and construction. Formaldehyde resins are also used in permanent press clothing to prevent wrinkling; therefore, launderers and workers in the textile industries may develop sensitization.[24] Formaldehyde releasers are preservatives that may release molecules of formaldehyde over time and are commonly found in cleansers, detergents, and

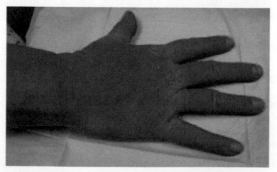

Fig. 2. ACD of the hands owing to rubber accelerator in gloves.

protective creams. People who do not handle these materials in their work may still be affected and can present with a diffuse dermatitis secondary to wearing clothing treated with formaldehyde or its resin.

Nickel is the most common contact allergen in North America[13] and is found in many workplaces, including those involving machines, office supplies, tools, electronics, uniforms, jewelry, keys, and coins.

Systemic Contact Dermatitis

ACD begins with sensitization through the skin. Systemic exposure to allergens (including transepidermal routes, intravenous or intramuscular routes, inhalation, and ingestion) that results in a cutaneous eruption is known as SCD.[25] SCD can manifest as a systemic exacerbation, reactivation of a previous dermatitis, vesicular hand eczema, or a flare-up reaction of the previous site of a positive patch test.[26] Studies have shown that, after clinical resolution of ACD, T cells may remain in the affected area.[27] Upon reexposure to the allergen via an alternative pathway, a rash can develop at a previous site of dermatitis or patch test.[26] The presentation of SCD is variable. The reactivation of a previously affected site can occur days after the exposure, making it difficult to identify and associate that exposure as the cause of the flare. In addition to an exacerbation of prior skin site reactions, SCD can present with dyshidrotic eczema on the hands, a generalized maculopapular or vesicular rash, erythema multiforme, and an entity known as the Baboon syndrome.[26] Baboon syndrome is characterized by a bright, erythematous eruption on the buttocks, and has been described more commonly with metals, balsam of Peru (BOP), and medications.[25] Several metals have been described to cause SCD, including nickel, mercury, cobalt, copper, chromium, gold, and zinc.[25] Numerous studies have shown oral ingestion of nickel in food resulting in worsening of dermatitis in nickel-allergic patients.[27–29]

Systemic contact allergy as it relates to metal implants has become of recent interest. Metals are frequently implanted into the human body, in the form of orthopedic, cardiac, gynecologic, and dental devices. As the metal wears down over time, free ions are released and may deposit around the prosthetic site or into other organs in the body.[29,30] Sensitization to metals increased by 6.5% after arthroplasty.[31] In patients with hip arthroplasty, sensitization to nickel, cobalt, or chromium was seen in 25% of well-functioning implants (>2× the general population) and 60% in failed or failing prosthesis (6× the general population).[32] A study of patients with total knee arthroplasty showed a metal sensitization rate of 20% in those with no implant, 48.1% in those with stable implant, and 59.6% in unstable implant group.[33]

Intravascular devices and prosthetic joints are typically made of stainless steel, nitinol, or vitallium (a chromium/cobalt alloy), all of which release varying amounts of nickel.[29,31] Joint failures, restenosis of cardiac stents, oral reactions to dental implants, and skin rashes including urticaria have all been attributed to ACD to implanted metals.[34,35] Because of the widespread exposure to metals in daily products and foods, it is often unclear what the role of the implant plays.

PEARLS AND PITFALLS OF PATCH TESTING

Patch testing is the only practical, scientific and objective method to confirm diagnosis of ACD.

Patch Test Allergens

A core or baseline series of patch test antigens includes those used by the North American Contact Dermatitis Group (NACDG), the T.R.U.E. Test panel, and the

Core Allergen Series outlined by the American Contact Dermatitis Society. Most of these allergens are dispersed in white petrolatum as its vehicle. Those that cannot be dispersed in white petrolatum owing to the chemical stability are supplied in aqueous form.

Studies have shown that approximately 23% to 25% of relevant allergens may be missed if supplementary allergens are not used..[13,36,37] Thus, consider using supplemental patch test allergens based on specific patient exposures, personal products, and workplace materials in addition to the core or baseline series of patch test allergens. Relying solely on these series in all patients is likely to lead to an underdiagnosis of ACD. Kits with allergen panels selected for a specific industry such as machinists, cosmetologists, or dental workers, or for specific exposures such as cosmetics, textiles, plastics, and glues, and medications and topical treatments may be obtained from different manufacturers. The American Contact Dermatitis Society recommends a screening panel of about 80 allergens,[38,39] but the current data suggest that even this number may not be sufficient to adequately screen a significant percentage of patients.

There are no head-to-head studies between the NACDG recommended series, the T.R.U.E. Test, or the American Contact Dermatitis Society core antigen panel. Hypothetically, if only the T.R.U.E. allergens were tested, the T.R.U.E. Test would detect 61.6% to 74.0% of reactions found by the NACDG screening series' results from January 1, 2015, to February 28, 2017.[13] Of the top 40 NACDG allergens, the following are not included in the T.R.U.E. Test and could be missed: MI, fragrance mix II, iodopropynyl butylcarbamate, propylene glycol, oleamidopropyl dimethylamine, 2-hydroxyethyl-methacrylate, dimethylaminopropylamine, decyl glucoside, ammoniumpersulfate, benzophenone-4, ethyl acrylate, cocamidopropyl betaine, methyl methacrylate, and amidoamine and propolis (used in homeopathic remedies).[13]

In certain distributions, such as in eyelid, lip, and facial dermatitis, it may be necessary to include the patient's personal products. In general, leave-on products (such as lipstick, blush, moisturizer, and foundation), clothing, and gloves can be tested as is. Rinse-off products (shampoo, conditioners, and antiperspirant) can be irritants and should be diluted.[26] Other nonstandardized allergens, household cleansers, and industrial products should only be tested by physicians with expertise in this type of testing after evaluating the material safety data sheets information. De Groot's Test Concentrations and Vehicles of 4350 Chemicals are available to help determine appropriate testing concentrations, vehicles, and controls.[40]

The standard and/or additional series of patch test allergens are sold by companies working in close connection with the International Contact Dermatitis Research Group and other international and national groups.

ALLERGENS CAUSING ALLERGIC CONTACT DERMATITIS

The most frequently positive allergic reactions in the most recent NACD Series report[13] included 2 metals—nickel sulfate (17.5%) and cobalt (6.2%); 2 antibiotics—neomycin (7.0%) and bacitracin (6.9%); 3 fragrances—fragrance mix I (11.3%), fragrance mix II (5.3%), and myroxylon pereirae (7.0%); 4 preservatives—MI [13.4%], methylchloroisothiazolinone (MCI)/MI (7.3%), formaldehyde 1% (6.4%) and 2% (8.4%); and iodopropynyl butylcarbamate (3.9%), propylene glycol (4.0%), p-phenylenediamine (PPD; 6.4%), lanolin alcohol (4.1%), and carba mix (4.6%; **Table 2**).

Table 2
Selected allergens and common sources of exposure

Allergen	Common Sources of Exposure
Fragrances	
BOP	Cosmetics, fragrances, dental hygiene products, topical medications, food
Fragrance mix I and II	Fragrances, scented household products
Formaldehyde and formaldehyde-releasing preservatives	
Formaldehyde	Fabric finishes, cosmetics
Quaternium-15	Preservative in cosmetics and skin care products
Diazolidinyl urea	Products for personal care, hygiene and hair care, cosmetics, pet shampoos
Imidazolidinyl urea	Products for personal care, hygiene and hair care, cosmetics, liquid soaps, moisturizers
2-Bromo-2-nitropropane-1,3-diol	Topical antibiotic/antifungal creams/ointments, finger paints, kitty litter, detergents, toiletries and cleansers, cleansing lotions, mouthwash, shampoos
DMDM hydantoin	Wipes, personal care/hygiene products, cosmetics, baby care products, polishes
Nonformaldehyde-releasing preservatives	
Parabens	Preservative in topical formulations, cosmetics, personal care products
MCI-MI	Baby products, personal care/hygiene products, cosmetics
Methyldibromoglutaronitrile-phenoxyethanol	Skin care products, sunscreens, baby care, personal hygiene products (moist toilet paper, shampoos, shower gel)
Iodopropynyl butylcarbamate	Baby care, personal care/hygiene products, cosmetics, hair dye, industry, lip products, paints, yard care
Surfactants	
Cocamidopropyl betaine	Hair and bath products, medicated ointments and creams, cosmetics, oral care
Oleamidopropyl dimethylamine	Cosmetics, conditioners, baby lotions, body lotions, deodorants
Decyl glucoside	Cosmetics, baby shampoo, body washes
Dimethylaminopropylamine	Personal care/hygiene products, medicated ointments and creams, cosmetics, hair detanglers
Amidoamine	Personal care/hygiene products, medicated ointments and creams, cosmetics, hair detanglers
Acrylates	
2-Hydroxyethyl-methacrylate	Possible exposure to acrylic compounds include nail polish, artificial finger nails, hair spray, paints, plastics, adhesives
Ethyl acrylate	Cross-link agent in rubber
Methyl methacrylate	Resin used in dentistry, bone cement, adhesive artificial nails
Metals	
Nickel	Buckles, snaps, jewelry, food
Cobalt	Metal plated utensils, keys, fasteners, paints, cobalt based pigments, vitamin B_{12} supplements
Gold sodium thiosulfate	Gold or gold plated jewelry, dental restorations

(continued on next page)

Table 2 *(continued)*	
Allergen	**Common Sources of Exposure**
Chemical additives integral to rubber manufacturing	
Carba mix	Rubber products, shampoo, disinfectants
Mercaptobenzothiazole	Rubber products, nitrile, neoprene, sports equipment
Thiuram	Rubber products, adhesives
Other allergens	
Propolis	Homeopathic remedies, food supplements, cosmetics, gum, medicated ointments/creams
Benzophenone-4	Chemical sunblock
Ammonium persulfate	Hair color allergen added to hydrogen peroxide
p-Phenylenediamine	Permanent or semipermanent hair dyes, cosmetics, printing ink, black henna tattoo
Propylene glycol	Vehicle in topical medications, personal care/hygiene products, auto care, cosmetics, foods, household cleaners, oral care, industry, sunscreens, wipes, yard care
Lanolin (wool alcohols)	Cosmetics, skin care products, personal hygiene items, facial masks, sunscreens, over-the-counter and prescription medications, pet grooming aids

Cosmetics and Personal Products

The term "cosmetic" is used synonymously with "make-up" in the general population. However, cosmetics include personal care products, hair care, nail products, and sunscreens. The number of cosmetic products available on the market today continues to increase together with the rates of adverse cutaneous reactions. The most common responsible cosmetic allergens are fragrances and preservatives.

Fragrances

It is important to keep in mind that many products labeled as unscented, hypoallergenic, or even fragrance free do, in fact, contain masking fragrances and many of the specific fragrance ingredients are considered trade secrets protected by the Fair Packaging and Labeling Act.

Balsam of Peru

BOP (myroxylon pereirae resin) is an aromatic fluid that consists of a mixture of potential contact allergens.[41] It is a complex mixture of many ingredients, including benzoyl cinnamate, benzoyl benzoate, benzoic acid, vanillin, and nerodilol. BOP chemicals can be found in fragrance in personal products such as cosmetics, perfumes, and medicinal products.

Although BOP extract itself is not commonly used in cosmetic products,[42] it is chemically related to many fragrances[43] and allergy to BOP is considered a marker for fragrance allergy.

Patients with contact allergy to BOP may also react to a number of substances that are well-known cross-reactants with BOP such as Balsam of Tolu, benzoin, benzyl acetate, benzyl alcohol, cinnamic alcohol/cinnamic aldehyde, cinnamon oil, clove oil, essential oils of orange peel, eugenol, and propolis.

BOP chemicals are also commonly found in spices, flavoring agents, food and drinks, as well as medications. For some patients allergic to BOP, topical avoidance of fragrance may not be enough to eliminate their dermatitis. Ingesting BOP-containing foods or beverages can also trigger SCD[44,45] and a diet containing low BOP may help. A BOP elimination diet avoids foods containing BOP constituents such as eugenol, cinnamates, vanillin, and benzoic acid derivatives. These potential allergens are commonly found in citrus fruits, sweets, tomatoes, certain spices, condiments, and some liquors (http://www.foodfacts.com, 2002–2012).

Fragrance mix I consists of 8 components: sorbitan sesquioleate, isoeugenol, eugenol, cinnamic aldehyde, cinnamic alcohol, hydroxycitronellal, geraniol, α-amyl-cinnamaldehyde, and oakmoss absolute. Fragrance mix II has 6 components: citral, hydroxyisohexyl 3-cyclohexene carboxaldehyde, farnesol, citronellol (0.5%),α-hexyl cinnamic aldehyde, and coumarin.[46] Currently, the 3 most common ingredients used to screen for fragrance allergy are BOP, Fragrance Mix I and Fragrance Mix II. Historically, it is estimated that most patients with fragrance allergy reacted to 1 or more of the 3 ingredients.[26]

Preservatives

Preservatives were identified as the most common cosmetic contact allergens in several recent studies. Preservatives can be further divided into formaldehyde preservatives, formaldehyde-releasers, and nonformaldehyde-releasing preservatives. Formaldehyde-releasing preservatives include quaternium-15, diazolidinyl urea, imidazolidinyl urea, 2-bromo-2-nitropropane-^{1,3}-diol, and DMDM hydantoin. Nonformaldehyde-releasing preservatives include parabens, MCI-MI, methyldibro-moglutaronitrile-phenoxyethanol, and iodopropynyl butylcarbamate.

Formaldehyde-sensitized individuals may also be allergic to any of the formaldehyde-releasing preservatives and may experience an exacerbation of ACD with a number of foods, including cod fish, caviar, coffee, shiitake mushrooms, smoked ham, maple syrup, and aspartame.[47] These reactions may manifest as SCD, distinguishable from an IgE-mediated type 1 hypersensitivity reaction to food.

Formaldehyde in both 1% and 2% aqueous solutions are very frequently positive on patch testing. Formaldehyde 2% aqueous solution has been shown to be a worthy screen for formaldehyde with little increase of irritant reaction[48,49]

The International Agency for Research on Cancer, a special agency of the World Health Organization, classified formaldehyde as a human carcinogen in 2004, and in 2011, the US Department of Health and Human Services, named formaldehyde as a known human carcinogen and it has thus been eliminated by many large companies from their products as a preservative.[50]

Methylchloroisothiazolinone/methylisothiazolinone and methylisothiazolinone

MCI and MI in a 3:1 combination (MCI/MI; trade names: Kathon CG, Euxyl K 400) is a widely used preservative in both industrial and consumer products. The rates of contact allergy to MCI/MI increased to levels of up to 8% when it was first introduced as a preservative in 1980.[51,52] This move prompted more strict use concentration recommendations from expert panels in both the European Union and the United States.

MCI is the more potent allergen in the combination MCI/MI. In 2005, MI was approved for use as a preservative in cosmetics and household products and sensitization to MI is increasing. MI can be found in baby products (lotion, oils, powders, and creams), bath products (soaps, detergents, and bubble baths), makeup (eyeliners, eye makeup remover, blushes, and face powders), hair care products (shampoos, conditioners, sprays, straighteners, rinses, and wave sets), hair-coloring products (dyes and colors, tints, and bleaches), nail care products, deodorants, shaving products (aftershaves and shaving creams), skin care products (cleansers, creams, lotions, and moisturizers), suntan products, and sunscreens, among others.

Patch testing to MCI/MI but not MI alone, could miss MI allergy in 33% to 60% of the cases. This is likely because of the low concentration of MI in the MCI/MI patch test substance (3:1). Testing MI alone at a higher concentration enables the detection of contact allergy more reliably.[53]

Nickel sulfate

Nickel retained its position as the most commonly positive allergen in the screening series, reaching a prevalence of 17.5%.[13] The European Union and institute regulations limit the levels of leachable nickel in items that are likely to have prolonged direct skin contact. In addition to its direct skin contact manifestation, nickel has been reported to cause SCD.

P-Phenylenediamine

The main source of exposure to PPD is hair dye. However, increasing exposure and sensitization have been reported from black henna tattoos.[54] PPD is added to temporary henna tattoos to darken the color and decrease the drying time.[55] Other sources of exposure to PPD include leather, fur, textiles, and industrial rubber products. ACD from PPD can manifest as a range of clinical patterns and can be severe, sometimes mimicking angioedema.

Cross-reactivity with other para-amino compounds such as benzocaine, para-aminobenzoic acid, sulfa drugs, aminoazobenzene, isopropyl-para-phenylenediamine and azo dyes has been reported.[56,57] Patients who test positive to PPD may try the semipermanent hair dye products such as Elumen (Goldwell, Linthicum Heights, MD), which is PPD free or Clairol Basic Instincts-Loving Care (The Proctor & Gamble Company, Cincinnati, OH), a semipermanent hair dye.[58]

Lanolin

Lanolin is a wax made of a mixture of esters, diesters, and hydroxyl esters of high-molecular-weight lanolin alcohols and high-molecular-weight lanolin acids.[59] Lanolin allergy is more common among patients with atopic dermatitis. Sources of exposure to lanolin include personal care products and toiletries, and clothing, as well as industrial sources. Lanolin is found in moisturizers, lipsticks, shampoos, and soaps. Lanolin is also found in ointment bases for topical medicaments such as antibiotics, corticosteroids, and analgesics.[60]

TREATMENT

The most important aspect of ACD treatment is avoidance of the offending allergen. Because many agents are found in everyday products, avoidance can be difficult, even if the allergen has been identified. Patients may find it difficult to read through ingredient lists of products, especially because many of the common contact allergens bear long, similar-looking chemical names. Many allergens cross-react with other allergens, further complicating avoidance. Two databases were developed to help patients identify and avoid products that contain the allergens to which they are sensitized as well as cross-reactive allergens. They are the American Contact Dermatitis Society database called the Contact Allergen Management Program (https://www.contactderm.org/resources/acds-camp) and the Contact Allergen Replacement Database (www.AllergyFreeSkin.com).

Both of these sites maintain a product database that can generate a list of safe products that is created for each patient by entering all positive results from patch testing. The list includes a wide variety of products, including hygiene products, cosmetics, and topical medications, that do not have the allergen to which the patient had patch tested positive.

In addition to avoidance, topical treatments can be used to alleviate symptoms. First-line medical treatment begins with topical corticosteroids (TCS). For acute ACD, mid- to high-potency corticosteroids can be used. If the dermatitis is especially severe, for example, with acute rhus dermatitis (poison ivy), systemic corticosteroids can provide quick relief.[26] For adults, 40 mg/d with a taper for a total course of 14 days is suggested.[26] Application of diphenhydramine topical preparations for pruritus should be avoided, because this practice can lead to cutaneous sensitization.[10]

For chronic ACD, systemic corticosteroids should be avoided if possible, because the course of dermatitis may be very long and its use can result in rebound flares. Low-potency TCS are preferred owing to the prolonged nature of use. Barrier creams and emollients can be helpful in treating chronic ACD and may decrease dryness and subsequent pruritus of the affected areas. Emollients should be fragrance free to avoid the risk of further sensitization.[10] Calcineurin inhibitors (tacrolimus, pimecrolimus) have not been approved for use in ACD, but are a reasonable alternative in chronic cases and those that involve delicate areas (face, eyelid, etc).[61] Phototherapy can be considered in the treatment of refractory cases.

Antihistamines have not been shown to be helpful in treating the intense pruritus associated with ACD.[26] They may prove helpful by acting as a sedative, however, to help patients sleep at night. Avoidance of wet work, excessive hand washing, hot water, soap, and sweating is advised.[62] Personal protective equipment is particularly important in cases of occupation-related ACD.[63]

If treatment with TCS does not improve or worsens the dermatitis, one should suspect ACD to the topical medication. Allergy to TCS has been described to affect 0.5%

Box 1
Corticosteroids cross-reactivity

Class A (hydrocortisone and tixocortol pivalate: has C17 or C21 short chain ester)
Hydrocortisone, hydrocortisone acetate, tixocortol, prednisone, prednisolone, prednisolone acetate, cloprednol, cortisone, cortisone acetate, fludrocortisone, methylprednisolone acetate

Class B (acetonides: has C16 C17 cis-ketal or –diol additions)
Triamcinolone acetonide, triamcinolone acetonide alcohol, budesonide, desonide, fluocinonide, fluocinolone acetonide, amcinonide, halcinonide

Class C (nonesterified betamethasone; C16 methyl group)
Betamethasone sodium phosphate, dexamethasone, dexamethasone sodium phosphate, fluocortolone

Class D1 (C16 methyl group and halogenated B ring)
Clobetasone 17-butyrate, clobetasone 17-propionate, bethamethasone valerate, bethamethasone dipropionate,
Aclometasone dipropionate, fluocortone caproate, fluocortone caproate pivalate, mometasone furoate

Class D2 (labile esters without C16 methyl nor B ring halogen substitution)
Hydrocortisone 17-butyrate, hydrocortisone 17-valerate, hydrocortisone 17-aceponate, hydrocortisone 17-buteprate, methylprednisolone aceponate

From Boguniewicz M, Aquino M, Fonacier L. Atopic Dermatitis and Contact Dermatitis. In: Adelman DC, Casale TB, Corren J, editors. Manual of Allergy and Immunology, 5th edition. Philadelphia: Wolters Kluwer Health/Lippincott Williams & Wilkins; 2012; with permission.

to 5.8% of patients.[64] The anti-inflammatory nature of TCS makes this an especially difficult diagnosis, with a high index of suspicion needed.[12] If suspected, the patient should undergo patch testing to the suspected medication and ingredients that are known to be contact sensitizers.[65] Additionally, there can be cross-reactivity between different corticosteroids based on similar chemical structures.[26] Corticosteroids are divided into groups A, B, C, and D (**Box 1**). Group D is subclassified into D1 (halogenated with C16 substitution) and D2 (labile esters without halogenation or C16 methyl group). Although these groups may predict cross-reactivity, many exceptions occur.[26]

Although corticosteroids are very effective in decreasing symptoms, they should be used with caution, especially when the dermatitis is located on a large portion of the body or regions of delicate skin (such as the intertriginous areas or face). Side effects of overuse can include atrophy of the skin, change in pigmentation, telangiectasia, and rebound dermatitis.

Contact allergy to nickel, as described elsewhere in this article, can present as an SCD. In this situation, a low nickel diet may prove helpful.[66] If the combination of nickel avoidance and a low nickel diet does not bring remission, disulfiram tablets have been reported to be effective.[26] Disulfiram works by binding to nickel and allowing for its excretion in urine and stool.

REFERENCES

1. Bolognia J, Jorizzo J, Schaffer J. Elsevier - dermatology 3rd edition. 3rd edition. Philadelphia: Saunders; 2012.

2. Rustemeyer T, van Hoogstraten IM, von Blomberg BME, et al. Contact dermatitis - mechanisms of irritant and allergic contact dermatitis. In: Johansen JD, Frosch PJ, Lepoittevin JP, editors. Contact Dermatitis. Berlin: Springer; 2011. p. 43–90.

3. Alinaghi F, Bennike NH, Egeberg A, et al. Prevalence of contact allergy in the general population: a systematic review and meta-analysis. Contact Dermatitis 2019;80(2):77–85.

4. Schnuch A, Carlsen BA. Contact dermatitis - genetics and individual predispositions in contact dermatitis. In: Frosch PJ, Johansen J, P, Lepoittevin J, editors. Berlin: Springer; 2011. p. 13–42.

5. Zack B, Arrandale VH, Holness DL. Preventing occupational skin disease: a review of training programs. Dermatitis 2017;28(3):169–82.

6. Friis UF, Menne T, Schwensen JF, et al. Occupational irritant contact dermatitis diagnosed by analysis of contact irritants and allergens in the work environment. Contact Dermatitis 2014;71(6):364–70.

7. Nicholson PJ, Llewellyn D, English JS, et al. Evidence-based guidelines for the prevention, identification and management of occupational contact dermatitis and urticaria. Contact Dermatitis 2010;63(4):177–86.

8. Lampel HP, Powell HB. Occupational and hand dermatitis: a practical approach. Clin Rev Allergy Immunol 2019;56(1):60–71.

9. Nethercott JR, Holness DL, Adams RM, et al. Patch testing with a routine screening tray in North America, 1985 through 1989 II. Gender and Response. Am J Contact Dermat 1991;2(2):130–4.

10. Adelman DC, Thomas, Corren J. Manual of allergy and immunology. 5th edition. Philadelphia: Wolters Kluwer Health/Lippincott Williams & WIlkins; 2012.

11. Sasseville D. Occupational contact dermatitis. Allergy Asthma Clin Immunol 2008;4(2):59–65.

12. Jacob SE, Steele T. Corticosteroid classes: a quick reference guide including patch test substances and cross-reactivity. J Am Acad Dermatol 2006;54(4): 723–7.
13. DeKoven JG, Warshaw EM, Zug KA, et al. North American Contact Dermatitis Group patch test results: 2015-2016. Dermatitis 2018;29(6):297–309.
14. Warshaw EM, Ahmed RL, Belsito DV, et al. Contact dermatitis of the hands: cross-sectional analyses of North American Contact Dermatitis Group Data, 1994-2004. J Am Acad Dermatol 2007;57(2):301–14.
15. Kedrowski DA, Warshaw EM. Hand dermatitis: a review of clinical features, diagnosis, and management. Dermatol Nurs 2008;20(1):17–25 [quiz 26].
16. Zirwas MJ. Contact dermatitis to cosmetics. Clin Rev Allergy Immunol 2019;56(1): 119–28.
17. Rietschel RL, Warshaw EM, Sasseville D, et al. Common contact allergens associated with eyelid dermatitis: data from the North American Contact Dermatitis Group 2003-2004 study period. Dermatitis 2007;18(2):78–81.
18. Gallo R, Marro I, Pavesi A. Allergic contact dermatitis from shellac in mascara. Contact Dermatitis 2005;53(4):238.
19. Le Coz CJ, Leclere JM, Arnoult E, et al. Allergic contact dermatitis from shellac in mascara. Contact Dermatitis 2002;46(3):149–52.
20. Saxena M, Warshaw E, Ahmed DD. Eyelid allergic contact dermatitis to black iron oxide. Am J Contact Dermat 2001;12(1):38–9.
21. Dejobert Y, Delaporte E, Piette F, et al. Eyelid dermatitis with positive patch test to coconut diethanolamide. Contact Dermatitis 2005;52(3):173.
22. Amin KA, Belsito DV. The aetiology of eyelid dermatitis: a 10-year retrospective analysis. Contact Dermatitis 2006;55(5):280–5.
23. Pesonen M, Jolanki R, Larese Filon F, et al. Patch test results of the European baseline series among patients with occupational contact dermatitis across Europe - analyses of the European Surveillance System on Contact Allergy network, 2002-2010. Contact Dermatitis 2015;72(3):154–63.
24. Reich HC, Warshaw EM. Allergic contact dermatitis from formaldehyde textile resins. Dermatitis 2010;21(2):65–76.
25. Jacob SE, Zapolanski T. Systemic contact dermatitis. Dermatitis 2008;19(1):9–15.
26. Fisher A. In: Rietschel R, Fowler J, editors. Fisher's contact dermatitis. 7th edition. USA: Walsworth; 2019. p. 76-79, 25-43, 323-326, 689-691.
27. Hindsen M, Bruze M, Christensen OB. Flare-up reactions after oral challenge with nickel in relation to challenge dose and intensity and time of previous patch test reactions. J Am Acad Dermatol 2001;44(4):616–23.
28. Veien NK. Ingested food in systemic allergic contact dermatitis. Clin Dermatol 1997;15(4):547–55.
29. Aquino M, Rosner G. Systemic contact dermatitis. Clin Rev Allergy Immunol 2018;56(1):9–18.
30. Cadosch D, Chan E, Gautschi OP, et al. Bio-corrosion of stainless steel by osteoclasts–in vitro evidence. J Orthop Res 2009;27(7):841–6.
31. Frigerio E, Pigatto PD, Guzzi G, et al. Metal sensitivity in patients with orthopedic implants: a prospective study. Contact Dermatitis 2011;64(5):273–9.
32. Hallab N. Metal Sensitivity in patients with orthopedic implants. J Clin Rheumatol 2001;7(4):215–8.
33. Granchi D, Cenni E, Tigani D, et al. Sensitivity to implant material in patients with total knee arthroplasties. Biomaterials 2008;29(10):1494–500.
34. Honari G, Ellis SG, Wilkoff BL, et al. Hypersensitivity reactions associated with endovascular devices. Contact Dermatitis 2008;59(1):7–22.

35. Raap U, Stiesch M, Reh H, et al. Investigation of contact allergy to dental metals in 206 patients. Contact Dermatitis 2009;60(6):339–43.
36. Warshaw EM, Belsito DV, Taylor JS, et al. North American Contact Dermatitis Group patch test results: 2009–2010. Dermatitis 2013;24(2):50–9.
37. Zug KA, Warshaw EM, Fowler JF Jr, et al. Patch-test results of the North American Contact Dermatitis Group 2005-2006. Dermatitis 2009;20(3):149–60.
38. Schalock PC, Dunnick CA, Nedorost S, et al. American contact dermatitis society core allergen series. Dermatitis 2013;24(1):7–9.
39. Schalock PC, Dunnick CA, Nedorost S, et al. American Contact Dermatitis Society Core Allergen Series: 2017 update. Dermatitis 2017;28(2):141–3.
40. DeGroot AC. Patch testing - test concentrations and vehicles for 4350 chemicals. 3rd edition. Wapserveen (The Netherlands): acdegroot publishing; 2008. p. 455.
41. Laguna C, de la Cuadra J, Martin-Gonzalez B, et al. Allergic contact dermatitis to cosmetics. Actas Dermosifiliogr 2009;100(1):53–60 [in Spanish].
42. Api AM. Only Peru Balsam extracts or distillates are used in perfumery. Contact Dermatitis 2006;54(3):179.
43. Hausen BM, Simatupang T, Bruhn G. Identification of new allergenic constituents and proof of evidence for coniferyl benzoate in Balsam of Peru. Am J Contact Dermat 1995;6(4):199–208.
44. Salam TN, Fowler JF Jr. Balsam-related systemic contact dermatitis. J Am Acad Dermatol 2001;45(3):377–81.
45. Veien NK, Hattel T, Laurberg G. Can oral challenge with balsam of Peru predict possible benefit from a low-balsam diet? Am J Contact Dermat 1996;7(2):84–7.
46. Frosch PJ, Pirker C, Rastogi SC, et al. Patch testing with a new fragrance mix detects additional patients sensitive to perfumes and missed by the current fragrance mix. Contact Dermatitis 2005;52(4):207–15.
47. E.C.c., Cosmetic products. Official Journal of the European Union, 2016. Amending Annex V to Regulation (EC) #1223/2009 of European Parliament and the European Parliament on Cosmetic Products: p. 2016/1198 of 22 July 2016.
48. Ponten A, Aalto-Korte K, Agner T, et al. Patch testing with 2.0% (0.60 mg/cm 2) formaldehyde instead of 1.0% (0.30 mg/cm 2) detects significantly more contact allergy. Contact Dermatitis 2013;68(1):50–3.
49. Ponten A, Bruze M. Formaldehyde. Dermatitis 2015;26(1):3–6.
50. Institute NC. Formaldehyde and cancer risk. Available at: https://www.cancer.gov/about-. Accessed January 15, 2019.
51. Fewings J, Menne T. An update of the risk assessment for methylchloroisothiazolinone/methylisothiazolinone (MCI/MI) with focus on rinse-off products. Contact Dermatitis 1999;41(1):1–13.
52. Mowad CM. Methylchloro-isothiazolinone revisited. Am J Contact Dermat 2000; 11(2):115–8.
53. Castanedo-Tardana MP, Zug KA. Methylisothiazolinone. Dermatitis 2013; 24(1):2–6.
54. Schnuch A, Lessmann H, Frosch PJ, et al. para-Phenylenediamine: the profile of an important allergen. Results of the IVDK. Br J Dermatol 2008;159(2):379–86.
55. Zapolanski T, Jacob SE. para-Phenylenediamine. Dermatitis 2008;19(3):E20–1.
56. Ho SG, Basketter DA, Jefferies D, et al. Analysis of para-phenylenediamine allergic patients in relation to strength of patch test reaction. Br J Dermatol 2005;153(2):364–7.
57. Saunders H, O'Brien T, Nixon R. Textile dye allergic contact dermatitis following paraphenylenediamine sensitization from a temporary tattoo. Australas J Dermatol 2004;45(4):229–31.

58. LaBerge L, Pratt M, Fong B, et al. A 10-year review of p-phenylenediamine allergy and related para-amino compounds at the Ottawa Patch Test Clinic. Dermatitis 2011;22(6):332–4.
59. Barnett G. Lanolin and derivatives. In: Cosmetics & toiletries science applied. 1986. p. 21–44.
60. Warshaw EM, Nelsen DD, Maibach HI, et al. Positive patch test reactions to lanolin: cross-sectional data from the North American Contact Dermatitis Group, 1994–2006. Dermatitis 2009;20(2):79–88.
61. Fonacier L, Noor I. Contact dermatitis and patch testing for the allergist. Ann Allergy Asthma Immunol 2018;120(6):592–8.
62. Lebwohl MG, Heymann WR, Berth-Jones J, editors. Treatment of skin disease: comprehensive therapeutic strategies. 5th edition. Elsevier Limited; 2018. p. 26–8.
63. NHS Plus, Royal College of Physicians. Faculty of Occupational Medicine. Dermatitis: occupational aspects of management. A national guideline. London: Royal College of Physicians; 2009.
64. Zmudzinska M, Czarnecka-Operacz M, Silny W. Contact allergy to glucocorticosteroids in patients with chronic venous leg ulcers, atopic dermatitis and contact allergy. Acta Dermatovenerol Croat 2008;16(2):72–8.
65. Fonacier L, Bernstein DI, Pacheco K, et al. Contact dermatitis: a practice parameter-update 2015. J Allergy Clin Immunol Pract 2015;3(3 Suppl):S1–39.
66. Mislankar M, Zirwas MJ. Low-nickel diet scoring system for systemic nickel allergy. Dermatitis 2013;24(4):190–5.

Approach to Patients with Allergic Rhinitis
Testing and Treatment

Linda Cox, MD[a,b,*]

KEYWORDS

- Allergen immunotherapy • Sublingual immunotherapy • Pharmacoeconomics
- Allergic rhinitis • Subcutaneous immunotherapy • Standard drug treatment
- Antihistamines • Nasal corticosteroids

KEY POINTS

- Allergic rhinitis (AR) is one the most common chronic conditions worldwide. It usually requires years of symptomatic treatment because allergies are chronic, beginning in childhood and lasting through late adulthood.
- There are considerable direct and indirect consequences and costs of poorly controlled AR.
- The clinical efficacy of allergen immunotherapy (AIT) in AR management seems to be equal, if not superior, to pharmacotherapy.
- AIT results in immunologic changes that can induce long-term allergen-specific tolerance.
- In contrast with pharmacotherapy, AIT can provide long-term clinical benefits after discontinuation of medications, which can translate into cost savings.
- AIT has been shown to prevent the progression of AR to asthma.
- Sustained improvement of symptoms, including prevention of asthma progression, and improvement of comorbid diseases has been shown to last longer with subcutaneous immunotherapy versus sublingual immunotherapy (SLIT), and some benefits with SLIT are specific to seasonal pollens, such as grass and birch, versus perennial allergens, such as house dust mite.

INTRODUCTION
Allergic Rhinitis Prevalence, Under-recognition, and Costs

Allergic rhinitis (AR) affects approximately 500 million people worldwide, with a higher incidence in westernized countries.[1] It is estimated that AR affects approximately 113 million people in Europe[2] and 30 to 60 million in the United States.[3,4] These approximations likely underestimate the true incidence of AR. Studies that have compared

---

[a] Department of Medicine, Nova Southeastern University, Davie, FL, USA; [b] Department of Medicine, University of Miami, Coral Gables, FL, USA
* 1108 South Wolcott Street, Casper, WY 82601.
E-mail addresses: lascoxmd@gmail.com; lindaswolfcox@msn.com

Med Clin N Am 104 (2020) 77–94
https://doi.org/10.1016/j.mcna.2019.09.001
0025-7125/20/© 2019 Elsevier Inc. All rights reserved.

clinically confirmed AR prevalence with questionnaire surveys suggest AR is frequently underdiagnosed.[5,6] In addition to being underdiagnosed, these studies indicate that AR is often undertreated and/or poorly controlled according to guideline recommendation.[7-9] One study designed to investigate the prevalence of AR undertreatment found that 83% of patients with moderate to severe rhinitis were undertreated according to guideline recommendations.[9] Other survey studies suggest that many AR patients remain untreated or self-treat with over-the-counter (OTC) medications. One telephone survey study found that only 50% of AR respondents received an AR prescription.[8] In an Internet/telephone survey, 52.6% of rhinitis respondents admitted to not seeing a medical professional in the past year. In this survey, medication costs were cited as the reason for not using allergy medications in 40.2% of the homeopathic or no-treatment respondents.[7]

The estimated direct cost of AR in 2005 was $11.5 billion according to the Medical Expenditure Panel Survey, a longitudinal survey that collects detailed information on health care use and expenditures in the United States.[10] At the time, prescription medications accounted for most of the treatment costs (59%). The costs of OTC medications were not this included in this survey, but were estimated at $1.2 billion to $1.7 billion in 2008.[11] Current OTC medications likely represent a significantly higher percentage of AR management costs because many effective medications have been moved from prescription to OTC status.

The AR indirect costs can be significantly greater than the direct costs.[12,13] In addition to OTC medications, indirect costs include treatment of comorbid illnesses as well as lost work productivity. In a survey of US employees, the total annual cost of lost productivity attributable to AR was significantly higher than the cost for any other condition assessed, including diabetes and coronary artery disease.[14]

Poorly controlled AR symptoms can result in impaired sleep, resulting in daytime fatigue, which can significantly affect patients' work or school performance and overall quality of life (QOL). AR can be associated with several comorbid conditions that may further impair QOL and add to the direct and indirect treatment costs.

AR has been identified as a risk factor for asthma. In a longitudinal study of 8275 children, AR was associated with a 2-fold to 7-fold increased risk of subsequent asthma in preadolescence, adolescence, or adult life.[15] In an international survey of patients and physicians on the management of AR, the 3 most common comorbidities were asthma, sinusitis, and conjunctivitis, which were reported in 32.7%, 49.9%, and 36.2% of patents, respectively.[16] In a birth cohort study investigating the association of otitis media with other allergic conditions, a significant association was only seen with AR (adjusted OR, 3.36; $P = .02$).[17]

AR treatment includes 3 components: allergen avoidance measures, pharmacotherapy, and allergen immunotherapy (AIT). In determining the optimal treatment plan, physicians should discuss the risks, benefits, and costs of each of these approaches. The discussion should include the evidence supporting each approach; that is, there is very little evidence supporting any single environmental control measure, as well as the magnitude of efficacy and long-term benefits of each approach. This discussion enables patients to make informed decisions regarding their treatment.

Evaluation of AR treatment strategies should also include the impact of the intervention on comorbid conditions and patient QOL. This article focuses on the role of AIT in the management of AR. The clinical efficacy, risks, and long-term benefits of AIT are compared with environmental control measures (avoidance) and pharmacotherapy. The cost-effectiveness of AIT compared with standard drug treatment (SDT) is also discussed.

Allergic Rhinitis Management: Environmental Controls and Pharmacotherapy

The ideal management approach to AR would be complete avoidance of the offending allergens. However, this is rarely achievable and there are limited data supporting the efficacy of environmental control interventions. In addition, there are very limited data that any single environmental control measure results in improved AR symptoms or other AR-related outcomes. A Cochrane systematic review of randomized controlled trials that compared the effectiveness of several bedroom environmental control measures in house dust mite (HDM) perennial AR (PAR) found that isolated use of HDM-impermeable bedding did not seem to be effective.[18] The investigators concluded that interventions that significantly reduced HDM load "… may offer some benefit in reducing rhinitis symptoms," but cautioned that the findings from these studies "need to be interpreted with care because of their methodological limitations."[18] An earlier Cochrane systematic review evaluating the effectiveness of environmental control measures in HDM asthma found there were no significant differences between the placebo and intervention groups in asthma symptoms, medication use, or peak expiratory flow rate.[19] The investigators concluded that "chemical and physical methods aimed at reducing exposure to house dust mite allergens cannot be recommended."[19]

Similarly, there is little evidence indicating that cat/dog removal from the household improves AR or asthma symptoms. This failure to improve after cat/dog removal may be caused by several factors, including persistence of airborne animal dander long after removal,[20] and the ubiquitous nature of animal dander.[21]

One study showed significant reductions in cockroach allergen levels after 6 months of a combined intervention program, which included pest management, professional cleaning, and patient education.[22] Decreased exposure to indoor allergens with an individualized, home-based, comprehensive environmental intervention program correlated with reduced complications of asthma.[23] A practice guideline series on "allergen environment assessment and exposure control" recommends a multifaceted approach using a combination of methods to reduce indoor allergen levels.[24–26] Restricting all activities to indoors would be the avoidance strategy for outdoor allergens, but this would counter the goal of normalizing the lifestyles of patients with AR or asthma.

In summary, although allergen avoidance would be the optimal treatment of AR, the evidence supporting this approach is sparse. It is likely that a combination of interventions sustained over time would be required to achieve any significant degree of clinical improvement.

There are several classes of effective allergy medication that treat different AR symptoms. The 2 most commonly prescribed AR medication classes, nasal corticosteroids (NCSs) and antihistamines, have several products available as OTC medications. OTC status may increase direct access to these medications but this also shifts more of the AR treatment costs to the patient. OTC medication may lessen the role of physicians and other health care professionals in AR management oversight, which may have several consequences; for example, delay in diagnosis and treatment of a frequent comorbid condition such as asthma or sinusitis. Physician guidance may also improve adherence to therapy. Although some patients may find intermittent allergy medication use effective, in general, effective pharmacotherapy requires regular use of medications. In addition, allergy medications provide relief of symptoms during use but provide no sustained benefits after discontinuation.[27,28]

Allergic Rhinitis Management: Allergen Immunotherapy

Unlike pharmacotherapy, AIT can provide symptomatic improvement that may continue for years after therapy discontinuation.[29,30] There is ample evidence that

AIT has a disease-modifying effect through favorable immunologic changes that induce sustained tolerance. The immunologic changes associated with AIT include changes in allergen-specific T-cell and B-cell responses, increase in allergen-specific immunoglobulin (Ig) G4, and suppression of allergen-specific IgE. Reductions in mast cell, eosinophil, and basophil activation, as well as end-organ sensitivity (eg, bronchial, nasal, or conjunctival) are also immunologic outcomes associated with AIT. The immunologic changes take place at different time points in the AIT course. Mast cell and basophil desensitization occurs early in the treatment course, followed by induction of the generation of T and B regulatory cells producing interleukin-10 and other cytokines that result in suppression of effector T-helper 1 (TH_1) and TH_2 cells.[31] These immunologic changes can result in disease modification, which can alter the progression of the allergic disease; for example, preventing AR progression to asthma and/or development of new allergen sensitizations.[30,32–34]

The 2 most commonly prescribed routes for AIT are subcutaneous immunotherapy (SCIT) and sublingual immunotherapy (SLIT). Because of the immunologic milieu of the allergen presentation site (sublingual vs subcutaneous), the 2 routes differ in initial allergen uptake and processing. However, once the allergen is systemically absorbed, their immunologic responses seem to be similar.[35] The clinical efficacy and safety of both routes in the treatment of AR has been established in numerous clinical trials, systematic reviews, and meta-analyses.[36–39] The 2 routes seem to have comparable efficacy, with most double-blind placebo-controlled (DBPC) controlled trials showing 20% to 30% greater improvement in combined symptom-medication score compared with placebo. Greater magnitudes of improvements have been seen in more symptomatic patient populations.[40,41]

The first DBPC trial showing SLIT efficacy was conducted nearly 75 years after the first report documenting SCIT efficacy in the treatment of AR.[42] Subsequently, the use of SLIT has increased significantly such that it is prescribed at least as frequently as SCIT, according to allergen extract manufacturers' sales data and expert opinion.[43] In some geographic locations, such as France and Italy, it is the predominant route for new AIT prescriptions.[44] To date, the AIT route most prescribed in the United States is SCIT, likely because there was no US Food and Drug Administration (FDA)–approved sublingual AIT formulation until 2014. Despite the absence of an FDA-approved SLIT formulation, there was a significant increase in the percentage of US physicians prescribing SLIT in 2011 (11.4%) compared with 2007 (5.9%; $P<.001$).[45,46] In early 2014, the FDA approved 3 sublingual tablets for pollen-induced AR/rhinoconjunctivitis (ARC); 5-grass combined (Oralair, Stallergenes, Anthony, France), short ragweed (Ragwitek, Merck & Co, Kenilworth, NJ), and timothy grass (Grastek, Merck & Co, Kenilworth, NJ).[47–49]

The specific indication in the prescribing information for the 3 FDA-approved SLIT tablet products is treatment of ragweed or grass pollen–induced AR with or without conjunctivitis confirmed by a positive skin test or in vitro testing for pollen-specific IgE antibodies.[47–49] Most SLIT studies were conducted in patients with ARC but the SLIT tablets' pivotal trials did include patients with controlled asthma. Neither the US agency–licensed nor the European Medicines Agency–licensed SLIT package inserts (PIs) include asthma alone as a clinical indication. The US-licensed allergen extract solutions PIs list similar indications, although some include asthma along with AR/ARC.[50] According to US practice guidelines, the primary indications for SCIT are ARC and asthma.[51]

There is emerging evidence that AIT is effective in patients with atopic dermatitis with aeroallergen sensitivities.[52,53] Investigations with oral and sublingual AIT for food allergy have shown some promising results in terms of desensitization during treatment.[54,55] However, sustained tolerance after discontinuation has only been shown in a minority of patients.[56] Many questions remain to be answered regarding long-term tolerance after discontinuation.[57,58] At present, food AIT is considered investigational.

SUBLINGUAL IMMUNOTHERAPY AND SUBCUTANEOUS IMMUNOTHERAPY SAFETY: HOW DO THEY COMPARE?

Both AIT routes can be associated with local or systemic adverse effects. Local reactions (LRs) are fairly common with both routes and have been reported in more than 70% of SCIT[59] and SLIT patients.[60] The LR clinical features vary with the route. SCIT LR presents as erythema, pruritus, and swelling at the injection site. SLIT LR usually manifests as oromucosal pruritus and/or swelling, but can include gastrointestinal symptoms as well. Most SLIT LRs occur shortly after treatment initiation and disappear within a few days to weeks without treatment or dose modification. However, some LR are severe enough to cause discontinuation of treatment. In addition, there have been case reports of eosinophilic esophagitis associated with SLIT.[61–63]

In addition to LRs, SCIT systemic reactions (SRs) can occur and range in severity from mild to life-threatening anaphylaxis. The incidence of SCIT SR varies depending on several factors, which include induction schedule, premeditation, and the degree of patient allergen hypersensitivity. The SR rate with traditional, nonaccelerated SCIT induction schedules is approximately 0.1% to 0.2% of injections and 2% to 5% of patients in most studies and surveys.[64,65] In a longitudinal AIT safety surveillance study that included more than 23.3 million injection visits, the reported SR rate was consistently 0.1% of injection visits.[65] Almost all of the SRs (97%) were classified as mild or moderate.[65,66] The incidence of severe SR was approximately 1 in 1 million injections, which is similar to previous surveys.[67] There were 2 confirmed SCIT fatalities in this survey. In previous surveys there were 3 to 4 SCIT-related fatalities a year, which translated into a fatality rate of 1 in 2 to 2.5 million SCIT injections.[68] Identified risk factors for SCIT SR include uncontrolled asthma, prior SCIT SR, and high degree of skin test reactivity.[51]

In contrast, SLIT systemic allergic reactions are very uncommon. In a comprehensive review of 104 SLIT studies published through October of 2005, the SLIT SR rate was 0.056% of doses administered, slightly more than half the rate of SCIT SR.[60] To date, there have been no confirmed reports of SLIT-related fatalities. However, SLIT anaphylaxis has been reported with SLIT.[69]

There are advantages and disadvantages of both routes. SLIT seems to have a clear advantage compared with SCIT in terms of treatment safety, which allows home administration, making it more convenient. In contrast, because of the risk of life-threatening anaphylaxis, practice guidelines recommend SCIT be administered in a medically supervised setting with a 30-minute postinjection observation period.[51,70] An SCIT treatment regimen may involve frequent visits during the initial updosing phase, all of which requires patient time and travel to the medical clinic. This phase is followed by a maintenance phase, during which the injections are administered at monthly intervals. In contrast, SLIT is administered in the home setting, but the maintenance dose frequency is usually daily. Despite their different patient time/travel requirements, both routes have been shown to have equally poor adherence,[71] likely because both routes require a multiyear treatment course (usually 3–5 years). The AIT adherence rate is similar to the poor adherence reported with long-term pharmacotherapy for many diseases.[72] Interventions such as more frequent clinic monitoring, telecommunication reminders, and educational programs may improve AIT adherence.[72–74]

In addition to efficacy and safety, several factors determine the AIT route selected, including availability of a regulatory body–approved allergen extract (eg, FDA approved), the patient's clinical allergy sensitization status (monosensitized vs poly-sensitized), treatment costs/insurance coverage status, and patient or physician preference.

To date, there continues to be no FDA-approved formulation for SLIT extract solution. However, studies are ongoing. A large patient population study that compared a US-licensed ragweed extract (N = 218) with placebo (N = 211) showed significant clinical efficacy with no significant adverse events.[75]

Allergen Immunotherapy in the Management of Allergic Rhinitis: How Does it Compare with Standard Drug Treatment in Terms of Clinical Efficacy?

In contrast with AR pharmacotherapy trials, virtually all AIT trials allow for rescue medication use. In essence, the placebo group in AIT clinical trials represents a pharmacotherapy-alone group. Thus, there are no randomized placebo controlled trials that compare AIT with a truly untreated control group. Despite the allowance for rescue allergy medications, virtually all of the systematic reviews and meta-analyses of SCIT and SLIT for AR and asthma have shown significant clinical efficacy compared with the placebo groups, which were allowed allergy medications.[36] A review of meta-analyses that included 5 or more randomized, DBPC trials of SCIT or SDT for seasonal AR provided indirect evidence that SCIT was at least as potent as SDT in controlling AR symptoms in the first treatment year.[76] There was a significantly greater improvement in nasal symptom scores with SCIT (relative clinical impact [RCI], −34.7% ± 6.8%), compared with 3 different medication classes (NCS, antihistamine, and a leukotriene antagonist; $P<.00001$); mometasone (RCI, −31.7% ± 16.7%), montelukast (RCI, −6.3% ± 3.0%), and desloratadine (RCI, −12.0% ± 5.1%).

PHARMACOECONOMICS OF ALLERGEN IMMUNOTHERAPY IN ALLERGIC RHINITIS MANAGEMENT

In evaluating the pharmacoeconomics of the different AR management options, consideration needs given to the long-term benefits of AIT, which may persist years or decades after treatment completion (**Tables 1–3** for summary of cost-effectiveness ratio of AIT vs SDT).[77,78] The AIT treatment costs can be offset by the reduction in the need for long-term symptomatic drug treatment, and its disease-modifying effect, which can prevent the development of asthma or new allergen sensitivities. These combined outcomes may translate the clinical efficacy of AIT into a significant economic benefit. This economic benefit has been confirmed in several studies that have compared SCIT and/or SLIT with SDT from several different perspectives, including societal, health care system, patient, and third-party payers.[79] The analysis designs used in these studies varied and included review of retrospective claims data and theoretic economic modeling. Outcomes assessed included real-life total health care costs and theoretic quality-adjusted life years (QALYs) gained or number of asthma cases prevented. In some studies, cost-effectiveness was based on the presumption of persistent efficacy for years after discontinuation or prevention of asthma. There was some variability across the studies in the AIT cost-effective or break-even time point. In a 6-year prospective study comparing a 3-year course of SCIT with SDT, the cost savings became significant in the third treatment year.[80]

Table 1
Studies comparing subcutaneous immunotherapy with standard drug treatment

Study	Comparators	Type	Perspective	Results
Schadlich,[90] 2000	Pollen or HDM SCIT for 3 y plus SDT as needed; SDT	CEA	Society, health care system, third-party payer	SCIT<SDT more than 10 y. Break-even point reached in the seventh year
Petersen,[91] 2005	Grass or HDM SCIT for 3–5 y plus SDT as needed; SDT	CEA	Society	Direct cost: SCIT>SDT If indirect costs of sick days included in the economic evaluation, SCIT costs <SDT
Ariano et al,[80] 2006	*Parietaria* SCIT for 3 y plus SDT as needed; SDT	CCA	Health care system, society	SCIT<SDT; 80% cost reduction found 3 y after stopping SCIT
Keiding,[92] 2007	Grass SCIT for 3 y plus SDT as needed; SDT	CEA CUA	Health care system, society	SCIT cost-effectiveness per QALY; in the range of €10,000–€25,000 per QALY from perspective of the health care system
Omnes,[93] 2007	HDM or pollen SCIT 3–4 y plus SDT as needed: SDT	CEA	Society	Cost-effective per incremental cost of asthma cases avoided (ICER)
Bruggenjurgen,[94] 2008	SCIT for 3 y plus SDT as needed; SDT	CUA	Third-party payer, society	Break-even point = 10 y. After 15 y, annual cost savings of €140 per SCIT-treated patient
Hankin et al,[83] 2008	Costs 6 mo before and 6 mo after SCIT	CCA	Health care system	Weighted mean 6-mo savings/patient: $401
Hankin et al,[82] 2010	SCIT for 18 mo plus SDT as needed; SDT as needed for 18 mo	CCA	Health care system	SCIT 18-mo total health care costs 33% reduction compared with SDT
Hankin et al,[81] 2013	SCIT plus SDT as needed for 18 mo; SDT as needed for 18 mo	CCA	Health care system	SCIT 18-mo total health care costs compared with SDT: Children: 42% reduction Adults: 30% reduction

Abbreviations: CCA, cost-consequence analysis; CEA, cost-effectiveness analysis; CUA, cost-utility analysis; ICER, incremental cost-effectiveness ratio; QALY, quality-adjusted life year.

From Cox L. Pharmacoeconomics of allergic diseases. In: Akdis CA, Agache I, editors. Global Atlas of Allergy. European Academy of Allergy and Clinical Immunology; 2014; with permission.

AIT cost savings reached 80% in the fourth year and was maintained through the 3 posttreatment years. In some studies, the cost-effective time point was reached several years after discontinuation, which likely reflects the time required for the sustained benefits of AIT to outweigh the AIT treatment costs.[79]

Two systematic reviews evaluating the cost-effectiveness of SLIT and/or SCIT found evidence favoring both more than SDT. One systematic review that identified

Table 2
Studies comparing sublingual immunotherapy with standard drug treatment

Study	Comparators	Type	Perspective	Results
Berto,[95] 2005	1 y of SDT before SLIT; SLIT for 3 y	CEA	Health care system, society	Cost savings with SLIT per health care system and society: • Year before SLIT: mean annual health care costs/annual total costs per patient were €506 and €2672, respectively • During SLIT: €224/d (health care costs) and €629/d (total cost)
Berto, 2006	Pollen SLIT for 3 y plus SDT as needed; SDT	CCA	Health care system, society	SCIT compared with SDT: • Greater 6-y mean savings from payer and societal perspective • More asthma cases avoided and patients improved
Bachert,[96] 2007	Grass SLIT for 3 y plus SDT as needed; SDT	CUA	Society	SLIT cost-effective cost per QALY; average 0.0287 QALYs per season compared with SDT
Beriot-Mathiot,[97] 2007	Grass SLIT for 3 y continuous or seasonal; SDT	CUA	Societal	Per ICER seasonal SLIT was cost-effective. Continuous SLIT was cost-effective if sustained effect for >2 y after treatment
Canonica,[98] 2007	Grass SLIT for 3 y plus SDT as needed; SDT	CUA	Society	SLIT cost-effective per QALY: average 0.0167 QALYs per season compared with SDT
Berto,[99] 2008	Grass SLIT for 1 y; SDT for 1 y	CCA	Third-party payer	Mean annual direct costs for SLIT greater than SDT €311.4 and €179.8, respectively
Nasser,[100] 2008	Grass SLIT for 3 y plus SDT as needed; SDT	CUA	Society	SLIT very cost-effective per QALY gained. QALY gained at 9 y = 0.197; equivalent to an extra 72 d of perfect health for patients treated with SLIT compared with those receiving placebo
Ariano,[101] 2009	SLIT for 3 y plus SDT as needed; SDT	CCA	Health care system	Health care costs greater for SLIT plus SDT in year 1, same in years 2 and 3, and significantly lower in years 4 and 5, compared with SDT
Ruggeri, 2013	SLIT for 3 y plus SDT as needed; SDT	CEA	Third-party payer, society	SLIT cost-effective per ICER; benefit of 0.127 QALYs in patients with medium AAdSS and 0.143 QALYs in patients with high AAdSS

[a]Included in the Meadows et al, systematic review.
[b]Included in the Hankin and colleagues systematic review.
[c]Included in both systematic review.
Abbreviation: AAdSS, adjusted average symptom score.
From Cox L. Pharmacoeconomics of allergic diseases. In: Akdis CA, Agache I, editors. Global Atlas of Allergy. European Academy of Allergy and Clinical Immunology; 2014; with permission.

14 economic evaluations published through April of 2011 concluded that both SCIT and SLIT may become cost-effective compared with SDT at around 6 years after beginning treatment.[77] The review found limited evidence that indicated SCIT may more beneficial and less costly than SLIT but the investigators noted the challenges

Table 3
Systematic reviews evaluating allergen immunotherapy health economics

Author, Year[a]	Economic Outcome Conclusion[b]	SCIT vs SDT[b]	SLIT Tablets vs SDT[b]	SLIT Drops vs SDT[b]	SCIT vs SLIT vs SDT[b]
Meadows et al,[77] 2013	14 Both SCIT and SLIT may be cost-effective from around 6 y	6 Cost-effective but varied in terms of payer perspective and time point	3 Cost-effective at ~6 y and various ICER	2 All favored SLIT	3 SCIT more cost-effective over time
Hankin & Cox,[78] 2014	23 favored AIT more than SDT	10 All favored SCIT	8 1 found higher costs with SLIT	1 reduced costs by year 4	4 All favored SLIT SLIT 48% cost savings from health care system perspective

[a] Included 3 studies that evaluated the total health care cost via claims analyses not included in the Meadows review.
[b] Number of studies evaluated.
From Cox L. The role of allergen immunotherapy in the management of allergic rhinitis. Am J Rhinol Allergy 2016;30(1):48-53; with permission.

in comparing and combining results across studies using different outcome measures and encouraged further research to "establish the comparative effectiveness of SCIT compared with SLIT and to provide more robust cost-effectiveness estimates."[77] All of the studies in this systematic review used a single allergen.

The other systematic review identified 24 studies that reported health economic outcomes associated with AIT comparing SLIT and/or SCIT with SDT or SCIT versus SLIT.[78] The review found that 23 of the 24 comparative cost studies provided "compelling evidence for the cost savings of AIT."[78] The review found that, in 4 of the 6 studies comparing SLIT and SCIT cost outcomes, the cost savings favored SLIT. Each study evaluated a different time period so this may affect results because it has been shown with SCIT that cost benefit may be delayed several years. With the exception of 3 Florida Medicaid retrospective claims analyses studies, all of these studies used single-allergen AIT.[81–83]

ALLERGEN IMMUNOTHERAPY IN THE MANAGEMENT OF ALLERGIC RHINITIS: UNMET NEEDS

There are several unmet needs regarding SLIT and SCIT.[36] Some unmet needs are more pertinent to 1 route, but in general they apply to both:

- Multiallergen AIT: there are very limited data on the effectiveness of multiallergen AIT with either route.[84] Almost all of the SCIT and SLIT randomized controlled, DBPC trials used single allergens.[85] Further studies are needed to determine the efficacy of multiallergen SCIT and SLIT.[86]

Table 4
Example of a cluster immunotherapy schedule

Visit	Dose (mL)	Concentration as Dilution of Maintenance Vial (v/v)
1	0.10	1:000
	0.40	1:1000
	0.10	1:100
2	0.20	1:100
	0.40	1:100
	0.07	1:10
3	0.10	1:10
	0.15	1:10
	0.25	1:10
4	0.35	1:10
	0.50	1:10
5	0.07	1:1
	0.10	1:1
6	0.15	1:1
	0.20	1:1
7	0.30	1:1
	0.40	1:1
8	0.50	1:1

Patients premedicated with a nonsedating antihistamine 2 hours before dosing. Injections administered at 30-minute intervals. Patients remain for observation in clinic for 1 hour after last injection each day.

Abbreviation: v/v, volume/volume.

Adapted from Cox L, Nelson H, Lockey R, et al. Allergen immunotherapy: a practice parameter third update. J Allergy Clin Immunol 2011;127(1 Suppl):S1-55; with permission.

- Optimal updosing and maintenance regimen: further research is needed to determine optimal dosing regimens for both routes. **Tables 4** and **5** and **Box 1** provide examples of cluster and conventional schedules and a schedule for dose adjustments for gaps in treatment. These forms can be downloaded from the www. aaaai.org Web site. The Web site also has patient instruction forms for SLIT as well as consent and instruction forms for SCIT and SLIT.
  - SCIT: the conventional updosing schedule for SCIT involves a single dose increase per administration visit. Accelerated schedules such as cluster and RUSH reduce the number of injection visits by administering multiple dose increases each visit, but they may be associated with higher risk of SR.[87] The optimal maintenance dosing frequency has not been studied in any controlled trials.
  - SLIT: many trials used no updosing schedule and began treatment at the maintenance dose. No updosing schedules seem to have similar safety to multiweek updosing SLIT protocols. A daily dosing regimen has been used in most recent clinical trials but comparative studies with less frequent dosing

Table 5
An example of a buildup schedule for weekly immunotherapy

Dilution (v/v)	Volume (mL)
1:1000	0.05
	0.10
	0.20
	0.40
1:100	0.05
	0.10
	0.20
	0.30
	0.40
	0.50
1:10	0.05
	0.07
	0.10
	0.15
	0.25
	0.35
	0.40
	0.45
	0.50
Maintenance concentrate	0.05
	0.07
	0.10
	0.15
	0.20
	0.25
	0.30
	0.35
	0.40
	0.45
	0.50

Dilutions are expressed as v/v from the maintenance concentrate.
Adapted from Cox L, Nelson H, Lockey R, et al. Allergen immunotherapy: a practice parameter third update. J Allergy Clin Immunol 2011;127(1 Suppl):S1-55; with permission.

Box 1

Example of immunotherapy dose adjustments for unscheduled gaps in allergen immunotherapy injection intervals

Buildup phase for weekly or biweekly injections (time intervals from missed injection):
- Up to 7 days, continue as scheduled (ie, if on weekly buildup then it would be up to 14 days after administered injection or 7 days after the missed scheduled injection)
- 8 to 13 days after missed scheduled injection; repeat previous dose
- 14 to 21 days after missed scheduled injection; reduce dose 25%
- 21 to 28 days after missed scheduled injection; reduce previous dose 50%

Then increase dose each injection visit as directed on the immunotherapy schedule until therapeutic maintenance dose is reached.

This suggested approach to modification of doses of allergen immunotherapy because of gaps between treatment during the buildup phase is not based on a retrospective or prospective published evidence, but it is presented as a sample for consideration. Individual physicians should use this or a similar protocol as a standard operating procedure for the specific clinical setting. A similar dose reduction protocol should be developed for gaps in maintenance immunotherapy.

Adapted from Cox L, Nelson H, Lockey R, et al. Allergen immunotherapy: a practice parameter third update. J Allergy Clin Immunol 2011;127(1 Suppl):S1-55; with permission.

regimens are lacking. Unmet needs more pertinent to SLIT include when to initiate treatment in terms of the allergy season and whether to treat year round or preseasonal.
- ○ Gaps in scheduled treatment: the unmet needs for the 2 routes differ in terms of addressing gaps in treatment:
  - ■ SCIT: the questions related to dose reductions (ie, how much after how long?)
  - ■ SLIT: the question is, how many days before requiring an intervention, such as contacting the health care professional?
- Effective allergen dose: there have been very few SCIT or SLIT allergen dose-response studies. Further research is needed to determine the effective dose for many allergens.
- Optimal duration of AIT: the optimal treatment duration for both routes has been suggested to be 3 years but there are very limited data to support this recommendation.[29,88] The optimal duration may vary depending on allergen-seasonal versus perennial, infrequent versus frequent intermittent exposure.[89]

The FDA PI of the approved SLIT tablets provides information and guidance on some of these issues. The Allergen Immunotherapy Practice Parameter also provides some consensus-based guidance on issues of SCIT unmet needs.[51]

SUMMARY

AIT is a well-established, proven effective treatment of AR that is unique in that it treats both AR symptoms and the underlying cause (an aberrant immune response) by inducing immunologic changes that produce allergen-specific immune tolerance. In addition, to improvement in AR symptoms and medication requirements, AIT has been shown to improve overall QOL. The 2 most commonly prescribed AIT routes, SCIT and SLIT, have shown comparable clinically efficacy. The safety profile of SLIT is superior to SCIT but both have been shown to have fairly poor adherence in real-life studies. The cost-effectiveness of both SCIT and SLIT compared with SDT has been shown in several studies and 2 systematic reviews. There is no conclusive evidence that either route is more cost-effective or clinically effective. More research using standardized outcome and reporting measures is needed is to establish the comparative effectiveness of SCIT and SLIT, as well as to assess the long-term cost-effectiveness of both AIT routes in terms of disease control and modification.

DISCLOSURE

Conflicts of interest: None.

REFERENCES

1. Ozdoganoglu T, Songu M. The burden of allergic rhinitis and asthma. Ther Adv Respir Dis 2012;6:11–23.
2. EFA book on respiratory allergies. In: Valovirta E, editor. Brussels, Belgium: European Federation of allergy and airways diseases patients associations. 2011.
3. Wallace DV, Dykewicz MS, Bernstein DI, et al. The diagnosis and management of rhinitis: an updated practice parameter. J Allergy Clin Immunol 2008;122: S1–84.
4. CDC Fast facts A-Z," vital health statistics, 2003. Available at: http://www.aafa.org/display.cfm?id=9&sub=30. Accessed May 22, 2011.
5. Bauchau V, Durham SR. Prevalence and rate of diagnosis of allergic rhinitis in Europe. Eur Respir J 2004;24:758–64.
6. Bunyavanich S, Soto-Quiros ME, Avila L, et al. Risk factors for allergic rhinitis in Costa Rican children with asthma. Allergy 2010;65:256–63.
7. Maurer M, Zuberbier T. Undertreatment of rhinitis symptoms in Europe: findings from a cross-sectional questionnaire survey. Allergy 2007;62:1057–63.
8. Sazonov V, Ambegaonkar BM, Bolge SC, et al. Frequency of diagnosis and treatment of allergic rhinitis among adults with asthma in Germany, France, and the UK: National Health and Wellness Survey. Curr Med Res Opin 2009; 25:1721–6.
9. Nolte H, Nepper-Christensen S, Backer V. Unawareness and undertreatment of asthma and allergic rhinitis in a general population. Respir Med 2006;100: 354–62.
10. Soni A. Medical expenditure Panel survey. Statistical brief #204: allergic rhinitis: trends in use and expenditures, 2000 and 2005. Bethesda (MD): Agency for Healthcare Research and Quality; 2008. Available at: meps.ahrq.gov/mepsweb/data_files/publications/st204/stat204.pdf. Accessed May 26, 2015.
11. Blaiss MS. Allergic rhinitis: direct and indirect costs. Allergy Asthma Proc 2010; 31:375–80.
12. Schultz AB, Chen CY, Edington DW. The cost and impact of health conditions on presenteeism to employers: a review of the literature. Pharmacoeconomics 2009;27:365–78.
13. Schoenwetter WF, Dupclay L Jr, Appajosyula S, et al. Economic impact and quality-of-life burden of allergic rhinitis. Curr Med Res Opin 2004;20:305–17.
14. Lamb CE, Ratner PH, Johnson CE, et al. Economic impact of workplace productivity losses due to allergic rhinitis compared with select medical conditions in the United States from an employer perspective. Curr Med Res Opin 2006;22: 1203–10.
15. Burgess JA, Walters EH, Byrnes GB, et al. Childhood allergic rhinitis predicts asthma incidence and persistence to middle age: a longitudinal study. J Allergy Clin Immunol 2007;120:863–9.

16. Baena-Cagnani CE, Canonica GW, Zaky Helal M, et al. The international survey on the management of allergic rhinitis by physicians and patients (ISMAR). World Allergy Organ J 2015;8:10.
17. Minto H, Hogan AD. Allergic rhinitis is associated with otitis media with effusion: a birth cohort study. Pediatrics 2013;132:S29–30.
18. Sheikh A, Hurwitz B, Nurmatov U, et al. House dust mite avoidance measures for perennial allergic rhinitis. Cochrane Database Syst Rev 2010;(7):CD001563.
19. Gotzsche PC, Johansen HK. House dust mite control measures for asthma. Cochrane Database Syst Rev 2008;(2):CD001187.
20. Wood RA, Chapman MD, Adkinson NF Jr, et al. The effect of cat removal on allergen content in household-dust samples. J Allergy Clin Immunol 1989;83: 730–4.
21. Arbes SJ Jr, Cohn RD, Yin M, et al. Dog allergen (Can f 1) and cat allergen (Fel d 1) in US homes: results from the National Survey of Lead and Allergens in Housing. J Allergy Clin Immunol 2004;114:111–7.
22. Arbes SJ Jr, Sever M, Archer J, et al. Abatement of cockroach allergen (Bla g 1) in low-income, urban housing: A randomized controlled trial. J Allergy Clin Immunol 2003;112:339–45.
23. Morgan WJ, Crain EF, Gruchalla RS, et al. Results of a home-based environmental intervention among urban children with asthma. N Engl J Med 2004; 351:1068–80.
24. Phipatanakul W, Matsui E, Portnoy J, et al. Environmental assessment and exposure reduction of rodents: a practice parameter. Ann Allergy Asthma Immunol 2012;109:375–87.
25. Portnoy J, Kennedy K, Sublett J, et al. Environmental assessment and exposure control: a practice parameter–furry animals. Ann Allergy Asthma Immunol 2012; 108:223.e1-15.
26. Portnoy J, Miller JD, Williams PB, et al. Environmental assessment and exposure control of dust mites: a practice parameter. Ann Allergy Asthma Immunol 2013; 111:465–507.
27. Guilbert TW, Morgan WJ, Zeiger RS, et al. Long-term inhaled corticosteroids in preschool children at high risk for asthma. N Engl J Med 2006;354:1985–97.
28. Strunk RC, Sternberg AL, Szefler SJ, et al. Long-term budesonide or nedocromil treatment, once discontinued, does not alter the course of mild to moderate asthma in children and adolescents. J Pediatr 2009;154:682–7.
29. Durham SR, Emminger W, Kapp A, et al. SQ-standardized sublingual grass immunotherapy: confirmation of disease modification 2 years after 3 years of treatment in a randomized trial. J Allergy Clin Immunol 2012;129:717–25.e5.
30. Marogna M, Spadolini I, Massolo A, et al. Long-lasting effects of sublingual immunotherapy according to its duration: a 15-year prospective study. J Allergy Clin Immunol 2010;126:969–75.
31. Akdis M, Akdis CA. Mechanisms of allergen-specific immunotherapy: multiple suppressor factors at work in immune tolerance to allergens. J Allergy Clin Immunol 2014;133:621–31.
32. Des Roches A, Paradis L, Menardo JL, et al. Immunotherapy with a standardized Dermatophagoides pteronyssinus extract. VI. Specific immunotherapy prevents the onset of new sensitizations in children. J Allergy Clin Immunol 1997;99: 450–3.
33. Jacobsen L, Niggemann B, Dreborg S, et al. Specific immunotherapy has long-term preventive effect of seasonal and perennial asthma: 10-year follow-up on the PAT study. Allergy 2007;62:943–8.

34. Novembre E, Galli E, Landi F, et al. Coseasonal sublingual immunotherapy reduces the development of asthma in children with allergic rhinoconjunctivitis. J Allergy Clin Immunol 2004;114:851–7.
35. Moingeon P. Update on immune mechanisms associated with sublingual immunotherapy: practical implications for the clinician. J Allergy Clin Immunol In Pract 2013;1:228–41.
36. Burks AW, Calderon MA, Casale T, et al. Update on allergy immunotherapy: American Academy of Allergy, Asthma & Immunology/European Academy of Allergy and Clinical Immunology/PRACTALL consensus report. J Allergy Clin Immunol 2013;131:1288–96.e3.
37. Canonica GW, Cox L, Pawankar R, et al. Sublingual immunotherapy: World Allergy Organization position paper 2013 update. World Allergy Organ J 2014; 7:6.
38. Radulovic S, Wilson D, Calderon M, et al. Systematic reviews of sublingual immunotherapy (SLIT). Allergy 2011;66:740–52.
39. Calderon MA, Alves B, Jacobson M, et al. Allergen injection immunotherapy for seasonal allergic rhinitis. Cochrane Database Syst Rev 2007;(1):CD001936.
40. Howarth P, Malling HJ, Molimard M, et al. Analysis of allergen immunotherapy studies shows increased clinical efficacy in highly symptomatic patients. Allergy 2012;67:321–7.
41. Varney VA, Gaga M, Frew AJ, et al. Usefulness of immunotherapy in patients with severe summer hay fever uncontrolled by antiallergic drugs. BMJ 1991; 302:265–9.
42. Noon L. Prophylactic inoculation against hay fever. Lancet 1911;1:1572–3.
43. Cox L. Sublingual immunotherapy for aeroallergens: Status in the United States. Allergy Asthma Proc 2014;35.34–42.
44. Cox L, Jacobsen L. Comparison of allergen immunotherapy practice patterns in the United States and Europe. Ann Allergy Asthma Immunol 2009;103:451–9 [quiz: 9–61], 95.
45. Sikora JM, Tankersley MS, Immunotherapy A, et al. Perception and practice of sublingual immunotherapy among practicing allergists in the United States: a follow-up survey. Ann Allergy Asthma Immunol 2013;110:194–7.e4.
46. Tucker MH, Tankersley MS. Perception and practice of sublingual immunotherapy among practicing allergists. Ann Allergy Asthma Immunol 2008;101: 419–25.
47. GRASTEK® (Timothy Grass Pollen Allergen Extract). Available at: http://www.fda.gov/downloads/BiologicsBloodVaccines/Allergenics/UCM393184.pdf date. Accessed December 14, 2014.
48. ORALAIR®(Sweet Vernal, Orchard, Perennial Rye, Timothy, and Kentucky Blue Grass Mixed Pollens Allergen Extract). 2014. Available at: http://www.fda.gov/downloads/BiologicsBloodVaccines/Allergenics/UCM391580.pdf date. Accessed A-pril 26, 2015.
49. RAGWITEKTM (Short Ragweed Pollen Allergen Extract) tablet for sublingual use prescribing information. 2014. Available at: http://www.merck.com/product/usa/pi_circulars/r/ragwitek/ragwitek_pi.pdf date. Accessed December 26, 2014.
50. Greer Standardized Mite Extracts Prescribing Information. Available at: http://www.greerlabs.com/files/DFU/L-505-Mites_w.pdf. Accessed May 24, 2015.
51. Cox L, Nelson H, Lockey R, et al. Allergen immunotherapy: a practice parameter third update. J Allergy Clin Immunol 2011;127:S1–55.
52. Schneider L, Tilles S, Lio P, et al. Atopic dermatitis: a practice parameter update 2012. J Allergy Clin Immunol 2013;131:295–9.e1-27.

53. Bae JM, Choi YY, Park CO, et al. Efficacy of allergen-specific immunotherapy for atopic dermatitis: a systematic review and meta-analysis of randomized controlled trials. J Allergy Clin Immunol 2013;132:110–7.

54. Narisety SD, Frischmeyer-Guerrerio PA, Keet CA, et al. A randomized, double-blind, placebo-controlled pilot study of sublingual versus oral immunotherapy for the treatment of peanut allergy. J Allergy Clin Immunol 2015;135:1275–82.e6.

55. Burks AW, Jones SM, Wood RA, et al. Oral immunotherapy for treatment of egg allergy in children. N Engl J Med 2012;367:233–43.

56. Burks AW, Wood RA, Jones SM, et al. Sublingual immunotherapy for peanut allergy: Long-term follow-up of a randomized multicenter trial. J Allergy Clin Immunol 2015;135(5):1240–8.e1-3.

57. Pajno GB, Cox L, Caminiti L, et al. Oral Immunotherapy for treatment of immunoglobulin E-mediated food allergy: the transition to clinical practice. Pediatr Allergy Immunol Pulmonol 2014;27:42–50.

58. Wood RA, Sampson HA. Oral immunotherapy for the treatment of peanut allergy: is it ready for prime time? J Allergy Clin Immunol In Pract 2014;2:97–8.

59. Coop CA, Tankersley MS. Patient perceptions regarding local reactions from allergen immunotherapy injections. Ann Allergy Asthma Immunol 2008;101:96–100.

60. Cox LS, Linnemann DL, Nolte H, et al. Sublingual immunotherapy: a comprehensive review. J Allergy Clin Immunol 2006;117:1021–35.

61. Béné J, Ley D, Roboubi R, et al. Eosinophilic esophagitis after desensitization to dust mites with sublingual immunotherapy. Ann Allergy Asthma Immunol 2016;116:583–4.

62. Sanchez-Garcia S, Rodriguez Del Rio P, Escudero C, et al. Possible eosinophilic esophagitis induced by milk oral immunotherapy. J Allergy Clin Immunol 2012;129:1155–7.

63. Miehlke S, Alpan O, Schroder S, et al. Induction of eosinophilic esophagitis by sublingual pollen immunotherapy. Case Rep Gastroenterol 2013;7:363–8.

64. Cox L, Larenas-Linnemann D, Lockey RF, et al. Speaking the same language: the World Allergy Organization subcutaneous immunotherapy systemic reaction grading system. J Allergy Clin Immunol 2010;125:569–74, 574.e1-7.

65. Epstein TG, Liss GM, Murphy-Berendts K, et al. AAAAI/ACAAI Surveillance study of subcutaneous immunotherapy, years 2008-2012: an update on fatal and nonfatal systemic allergic reactions. J Allergy Clin Immunol In Pract 2014;2:161–7.e3.

66. Bernstein DI, Epstein T, Murphy-Berendts K, et al. Surveillance of systemic reactions to subcutaneous immunotherapy injections: year 1 outcomes of the ACAAI and AAAAI collaborative study. Ann Allergy Asthma Immunol 2010;104:530–5.

67. Amin HS, Liss GM, Bernstein DI. Evaluation of near-fatal reactions to allergen immunotherapy injections. J Allergy Clin Immunol 2006;117:169–75.

68. Cox L, Aaronson D, Casale TB, et al. Allergy immunotherapy safety: location matters! J Allergy Clin Immunol In Pract 2013;1:455–7.

69. Calderon MA, Simons FE, Malling HJ, et al. Sublingual allergen immunotherapy: mode of action and its relationship with the safety profile. Allergy 2012;67:302–11.

70. Alvarez-Cuesta E, Bousquet J, Canonica GW, et al. Standards for practical allergen-specific immunotherapy. Allergy 2006;61(Suppl 82):1–20.

71. Cox LS, Hankin C, Lockey R. Allergy immunotherapy adherence and delivery route: location does not matter. J Allergy Clin Immunol In Pract 2014;2:156–60.

72. Bender BG, Oppenheimer J. The special challenge of nonadherence with sublingual immunotherapy. J Allergy Clin Immunol In Pract 2014;2:152–5.
73. Incorvaia C, Rapetti A, Scurati S, et al. Importance of patient's education in favouring compliance with sublingual immunotherapy. Allergy 2010;65:1341–2.
74. Vita D, Caminiti L, Ruggeri P, et al. Sublingual immunotherapy: adherence based on timing and monitoring control visits. Allergy 2010;65:668–9.
75. Creticos PS, Esch RE, Couroux P, et al. Randomized, double-blind, placebo-controlled trial of standardized ragweed sublingual-liquid immunotherapy for allergic rhinoconjunctivitis. J Allergy Clin Immunol 2014;133:751–8.
76. Matricardi PM, Kuna P, Panetta V, et al. Subcutaneous immunotherapy and pharmacotherapy in seasonal allergic rhinitis: a comparison based on meta-analyses. J Allergy Clin Immunol 2011;128:791–9.e6.
77. Meadows A, Kaambwa B, Novielli N, et al. A systematic review and economic evaluation of subcutaneous and sublingual allergen immunotherapy in adults and children with seasonal allergic rhinitis. Health Technol Assess 2013;17:vi, xi-xiv, 1-322.
78. Hankin CS, Cox L. Allergy immunotherapy: what is the evidence for cost saving? Curr Opin Allergy Clin Immunol 2014;14:363–70.
79. Cox L. Allergy immunotherapy in reducing healthcare cost. Curr Opin Otolaryngol Head Neck Surg 2015;23:247–54.
80. Ariano R, Berto P, Tracci D, et al. Pharmacoeconomics of allergen immunotherapy compared with symptomatic drug treatment in patients with allergic rhinitis and asthma. Allergy Asthma Proc 2006;27:159–63.
81. Hankin CS, Cox L, Bronstone A, et al. Allergy immunotherapy: Reduced health care costs in adults and children with allergic rhinitis. J Allergy Clin Immunol 2013;131:1084–91.
82. Hankin CS, Cox L, Lang D, et al. Allergen immunotherapy and health care cost benefits for children with allergic rhinitis: a large-scale, retrospective, matched cohort study. Ann Allergy Asthma Immunol 2010;104:79–85.
83. Hankin CS, Cox L, Lang D, et al. Allergy immunotherapy among Medicaid-enrolled children with allergic rhinitis: patterns of care, resource use, and costs. J Allergy Clin Immunol 2008;121:227–32.
84. Nelson HS. Multiallergen immunotherapy for allergic rhinitis and asthma. J Allergy Clin Immunol 2009;123:763–9.
85. Calderon MA, Cox L, Casale TB, et al. Multiple-allergen and single-allergen immunotherapy strategies in polysensitized patients: looking at the published evidence. J Allergy Clin Immunol 2012;129:929–34.
86. Calderon MA, Cox LS. Monoallergen sublingual immunotherapy versus multiallergen subcutaneous immunotherapy for allergic respiratory diseases: a debate during the AAAAI 2013 Annual Meeting in San Antonio, Texas. J Allergy Clin Immunol In Pract 2014;2:136–43.
87. Copenhaver CC, Parker A, Patch S. Systemic reactions with aeroallergen cluster immunotherapy in a clinical practice. Ann Allergy Asthma Immunol 2011;107:441–7.
88. Durham SR, Walker SM, Varga EM, et al. Long-term clinical efficacy of grass-pollen immunotherapy. N Engl J Med 1999;341:468–75.
89. Cox L, Cohn JR. Duration of allergen immunotherapy in respiratory allergy: when is enough, enough? Ann Allergy Asthma Immunol 2007;98:416–26.
90. Schadlich PK, Brecht JG. Economic evaluation of specific immunotherapy versus symptomatic treatment of allergic rhinitis in Germany. Pharmacoeconomics 2000;17:37–52.

91. Petersen KD, Gyrd-Hansen D, Dahl R. Health-economic analyses of subcutaneous specific immunotherapy for grass pollen and mite allergy. Allergol Immunopathol (Madr) 2005;33:296–302.
92. Keiding H, Jorgensen KP. A cost-effectiveness analysis of immunotherapy with SQ allergen extract for patients with seasonal allergic rhinoconjunctivitis in selected European countries. Curr Med Res Opin 2007;23:1113–20.
93. Omnes LF, Bousquet J, Scheinmann P, et al. Pharmacoeconomic assessment of specific immunotherapy versus current symptomatic treatment for allergic rhinitis and asthma in France. Eur Ann Allergy Clin Immunol 2007;39:148–56.
94. Bruggenjurgen B, Reinhold T, Brehler R, et al. Cost-effectiveness of specific subcutaneous immunotherapy in patients with allergic rhinitis and allergic asthma. Ann Allergy Asthma Immunol 2008;101:316–24.
95. Berto P, Bassi M, Incorvaia C, et al. Cost effectiveness of sublingual immunotherapy in children with allergic rhinitis and asthma. Allerg Immunol (Paris) 2005;37:303–8.
96. Bachert C, Vestenbaek U, Christensen J, et al. Cost-effectiveness of grass allergen tablet (GRAZAX(R)) for the prevention of seasonal grass pollen induced rhinoconjunctivitis - a Northern European perspective. Clin Exp Allergy 2007;37:772–9.
97. Beriot-Mathiot A, Vestenbaek U, Bo Poulsen P. Influence of time horizon and treatment patterns on cost-effectiveness measures: the case of allergen-specific immunotherapy with Grazax. J Med Econ 2007;10:215–28.
98. Canonica GW, Poulsen PB, Vestenbaek U. Cost-effectiveness of GRAZAX for prevention of grass pollen induced rhinoconjunctivitis in Southern Europe. Respir Med 2007;101:1885–94.
99. Berto P, Frati F, Incorvaia C, et al. Comparison of costs of sublingual immunotherapy and drug treatment in grass-pollen induced allergy: results from the SIMAP database study. Curr Med Res Opin 2008;24:261–6.
100. Nasser S, Vestenbaek U, Beriot-Mathiot A, et al. Cost-effectiveness of specific immunotherapy with Grazax in allergic rhinitis co-existing with asthma. Allergy 2008;63:1624–9.
101. Ariano R, Berto P, Incorvaia C, et al. Economic evaluation of sublingual immunotherapy vs. symptomatic treatment in allergic asthma. Ann Allergy Asthma Immunol 2009;103:254–9.

Asthma in Adults

Anil Nanda, MD[a,b,c],*, Anita N. Wasan, MD[d]

KEYWORDS

- Asthma • Adult • Allergy • Cough • Rhinitis • Sinusitis • COPD • ACO

KEY POINTS

- The diagnosis of asthma is a clinical one, but objective measures, such as pulmonary function testing, can be used to aid in the diagnosis.
- There are multiple associated comorbidities with asthma, including rhinitis, sinusitis, gastroesophageal reflux disease, obstructive sleep apnea, and depression.
- Pharmacologic therapies include inhaled corticosteroids (ICS), ICS–long-acting ß-agonist combinations, leukotriene antagonists, long-acting muscarinic antagonists, and short-acting ß-agonists. The latest therapies are biologic medications for severe asthma.
- Special populations include pregnant adults with asthma, patients with exercise-induced asthma/bronchoconstriction, older adults with asthma, and patients with occupational asthma.
- Individualized and precision therapy for each patient is essential.

INTRODUCTION

Asthma affects approximately 300 million people worldwide and approximately 7.5% of adults in the United States.[1,2] Among adults, asthma results in about 10.5 million physician office visits per year and affects approximately 8.7% of blacks, 7.6% of whites, and 5.8% of Hispanics.[2] Asthma is characterized by inflammation of airways, variable airflow obstruction, and bronchial hyperresponsiveness.[3] It is a heterogeneous condition that is diagnosed clinically.[2] A detailed history and physical examination are essential, but objective measures, such as pulmonary function testing (PFT), methacholine challenge, and fractional exhaled nitric oxide (FeNO), can aid in the diagnosis. Comorbidities of asthma include rhinitis, sinusitis, gastroesophageal reflux disease (GERD), obstructive sleep apnea (OSA), and depression.[3] It is vital to understand that asthma can initially occur at any age, even in older adults. Adult-onset asthma is often misdiagnosed as chronic obstructive pulmonary disease (COPD).

Disclosure Statement: The authors have nothing to disclose.
[a] Asthma and Allergy Center, 724 West Main Street, Suite 160, Lewisville, TX 75067, USA;
[b] Asthma and Allergy Center, 4900 Long Prairie Road, Suite 100, Flower Mound, TX, USA;
[c] Division of Allergy and Immunology, University of Texas Southwestern Medical Center, Dallas, TX, USA; [d] Allergy and Asthma Center, 6824 Elm Street, Suite 120, McLean, VA 22101, USA
* Corresponding author. 724 West Main Street, Suite 160, Lewisville, TX 75067.
E-mail address: anilnanda@yahoo.com

Med Clin N Am 104 (2020) 95–108
https://doi.org/10.1016/j.mcna.2019.08.013
0025-7125/20/© 2019 Elsevier Inc. All rights reserved.

COPD shares some features of asthma, and these conditions can overlap (asthma-COPD overlap, or ACO). Asthma can be allergic, nonallergic, or both. Nonpharmacologic therapies for asthma include patient education on inhaler technique and asthma action plan. Pharmacologic therapies include inhaled corticosteroids (ICS), inhaled corticosteroid-long-acting ß-agonist combinations (ICS-LABA), leukotriene antagonists, long-acting muscarinic antagonists (LAMA), and short-acting ß-agonists, as well as several biologics. Special populations include pregnant adults with asthma, patients with exercise-induced asthma/bronchoconstriction, older adults with asthma, and patients with occupational asthma.

PATHOPHYSIOLOGY OF ASTHMA

Airway inflammation is a hallmark of asthma, with eosinophils, mast cells, and most type 2 helper T lymphocytes (Th2, or T2, cells) involved.[3] The specific cells involved in mild, moderate, or severe asthma can be variable, including T2 cells, type 1 helper lymphocytes (Th1, or T1 cells), eosinophils, and neutrophils.[3] Cytokines associated with severe asthma include interleukin-17 (IL-17), IL-12, and IL-23.[2] Inflammatory cytokines associated with a Th2 response include IL-3, IL-4, IL-5, IL-13, and granulocyte-macrophage colony stimulating factor.[3] A mixed pattern may predominate also, depending on exacerbating factors or severity.[2,3]

Structural changes in the airway include mucous hypersecretion and an increase in the number of goblet cells and secretory glands.[3] There may be evidence of epithelial damage, subepithelial fibrosis, and increased airway smooth muscle.[3]

DIAGNOSIS OF ASTHMA

The diagnosis of asthma is clinical and relies heavily on the history and physical examination, yet judicious use of diagnostic testing can assist in the diagnosis. Symptoms of asthma include cough, wheezing, and shortness of breath.[4] Physical examination may display wheezing, hyperinflation, prolonged expiratory time, and increased labor of breathing.[3,5] In severe exacerbations, cyanosis and use of accessory muscles of respiration may be evident.[2] However, some patients with severe asthma at baseline may not show the typical acute symptoms. For example, in patients with cough-predominant asthma, there may just be an inhalational cough. Atypical asthma presentations may lead to a misdiagnosis. Symptoms can be triggered by exercise, cold air, inhaled allergens, irritants, or stresses.[3] However, examination is usually normal, because patients are often in between exacerbations.[5] Imaging, including chest radiography, in asthma is usually normal, but bronchial thickening can occasionally be noted. Another test is allergy skin prick testing or measurement of specific immunoglobulin E (IgE) to determine if there is allergic asthma.[6]

In terms of diagnostic testing, spirometry is a PFT that measures the volume (amount) and flow (speed) of air that can be exhaled and inhaled and which can be done in the office setting.[6] The forced expiratory volume in the first second of exhalation (FEV_1) is measured and is also compared with the forced vital capacity (FVC), the complete volume of air that can be exhaled in a forced attempt.[6] A reduced FEV_1/FVC ratio (<0.75) demonstrates airflow obstruction.[7] FEV_1 is often variable and coincides with a deterioration of improvement in symptoms.[7] The predicted FEV_1 is calculated based on a variety of factors, including age, gender, weight, and ethnicity. There is usually a bronchodilator response to asthma with a 12% or greater than 200-mL increase of baseline FEV_1 about 10 to 15 minutes following administration of a short-acting ß-agonist.[6] However, some patients with a baseline FEV_1 of higher than 80%

may have a clinically significant bronchodilator response.[7] Peak flow meters are less accurate than spirometers in the diagnosis of asthma.[6]

Measuring airway, or bronchial, hyperresponsiveness can also aid in the diagnosis of asthma.[8] Traditionally, methacholine challenge has been used.[8] Methacholine directly stimulates the constriction of airway smooth muscle, resulting in a discernible change in spirometry.[8] Progressively increasing concentrations of methacholine are inhaled, and FEV_1 is serially measured.[8] The concentration of methacholine that induces a decrease in FEV_1 of 20% is called the provocative dose, or PC_{20}.[6] Typically, a PC_{20} <1 mg/mL is moderate-severe bronchial hyperresponsiveness; a value between 1 and 4 mg/mL is mild bronchial hyperresponsiveness, and a value between 4 and 16 mg/mL is borderline responsiveness.[9] A value greater than 16 mg/mL demonstrates normal bronchial hyperresponsiveness, essentially ruling out asthma.[2] However, the presence of bronchial (airway) hyperresponsiveness does not definitively diagnose asthma. For example, some patients with allergic rhinitis may have airway hyperresponsiveness during specific pollen seasons.[10]

Exhaled nitric oxide can also be used as a measure of eosinophilic airway inflammation. This method is less invasive than other methods of quantifying airway eosinophil levels and can be done in the office.[6] Elevated FeNO levels (for example, >50 parts per billion) may predict an improved clinical response to ICS therapy.[7]

DIFFERENTIAL DIAGNOSIS OF ASTHMA AND ASSOCIATED COMORBIDITIES

The differential diagnosis of asthma is vast (**Box 1**). Conditions affecting multiple organ systems can present with symptoms similar to asthma. There are also multiple comorbid conditions associated with asthma. Upper respiratory tract conditions include vocal cord dysfunction, rhinitis and sinusitis, and OSA.[2] GERD is also associated with asthma. Other conditions in the differential diagnosis of asthma include congestive heart failure, pulmonary hypertension, and chronic thromboembolic pulmonary disease. Chest radiograph, computed tomography (CT) chest scan, and echocardiography can narrow down the diagnosis between these cardiovascular conditions. Foreign body airway obstruction and medication-related cough (such as

---

Box 1
Differential diagnosis of asthma

Vocal cord dysfunction

Rhinitis and sinusitis

OSA

Congestive heart failure

Pulmonary hypertension

Thromboembolic pulmonary disease

Foreign body airway obstruction

Medications (ACE inhibitors)

COPD

GERD

The above list depicts some conditions in the differential diagnosis of asthma, but is not intended to be an exhaustive list.

angiotensin-converting enzyme inhibitors [ACE inhibitors]) are also in the differential.[7] COPD and ACO are discussed in subsequent sections of this article.

Vocal cord dysfunction is a "paradoxic movement of the vocal cords."[11] Prevalence may be as high as 50% in severe asthma patients.[11] If a patient is not responding to typical asthma therapies, including ICSs, or symptoms appear to be more severe than spirometry indicates, vocal cord dysfunction should be considered. There is adduction of vocal cords, resulting in airflow limitation.[11] Potential triggers of vocal cord dysfunction attacks include exercise and anxiety. Symptoms include hoarseness, throat tightness, cough, dyspnea, and wheezing.[11] Diagnosis is made by laryngoscopy during exacerbations.[11] On spirometry, truncation of the inspiratory loop can occur.[11] Treatment is with speech therapy with specific breathing exercises. Similar to vocal cord dysfunction, exercise-induced laryngeal obstruction occurs when there is swelling of the aryepiglottic folds at the peak of exercise, with prompt resolution following exercise completion.[11]

GERD is more common in patients with asthma, with prevalence rates as high as 74%.[11] GERD can present with chronic cough, as can asthma.[12] Of note, many patients may not have the "typical" symptoms of GERD, such as heartburn or dyspepsia. Treatment with lifestyle changes and daily proton pump inhibitors can be initiated.[12] The treatment of GERD has shown variable effects on asthma outcomes, but quality of life of asthma patients has been shown to be improved in some studies.[11]

Rhinitis and sinusitis are common in patients with asthma. Both allergic and nonallergic rhinitis cause similar symptoms.[13] Most patients with severe asthma are sensitized (have allergen-specific IgE to aeroallergens), and early onset of severe asthma is associated with allergic rhinitis and allergic conjunctivitis.[11] Patients with allergic rhinitis have worse asthma control with increase in number of exacerbations and emergency room visits.[14] Approximately 48% of patients with chronic rhinosinusitis with nasal polyps have asthma.[15] Therapies for rhinitis and chronic sinusitis include nasal saline rinses, intranasal corticosteroids, intranasal antihistamines, leukotriene inhibitors, and in the case of allergic rhinitis, allergen immunotherapy. Sinus surgery can also be an option for rhinitis and sinusitis with or without nasal polyps.[16] In fact, difficult-to-control asthma in patients with sinusitis with or without nasal polyps can be an indication for surgery.[16] Studies involving biologic medications are ongoing.

A subset of chronic rhinosinusitis patients with nasal polyps has a condition called aspirin-exacerbated respiratory disease.[17] Classically, it is a triad of asthma, eosinophilic nasal polyps, and respiratory reactions caused by aspirin, nonsteroidal anti-inflammatory drugs (NSAID), and other cyclooxygenase 1 inhibitors.[17] The respiratory reactions typically occur within 30 to 120 minutes of NSAID intake and induce asthma as well as rhinitis symptoms of rhinorrhea and nasal congestion.[17] Aspirin desensitization, consisting of delivering gradual doses of aspirin and treating symptoms resulting from the provocative dose, can be performed until a concentration of 325 mg is reached.[17] The patient then is maintained on high-dose aspirin therapy at 325 mg or 650 mg twice daily to maintain desensitization.[17] Aspirin desensitization has been shown to decrease use of systemic corticosteroids and hospitalizations for asthma as well as improve sinusitis symptoms.[13]

OSA is frequently associated with asthma.[18] OSA is characterized by episodes of apnea during sleep, and this is associated with upper airway obstruction and upper airway resistance.[11] Symptoms include daytime sedation and poor quality of sleep.[11] There is a higher frequency of OSA symptoms or polysomnography-diagnosed OSA in patients with asthma.[18] Treatment of OSA (with continuous positive airway pressure or mechanical devices/surgery) improves asthma symptoms, bronchodilator use, and asthma-specific quality of life.[18] One study showed that OSA risk may be associated with neutrophilic asthma.[18] Again, concomitant rhinitis should also be treated, because rhinitis can be a major contributor to upper airway resistance.[19] Rhinitis, both allergic and nonallergic, may contribute to upper airway resistance syndrome.[19] There appears to be a connection between upper and lower airways, involving a unified airway.[19] Treatment of both the upper and the lower airways is paramount, rather than focusing on either one alone.[19]

Obesity is another comorbid condition associated with asthma. Obesity is correlated with increased asthma incidence, prevalence, and severity.[20] One study involving more than 10,000 adult asthma patients in the United States found a positive correlation between elevated body mass index and asthma exacerbations.[20] Another study showed that patients with increased abdominal visceral adiposity were associated with decreased asthma quality of life.[21]

Infections, including viral, bacterial, and fungal causes, are often comorbid conditions associated with asthma exacerbations.[3] Allergic bronchopulmonary aspergillosis (ABPA) is a particular condition with diagnostic criteria, including asthma (or cystic fibrosis [CF]) with worsening lung function (FEV_1), Aspergillus mold sensitivity (positive specific IgE and IgG to Aspergillus), total serum IgE greater than 1000 ng/mL (416 IU/mL), and infiltrates on chest radiography.[22] The main therapy consists of oral corticosteroids with antifungal therapies as an adjunct.[22] Allergic fungal rhinosinusitis is a subcategory of rhinosinusitis with nasal polyps.[23] It is associated with mucus-containing eosinophils and allergy to fungus in the sinusitis.[23] Fungi involved are usually Aspergillus, Bipolaris, and Alternaria species.[23] Soft tissue densities are commonly found on CT scan of sinuses.[23] The main therapy for allergic fungal rhinosinusitis is functional endoscopic sinus surgery, and medical therapy with corticosteroids and antifungal agents can be adjuvant therapy.[23] One vasculitis in the differential diagnosis of asthma is eosinophilic granulomatosis with polyangiitis, typified by asthma, sinusitis, eosinophilia, pulmonary infiltrates, evidence of eosinophilic vasculitis, and peripheral neuropathy.[11]

Depression is associated with asthma; however, the exact mechanisms are unknown.[24] Behavioral, affective, and cognitive dysfunction can influence medication use and inhaler technique.[24] One recent study revealed that depression was related to reduced bronchodilator use in asthma patients.[25] In the study, major depression was increased among patients with asthma (8.9%) compared with nonasthmatic patients (2.5%).[25] Controller medication underuse was linked to depression in asthma patients .[24] In 1 study of older adults, elevated depression scores correlated with decreased asthma control levels and reduced quality of life.[26]

CF, a genetic disease owing to mutations in the CF transmembrane conductance regulator, is associated with respiratory exacerbations that can be similar to asthma.[27,28] ABPA can also occur with CF, and its presentation may be indistinguishable from a CF exacerbation (shortness of breath, infiltrate on chest radiograph).[27,28] Early recognition of both conditions is imperative, and ABPA should be considered in any CF patient with an exacerbation unresponsive to antibiotics.

TREATMENT OF ASTHMA

The main care components for asthma include assessment and monitoring, patient education, addressing environmental controls and comorbid conditions, and pharmaceutical therapy.[29] Assessment of asthma control is subdivided into impairment and risk.[30] The impairment component includes symptoms, nighttime awakenings, use of short-acting ß-agonists, and pulmonary function.[30] Risk component includes exacerbations (such as requiring systemic corticosteroids), progressive loss of lung function, and pharmaceutical side effects.[30] Tools for assessing asthma symptom control include the Asthma Control Questionnaire (ACQ) and Asthma Control Test (ACT), a 5-question test that is easy to access on the Internet and very practical to use at an office visit, taking less than a minute for a patient to complete.[31–35] Scores on the ACQ from 0.0 to 0.75 indicate well-controlled asthma, and scores greater than 1.5 indicate poorly controlled asthma.[31,32] Scores on the ACT of 20 to 25 indicate well-controlled asthma; 16 to 19 indicate not well-controlled asthma, and 5 to 15 indicate poorly controlled asthma.[33–35] Patient education is paramount in the treatment of asthma because this is an outpatient disease, and patient adherence is increased with greater understanding of controller medication and exacerbation prevention. Patient adherence and inhaler technique are essential.[29] At every health care office visit, patient education should be emphasized. In addition, if there is evidence of allergic asthma, environmental controls, including reducing pet and dust mite exposure, may be implemented as well as treatment of allergic rhinitis.[29]

PHARMACOLOGIC THERAPY FOR ASTHMA

Asthma severity can be further divided into intermittent and persistent, and these severities (including uncontrolled, partially controlled, and controlled) correspond with various steps of therapy (**Table 1**).[29,30] Persistent asthma can be subdivided into mild, moderate, and severe and is treated with controller medications.[29,30] Controller medications include ICSs, leukotriene inhibitors, combination ICS/LABA, LAMA, methylxanthines, cromolyn, and biologic medications.[29,36] Allergen immunotherapy is also an option.[36] Reliever medications are rapid acting and include short-acting β_2-agonists, such as albuterol and levalbuterol, as well as muscarinic cholinergic antagonists (anticholinergics), such as ipratropium bromide.[29]

ICSs are the foundation of therapy for asthma-improving condition-related outcomes associated with both impairment and risks.[29,36] The mechanisms of their

Table 1 Asthma severity				
Impairment	Intermittent	Mild Persistent	Moderate Persistent	Severe Persistent
Symptoms	≤2 d/wk	>2 d/wk	Daily	Multiple times per day
Night-time Awakenings	≤2/mo	3–4/mo	>1/wk	Daily
Short-acting inhaler use (β-agonist)	≤2 d/wk	>2 d/wk	Daily	Multiple times per day
Lung function	FEV₁ >80% predicted	FEV₁ >80% predicted	FEV₁ >60% but <80%	FEV₁ <60%
Exacerbations (requiring oral corticosteroids)	0–1/y	≥2/y	≥2/y	≥2/y
	Step 1	Step 2	Step 3 and/or 4	Step 5 and/or 6

Adapted from Durrani SR, Busse WW. Management of Asthma in Adolescents and Adults. In: Adkinson NF, Bochner BS, Burks AW, et al., editors. Middleton's allergy principles and practice, 8th edition. Philadelphia: Saunders; 2014; and National Asthma Education and Prevention Program. Expert Panel Report 3 (EPR-3): Guidelines for the diagnosis and management of asthma-Summary Report 2007. J Allergy Clin Immunol 2007;120(5 Suppl):s94-s138; with permission.

actions include inhibition of inflammatory cell activation and migration.[29] Side effects are much lower than systemic corticosteroids, the long-term use of which is associated with the development of numerous conditions, including diabetes, osteoporosis, and decreased immunity. Low-dose inhaled steroids are recommended as first-line therapy for asthma.[36] Medium and higher doses of ICSs are also used.[36] Examples of low-dose inhaled daily corticosteroid therapies include fluticasone propionate 100 to 250 μg, budesonide 200 to 400 μg, and mometasone 110 to 220 μg.[7] Medium-dose therapies include fluticasone propionate 250 to 500 μg, budesonide 400 to 800 μg, and mometasone 220 to 440 μg.[7] Higher-dose therapies include fluticasone propionate 500 to 1000 μg, budesonide greater than 800 μg, and mometasone greater than 440 μg.[7]

The leukotriene pathway of inflammation involves the cysteinyl leukotrienes, and these are potent inflammatory lipid mediators.[37] Leukotriene receptor antagonists include montelukast and zafirlukast, and zileuton is in a similar medication class, because it modifies the 5-lipoxygenase pathway.[29] These medications are not as effective as ICS medications, but can be added on to inhaled steroid therapy.[36] They are less effective than combination ICS/LABA therapies.[36] Side effects in adults are minimal.[36]

Combination ICS/LABA therapies are effective and are the preferred agents in adults whose asthma is not well controlled on low-dose ICS therapy.[36] The black-box warning of increased mortality in asthma patients taking LABA therapy, subsequently transferred to ICS/LABA therapy, was removed by the Food and Drug Administration owing to multiple safety trials.[38]

LAMA, or anticholinergics, provide additional bronchodilation.[39,40] LAMA medications, such as tiotropium, when added to ICS/LABA therapy, have been shown to reduce asthma exacerbations, and when added to ICS monotherapy, have improved asthma symptoms and lung function.[40,41]

Methylxanthines, such as theophylline, provide bronchodilation with some anti-inflammation.[36] However, because of a narrow therapeutic window and common adverse events, such as nausea, vomiting, diarrhea, cardiac arrhythmias, and seizures, use of these medications should be for patients who cannot tolerate other therapies or who are still symptomatic despite other therapies.[36] Mast cell release inhibitors include cromolyn sodium, and these are safe; however, ICSs have better efficacy.[29] Long-term macrolide therapy has been proposed for severe asthma, but there has been inadequate evidence.[42] In bronchial thermoplasty, radiofrequency pulses are used to treat the airway smooth muscle in patients with severe asthma; however, it is still unclear which patients should be selected for this procedure.[36,42]

There is a prominent role of allergy in asthma, and patients with persistent asthma should be evaluated for contributing allergies. For allergic asthma in patients who are sensitized to inhaled allergens (aeroallergens), allergen immunotherapy has been shown to reduce asthma symptoms and the use of asthma medications.[7,43] Airway hyperresponsiveness has also been improved.[43] Both subcutaneous and sublingual allergen immunotherapy have been shown to benefit asthma.[42,44] The treatment of the upper airway, including rhinitis and chronic sinusitis, with medical therapies, such as intranasal corticosteroids, and if indicated, allergen immunotherapy, is also of paramount importance. In addition, comorbid conditions, such as GERD and sinusitis, must be considered and treated, especially in patients with poorly controlled asthma.

The newest agents for asthma are the biologic therapies. These agents are usually reserved for moderate to severe asthma patients. Currently approved biologics for asthma involve anti-IgE, anti-IL-5, and anti-IL-4/anti-IL-13 antibodies. Omalizumab is a monoclonal antibody that attaches to free IgE and prevents activation of cells involved in the allergic inflammatory response, such as mast cells and basophils.[42] Criteria for treating patients with omalizumab include positive IgE (skin test or serum-specific IgE) to an aeroallergen and elevated IgE levels (allergic asthma).[42] Omalizumab, a subcutaneous injection, has been shown to reduce severe exacerbations and hospitalizations owing to asthma as well as reduce the dose of ICSs.[42] Mepolizumab is a monoclonal antibody against IL-5, which reduces the number of eosinophils in both blood and sputum.[45] Mepolizumab, a subcutaneous injection, has been shown to reduce emergency room visits and hospitalizations owing to asthma.[45] Reslizumab, an intravenous agent, is also a monoclonal antibody to IL-5 and has also been shown to reduce asthma exacerbations.[46] Benralizumab, a subcutaneous injection, is a monoclonal antibody that attaches to the alpha-subunit of the IL-5 receptor, inducing a natural killer cell and antibody-mediated depletion of eosinophils.[47] It has also been shown to reduce oral glucocorticoid doses in patients with severe asthma as well as lower asthma exacerbation rates.[47] The most recent biologic approved for asthma is dupilumab, which had been previously approved for the treatment of atopic dermatitis. Dupilumab, a subcutaneous injection, is an anti-IL-4 receptor alpha-subunit monoclonal antibody that blocks both IL-4 and IL-13 signaling.[48] IL-4 and IL-13 are involved in Th2 inflammation.[48] Dupilumab has been shown to decrease severe asthma exacerbations and improved asthma control and lung function.[48] Dupilumab also has been shown to reduce oral corticosteroid use in severe asthma.[49]

The overall treatment of asthma using the above therapies is indicated in **Table 2**.[29,30] **Tables 1** and **2**, using step therapies, are only guides, and individualized patient assessment and therapy are essential. In addition, therapy can be "stepped up" or "stepped down" depending on the clinical situation.

Table 2
Treatment of asthma

	Intermittent	Mild Persistent	Moderate Persistent	Moderate Persistent	Severe Persistent
Step	Step 1	Step 2	Step 3	Step 4	Step 5 and Step 6
Treatment	Short-acting ß-agonist as needed	Low-dose ICS	Medium-dose ICS Or Low-dose ICS-LABA	Medium-dose ICS-LABA	High-dose ICS-LABA LAMA May also consider biologic therapies
Alternative		Leukotriene antagonist	Low-dose ICS and leukotriene antagonist	Medium-dose ICS and leukotriene antagonist LAMA may be added	Oral prednisone may need to be added

Allergen immunotherapy can also be considered for allergic asthma.
Adapted from Durrani SR, Busse WW. Management of Asthma in Adolescents and Adults. In: Adkinson NF, Bochner BS, Burks AW, et al., editors. Middleton's allergy principles and practice, 8th edition. Philadelphia: Saunders; 2014; and National Asthma Education and Prevention Program. Expert Panel Report 3 (EPR-3): Guidelines for the diagnosis and management of asthma-Summary Report 2007. J Allergy Clin Immunol 2007;120(5 Suppl):s94-s138; with permission.

TREATMENT OF ACUTE ASTHMA EXACERBATIONS

Usually, with regular therapy and education, asthma exacerbations requiring emergency department visits or hospitalization can be avoided; however, 12 million people in the United States per year suffer from acute asthma exacerbations, with approximately 3 million hospitalized.[1] Severe asthma signs include tachypnea, tachycardia, use of accessory muscles of respiration, diaphoresis, wheezing (although lack of airflow or diminished breath sounds may also indicate severe asthma), and difficulty in lying down.[1] However, in severe, chronic asthmatics, these signs may not be seen. Bradycardia can be a sign of imminent respiratory failure.[1] Risk factors for fatal asthma or near-fatal asthma include multiple hospitalizations or emergency room visits, intensive care unit admission or intubation/mechanical ventilation, excessive short-acting ß-agonist use, and allergy to the mold, *Alternaria*.[1] Spirometry can be used, measuring FEV_1 as well as peak flow, to assess change from baseline.[1] Laboratory evaluation or chest radiographs are usually not required, unless there are co-morbid conditions or the diagnosis is uncertain.[1] Arterial blood gases can be considered in acutely ill patients, including patients with oxygen saturation of less than 92% on room air.[1] Arterial blood gases can give information on respiratory status, impending respiratory fatigue, and respiratory failure.[1]

Treatment consists of short-acting ß-agonists, such as albuterol, either by metered dose inhaler or by nebulized therapy, with continued treatments until the patient has become stable.[1] Ipratropium bromide, an anticholinergic, can also be added.[1] Corticosteroids are also vital concomitant therapies. In the outpatient setting, ICSs can be considered for mild asthma exacerbations, usually quadrupling the recommended dose of the ICS.[1] Short courses of oral corticosteroids can also be effective, with no tapering required if less than 3 weeks of treatment.[1] In the acute setting, such as the emergency room, systemic corticosteroids should be used (either oral, intravenous, or intramuscular).[1] Oral steroids are recommended after emergency room discharge.[1]

Failure to respond to the above therapies requires hospitalization.[1] Noninvasive positive pressure ventilation can be attempted in patients at an increased rate of respiratory failure; however, intubation should not be delayed once it is thought to be clinically necessary.[1] High ventilator pressures should be avoided to avoid the risk of barotrauma.[1] Upon discharge, patient education should be emphasized with appropriate follow-up with an asthma specialist, such as an allergist/immunologist.[1]

ASTHMA IN PREGNANCY

Approximately 8% of pregnant women report asthma, which incurs higher risks of pregnancy complications, including preeclampsia and preterm birth.[50] Improved asthma control can lead to improved pregnancy outcomes.[50] Asthma can worsen, improve, or remain the same during pregnancy.[50] Most patients have a diagnosis of asthma before pregnancy, but new onset pulmonary symptoms during pregnancy should be evaluated.[50] Spirometry and allergy testing (through use of specific IgE, and not allergy skin testing) can be used to evaluate symptoms, if necessary, but methacholine testing is contraindicated in pregnant patients because of lack of safety data.[50]

Comorbid conditions should be treated, including rhinitis (both allergic and nonallergic), sinusitis, and GERD.[50] Pregnant patients with well-controlled asthma should continue the medications.[50] Rapid-acting therapy includes short-acting ß-agonists, including albuterol.[50] Among controller medications, ICSs are the most effective medications.[50] Budesonide is a pregnancy medication class category B corticosteroid.[50] It is recommended for women on controller medication to be seen on a monthly basis.[50] Most data on adverse effects of medications for asthma are from observational studies, but most data are reassuring.[50]

Asthma exacerbations should be treated with short-acting ß-agonists, anticholinergic medications, and systemic corticosteroids.[50] Fetal assessment is contingent on pregnancy stage.[50] Asthma medications should be continued during labor and delivery.[50]

ASTHMA AND EXERCISE-INDUCED BRONCHOCONSTRICTION IN ADULTS

Exercise-induced bronchoconstriction (EIB) refers to the momentary narrowing of the airways after exercise.[51] EIB occurs among adults who may not even have asthma symptoms otherwise.[51] Asthma is more common among endurance athletes, such as winter-sports athletes and swimmers.[51] The mechanism may involve airway dehydration during increased ventilation on exercise, and this increases osmolarity of fluid lining the airways.[51] The resulting release of mediators causes airway bronchoconstriction.[51]

EIB usually occurs within 15 minutes after 5 to 8 minutes of intensive aerobic training and usually resolves within 60 minutes.[52] Symptoms alone are not enough for diagnosis.[51] Objective testing includes exercise challenge, eucapnic voluntary hyperpnea (EVH), and mannitol challenges.[53] In adult recreational or elite athletes suspected of having EIB who have normal lung function and no clinical history of asthma, an indirect, ungraded challenge (exercise or EVH) can be performed.[53,54] As an example, during an exercise challenge, a 10% or greater decrease in FEV_1 compared with preexercise baseline at any 2 consecutive time points during challenge is diagnostic of EIB.[53] Vocal cord dysfunction, discussed previously, is important to consider in the differential.[51]

Nonpharmacologic therapies include addressing environment (such as improving ventilation in indoor pools), using face masks to decrease cold air exposure, and using a preexercise warmup.[51] Treating underlying asthma in athletes, with therapies noted previously (such as ICSs), is important. Pharmacologic therapies for EIB include the use of short-acting ß-agonists 5 to 10 minutes before exercise, but overuse can cause tolerance.[51] Leukotriene antagonists also decrease EIB and can be considered as well as cromolyn products as alternative therapies.[51] Exercise challenge can be difficult to perform in the outpatient setting, so a trial of a ß-agonist before exercise is a prudent first step. If there is no improvement in symptoms, conditions such as uncontrolled asthma and vocal cord dysfunction can be further considered.

ASTHMA IN OLDER ADULTS

It is estimated that there is an approximate 7.8% prevalence of asthma among people 65 to 74 years old and a 6% prevalence in people 75 years and older.[55] Diagnosing asthma in adults can be more difficult because of multiple comorbid conditions, and management can be more challenging because of medication side effects and diminished cognition.[55] Again, asthma education is a critical component; however, there are some unique circumstances regarding older adults.[55] Arthritis, affecting many older adults, can lead to difficulty in using inhalers, especially metered dose inhalers.[55] In addition, polypharmacy is common in the older adult population.[55] Depression also is common and should be addressed.[55]

ASTHMA CHRONIC OBSTRUCTIVE PULMONARY DISEASE OVERLAP

Like asthma, COPD is an inflammatory condition of the airway, but is generally associated with tobacco smoking and older patients.[56] Patients have airflow limitation, and the condition is usually progressive.[56] Forms of COPD include emphysema and chronic bronchitis.[56] COPD has been considered a neutrophilic, rather than eosinophilic inflammatory disease; however, there is evidence that both COPD and asthma can have eosinophilic and neutrophilic pathologies.[56] ACO refers to a combination of asthma and COPD features.[56] Bronchial hyperresponsiveness, thought to be a trademark of asthma, occurs in COPD patients also, and many asthma patients have a significant smoking history also.[56] Treatment of ACO consists of ICSs, LAMAs, and long-acting ß-agonists, which are currently used in the therapy for both asthma and COPD.[56] However, there is still no firm consensus for either the diagnosis or the exact treatment of ACO.

OCCUPATIONAL ASTHMA

Occupational asthma occurs when an agent at a workplace causes the asthma.[57] Atopy (presence of IgE antibodies) to inhaled allergens is associated with the development of asthma to high-molecular-weight agents.[57] Some examples of more common high-molecular-weight agents include flour (wheat, rye with bakers), latex (gloves in health care workers), and animal proteins (mice, rat dander in laboratory workers).[57] Low-molecular-weight agents include isocyanates, metals, acid anhydrides, acrylates, and wood dusts and are common in the manufacturing industries.[57] In addition to the history and physical examination, diagnosis includes specific IgE testing, bronchial responsiveness challenge (such as methacholine challenge), and laboratory challenges with a suspected occupational agent.[57] Avoidance of the causative agent is the ideal treatment.[57]

SUMMARY

Asthma is a relatively common condition and can be frequently underdiagnosed or misdiagnosed. Today's internist will encounter patients with this condition frequently.

Asthma is also associated with multiple comorbid conditions, which may exacerbate asthma if not also controlled. New therapies include biologics, and there are multiple new modalities of treatment in the pipeline. Referral to an asthma specialist, such as an allergist/immunologist, should be considered if the diagnosis is in doubt, if initial treatment is ineffective, or if there are multiple comorbidities. Individualized and precision therapy for each patient is essential.

REFERENCES

1. Fergeson J, Patel S, Lockey R. Acute asthma, prognosis, and treatment. J Allergy Clin Immunol 2017;139:438–47.
2. McCracken J, Veeranki S, Ameredes B, et al. Diagnosis and management of asthma in adults. JAMA 2017;318:279–90.
3. Boulet L-P. In: Adkinson NF, Bochner BS, Burks AW, et al, editors. Diagnosis of asthma in adults in Middleton's allergy: principles and practice. Philadelphia, PA: Elsevier; 2014. p. 892–901.
4. Lowhagen O. Diagnosis of asthma-new theories. J Asthma 2015;52:538–44.
5. Tarasidis G, Wilson K. Diagnosis of asthma: clinical assessment. Int Forum Allergy Rhinol 2015;5:s23–6.

6. McCormack M, Enright P. Making the diagnosis of asthma. Respir Care 2008;53: 583–92.
7. GINA Reports. Available at: https://ginasthma.org/gina-reports/. Accessed September 20, 2018.
8. Davis B, Blais C, Cockcroft D. Methacholine challenge testing: comparative pharmacology. J Asthma Allergy 2018;11:89–99.
9. Crapo R, Casaburi R, Coates A, et al. for the American Thoracic Society. Guidelines for methacholine and exercise challenge testing–1999. Am J Respir Crit Care Med 2000;161:309–29.
10. Thomas M. Allergic rhinitis: evidence for impact on asthma. BMC Pulm Med 2006; 6:s1–4.
11. Porsbjerg C, Menzies-Gow A. Co-morbidities in severe asthma: clinical impact and management. Respirology 2017;22:651–61.
12. Smith J, Woodcock A. Chronic cough. N Engl J Med 2016;375:1544–51.
13. Ocampo C, Grammer L. Chronic rhinosinusitis. J Allergy Clin Immunol Pract 2013;1:205–11.
14. Bousquet J, Gaugris S, Kocevar V, et al. Increased risk of asthma attacks and emergency visits among asthma patients with allergic rhinitis: a subgroup analysis of the improving asthma control trial. Clin Exp Allergy 2005;35:723–7.
15. Stevens W, Peters A, Hirsch A, et al. Clinical characteristics of patients with chronic rhinosinusitis with nasal polyps, asthma, and aspirin exacerbated respiratory disease. J Allergy Clin Immunol Pract 2017;5:1061–70.
16. Ragab S, Scadding GK, Lund VJ, et al. Treatment of chronic rhinosinusitis and its effects on asthma. Eur Respir J 2006;28:68–74.
17. Laidlaw T, Cahill K. Current knowledge and management of hypersensitivity to aspirin and NSAIDs. J Allergy Clin Immunol Pract 2017;5:537–45.
18. Teodorescu M, Broytman O, Curran-Everett D, et al. Obstructive sleep apnea risk, asthma burden, and lower airway inflammation in adults in the severe asthma research program, (SARP) II. J Allergy Clin Immunol Pract 2015;3:566–75.
19. Giavina-Bianchi P, Aun M, Takejima P, et al. United airway disease: current perspectives. J Asthma Allergy 2016;9:93–100.
20. Schatz M, Zeiger R, Yang S, et al. Prospective study on the relationship of obesity to asthma impairment and risk. J Allergy Clin Immunol Pract 2015;3:560–5.
21. Goudarzi H, Konno S, Kimura H, et al. Impact of abdominal visceral adiposity on adult asthma symptoms. J Allergy Clin Immunol Pract 2019;4(7):1222–9.e5.
22. Greenberger P, Bush R, Demain J, et al. Allergic bronchopulmonary aspergillosis. J Allergy Clin Immunol Pract 2014;2:703–8.
23. Dykewicz M, Rodrigues J, Slavin R. Allergic fungal rhinosinusitis. J Allergy Clin Immunol 2018;142:341–51.
24. Gerald J, Moreno F. Asthma and depression. J Allergy Clin Immunol Pract 2016; 4:74–5.
25. Han Y, Forno E, Marsland A, et al. Depression, asthma and bronchodilator response in a nationwide study of US adults. J Allergy Clin Immunol Pract 2016;4:68–73.
26. Ross J, Yang Y, Song P, et al. Quality of life, health care utilization, and control in older adults with asthma. J Allergy Clin Immunol Pract 2013;1:157–62.
27. Chapron J, Zuber B, Kanaan R, et al. Management of acute and severe complications in adults with cystic fibrosis. Rev Mal Respir 2011;28:503–16.
28. King C, Brown A, Aryal S, et al. Critical care of the adult patient with cystic fibrosis. Chest 2019;155:202–14.

29. Durrani S, Busse W. In: Adkinson NF, Bochner BS, Burks AW, et al, editors. Management of asthma in adolescents and adults in Middleton's allergy: principles and practice. Philadelphia, PA: Elsevier; 2014. p. 902–22.

30. Busse W, et al. Expert Panel Report 3 (EPR-3): guidelines for the diagnosis and management of asthma–Summary Report 2007. J Allergy Clin Immunol 2007;120: S94–138.

31. Juniper E, O'Byrne P, Guyatt G, et al. Development and validation of a questionnaire to measure asthma control. Eur Respir J 1999;14:902–7.

32. Juniper E, Svennson K, Mork A, et al. Measurement properties and interpretation of three shortened versions of the asthma control questionnaire. Respir Med 2005;99:553–8.

33. Thomas M, Kay S, Pike J, et al. The Asthma Control Test (ACT) as a predictor of GINA guideline-defined asthma control: analysis of a multinational cross-sectional survey. Prim Care Respir J 2009;18:41–9.

34. Nathan R, Sorkness C, Kosinski M, et al. Development of the asthma control test: a survey for assessing asthma control. J Allergy Clin Immunol 2004;113:59–65.

35. Schatz M, Kosinski M, Yarlas A, et al. The minimally important difference of the Asthma Control Test. J Allergy Clin Immunol 2009;124:719–723 e1.

36. Quirt J, Hildebrand K, Mazza J, et al. Asthma. Allergy Asthma Clin Immunol 2018; 14:15–30.

37. Singh R, Tandon R, Dastidar S, et al. A review on leukotrienes and their receptors with reference to asthma. J Asthma 2013;50:922–31.

38. Seymour S, Lim R, Xia C, et al. Inhaled corticosteroids and LABAs–removal of the FDA's boxed warning. N Engl J Med 2018;378:2461–3.

39. Bel E. Tiotropium for asthma-promise and caution. N Engl J Med 2012;367: 1257–9.

40. Kerstjens H, Engel M, Dahl R, et al. Tiotropium in asthma poorly controlled with standard combination therapy. N Engl J Med 2012;367:1198–207.

41. Peters S, Kunselman S, Ictovic N, et al. Tiotropium bromide step-up therapy for adults with uncontrolled asthma. N Engl J Med 2010;363:1715–26.

42. Israel E, Reddel H. Severe and difficult-to-treat asthma in adults. N Engl J Med 2017;377:965–76.

43. Abramson M, Puy R, Weiner J. Injection allergen immunotherapy for asthma. Cochrane Database Syst Rev 2010;8:001186.

44. Calamita Z, Saconato H, Pela A, et al. Efficacy of sublingual immunotherapy in asthma: systematic review of randomized clinical trials using the Cochrane Collaboration method. Allergy 2006;61:1162–72.

45. Ortega H, Liu M, Pavord I, et al. Mepolizumab treatment in patients with severe eosinophilic asthma. N Engl J Med 2014;371:1198–207.

46. Cardet J, Israel E. Update on reslizumab for eosinophilic asthma. Expert Opin Biol Ther 2015;15:1531–9.

47. Nair P, Wenzel S, Rabe K, et al. Oral glucocorticoid-sparing effect of benralizumab in asthma. N Engl J Med 2017;376:2448–58.

48. Castro M, Corren J, Pavord ID, et al. Dupilumab efficacy and safety in moderate-to-severe uncontrolled asthma. N Engl J Med 2018;378:2486–95.

49. Rabe K, Nair P, Brusselle G, et al. Efficacy and safety of dupilumab in glucocorticoid-dependent severe asthma. N Engl J Med 2018;378:2475–85.

50. Schatz M, Dombrowski M. Asthma in pregnancy. N Engl J Med 2009;360:1862–9.

51. Boulet L, O'Byrne P. Asthma and exercise-induced bronchoconstriction in athletes. N Engl J Med 2015;372:641–8.

52. Bonini M, Silvers W. Exercise-induced bronchoconstriction: background, prevalence, and sport considerations. Immunol Allergy Clin N Am 2018;38:205–14.
53. Weiler J, Brannan J, Randolph C, et al. Exercise-induced bronchoconstriction update–2016. J Allergy Clin Immunol 2016;138:1292–5.
54. Brannan J, Posbjerg C. Testing for exercise-induced bronchoconstriction. Immunol Allergy Clin N Am 2018;38:215–29.
55. Nanda A, Baptist A, Divekar R, et al. Asthma in the older adult. J Asthma 2019;1–12 [Epub ahead of print].
56. Desai M, Oppenheimer J, Tashkin D. Asthma-chronic obstructive pulmonary disease overlap syndrome. Ann Allergy Asthma Immunol 2017;118:241–5.
57. Lemiere C, Vandenplas O. In: Adkinson NF, Bochner BS, Burks AW, et al, editors. Occupational allergy and asthma in Middleton's allergy: principles and practice. Philadelphia, PA: Elsevier; 2014. p. 970–85.

Drug Hypersensitivity Reactions

Mark S. Dykewicz, MD[a],*, Jason K. Lam, DO[a]

KEYWORDS

- Adverse drug reaction • Drug hypersensitivity reaction • Drug allergy • Drug rash
- Skin testing • Graded challenge • Desensitization

KEY POINTS

- Drug hypersensitivity reactions (DHRs) may be classified based on timing (immediate vs delayed), mechanisms (allergic vs nonallergic), and pattern of clinical manifestations. Classifying DHR based on these characteristics may aid in diagnosis and management.
- Drug allergy management may include selection of alternative, non–cross-reactive agents, drug allergy testing, graded challenge, and/or desensitization.
- Diagnostic tools for DHR are limited. Immediate-type skin testing evaluates only for immediate allergic reactions, not delayed allergic reactions.
- Graded challenge is used when drug allergy suspicion is low. It involves administering several graduated doses and if tolerated, indicates no drug allergy.
- Desensitization is used when suspicion for drug allergy is high. It involves many more steps than graded challenge and induces a temporary state of tolerance that is maintained only so long as the drug is continued.

DEFINITIONS

Adverse drug reactions (ADRs) are defined as any noxious and unintended response to a drug. ADRs may be predictable, based on known pharmacologic properties of a drug, or unpredictable, related to immunologic response or genetic differences in patients.[1] A subset of ADRs is drug hypersensitivity reactions (DHRs), reactions that resemble immunologic reactions (whether or not there is demonstration of immune responses such as drug-specific antibodies or T cells). Drug allergies are DHRs for which an immunologically mediated mechanism is demonstrated.[2]

---

[a] Section of Allergy and Immunology, Division of Infectious Diseases, Allergy and Immunology, Department of Internal Medicine, Saint Louis University School of Medicine, Saint Louis University Allergy & Immunology, 1402 South Grand Boulevard Room M 157, St Louis, MO 63104, USA
* Corresponding author.
E-mail address: mark.dykewicz@health.slu.edu

Med Clin N Am 104 (2020) 109–128
https://doi.org/10.1016/j.mcna.2019.09.003
0025-7125/20/© 2019 Elsevier Inc. All rights reserved.

medical.theclinics.com

EPIDEMIOLOGY

ADRs are estimated to account for 3% to 6% of all hospital admissions and to occur in 10% to 15% of hospitalized patients.[3] DHRs comprise up to 15% of all ADRs.[4]

RISK FACTORS

Important risk factors for DHRs include chemical properties of the drug and host factors. Large molecular weight agents such as proteins and some polysaccharides may be more likely to induce antibody-mediated reactions. Specific structural moieties in smaller molecular weight ($\leq$1000 kD) nonprotein agents (eg, antibiotics) and/or their metabolic products may be more likely to covalently react with self-proteins to produce immunogenic hapten-protein conjugates.

Host risk factors for DHRs include female gender, history of drug allergy, recurrent exposure to drugs, concurrent disease state, and genetic factors.[3] Patients with cystic fibrosis who require recurrent courses of same or similar antibiotics are more prone to have DHRs, probably reflecting the frequency of drug exposure.[5] Patients with Epstein–Barr virus (EBV) infections are more prone to developing DHR rashes to aminopenicillin antibiotics.[6] These rashes are usually nonpruritic and may be due to transient immune-stimulation by EBV.[7] Patients with a history of nonpruritic, EBV-associated rashes are not at increased risk of life-threatening reactions and most will tolerate future courses of aminopenicillins.[7,8] Patients with human immunodeficiency virus (HIV) infections are more prone to have reactions to sulfonamides as well as other drugs.[9]

Genetics and Polymorphisms in Drug Metabolism

As examples of genetic risk factors, patients with certain human leukocyte antigen (HLA) alleles have significant increased risk of severe cutaneous drug reactions (SCARs) to certain drugs, for example, HLA B 1502 (carbamazepine) and HLA B 5701 (abacavir).[10] Prospective pharmacogenetic screening for HLA B 5701 and use of alternative agents in patients with HLA-B 5701 has nearly eliminated SCARs to abacavir. Patients who are slow acetylators are twice as likely to have sulfonamide antibiotic DHRs, as they have increased metabolism of sulfonamides through an alternative oxidative pathway that generates production of reactive metabolites that can then elicit an immune response.[11]

Multiple Drug Hypersensitivity Syndrome

An estimated 1% to 10% of patients have DHRs to multiple chemically unrelated, non–cross-reactive drugs. This should be distinguished from patients who reacts to multiple drugs because of (1) cross-reactivity to drugs due to structural similarities, common metabolic pathways, or pharmacologic mechanisms; (2) flare-up reactions (exacerbation of an existing drug allergy by the early switch of therapy to a novel drug); and (3) multiple drug intolerance syndrome in which there is no confirmation after evaluation and which may be driven by patient anxiety.

CHRONOLOGY, CLINICAL PRESENTATIONS, AND MECHANISMS

Classifying drug reactions based on chronology, patterns of clinical manifestations, and mechanisms may aid in evaluation and management.

Chronology and Clinical Presentations

DHRs may be classified as immediate or delayed, based on the timeline from exposure to onset of clinical reaction. DHRs may also be classified mechanistically as allergic (immunologically mediated by antibody or T-cell mechanisms) or nonallergic (mediated by nonimmunological mechanisms) (**Table 1**).

Mechanisms

Immediate reactions

Signs and symptoms from immediate DHRs occur within 1 to 6 hours of drug exposure and may include cutaneous (flushing, pruritus, urticaria, angioedema, laryngeal edema), respiratory (bronchospasm, rhinoconjunctivitis), cardiovascular (hypotension, tachycardia), gastrointestinal symptoms (nausea, vomiting, diarrhea, abdominal pain or cramping), or anaphylaxis.[12] In contrast to anaphylaxis, vasovagal reactions are

Table 1
Immediate and delayed drug hypersensitivity reactions

Timing	Signs and Symptoms	Mechanisms
Immediate (occurring within 1–6 h from drug administration)	• Urticaria • Angioedema • Rhinitis • Conjunctivitis • Bronchospasm • Gastrointestinal symptoms (nausea, vomiting, diarrhea, abdominal pain) • Anaphylaxis	Allergic (IgE antibody mediated) Or Nonallergic (examples) • Direct stimulation of mast cell and/or basophils (opiates) • Complement activation • Alterations in metabolic pathways (aspirin and nonsteroidal antiinflammatory drugs through cyclo-oxygenase 1 inhibition)
Delayed (occurring >6 h from drug administration)	Skin ± organ involvement: • Delayed urticaria • Maculopapular eruptions (morbilliform) • Fixed drug eruptions • Vasculitis • SJS/TEN • DiHS/DRESS • AGEP • Symmetric drug-related intertriginous and flexural exanthems Internal organ involvement may include • Hepatitis • Renal failure • Pneumonitis • Anemia • Neutropenia • Thrombocytopenia	*Allergic:* immunologically mediated by antibodies or T cells ± neutrophils, eosinophils, monocytes

Abbreviations: AGEP, acute generalized exanthematous pustulosis; DiHS/DRESS, drug-induced hypersensitivity syndrome/drug reaction with eosinophilia and systemic symptoms; SJS/TEN, Stevens-Johnson syndrome/toxic epidermal necrolysis.

Data from Demoly P, Adkinson NF, Brockow K, et al. International consensus on drug allergy. Allergy 2014;69(4):420-437.

typically characterized by pallor and bradycardia rather than flushing and tachycardia seen in anaphylaxis.

Signs and symptoms are typically due to massive and sudden release of mediators from mast cells and basophils via immunoglobulin E (IgE) or non–IgE-mediated mechanisms.[2,13,14] Non-IgE mechanisms may include direct stimulation of mast cell and/or basophils (eg, many reactions from radiocontrast media, vancomycin), complement activation, and cyclooxygenase (COX-1) inhibition.[2] Phototoxic skin reactions may also occur in an immediate time frame.

Delayed reactions

By definition, delayed-onset DHRs occur 6 or more hours after drug exposure.[13] However, most delayed-onset reactions occur days to weeks after allergen exposure and can involve multiple organs. Mechanisms include T-cell–mediated reactions or development of toxic metabolites in a genetically predisposed person.

Cutaneous reactions are the most common manifestation of delayed DHRs. Drug eruptions usually occur within 5 to 14 days of drug initiation but may develop within 1 to 2 days in previously sensitized patients. In patients taking antibiotics, drug eruptions may occur up to 2 weeks after treatment has been stopped.[15]

Drug-induced exanthems often present with erythematous macules and papules (morbilliform rash) and rarely with pustules or bullae. Rashes are usually pruritic and in a centrifugal pattern, starting with trunk and spreading distally to extremities in a symmetric manner.[16] Systemic manifestations include fever, lymphadenopathy, eosinophilia, and organ dysfunction (primarily liver, bone narrow, and/or kidneys).[17] Photosensitivity rashes may be phototoxic or photoallergic. Phototoxic rashes are more common, may present within minutes to hours of sunlight exposure, and present as an exaggerated sunburn that desquamates within several days. Vesicles and bullae may occur in more severe cases. Mechanistically, drugs absorb ultraviolet light and release excessive energy, causing cell damage. Tetracyclines, especially doxycycline, and nonsteroidal antiinflammatory drugs (NSAIDs) are some of the more common causal drugs. In contrast, photoallergic rashes are T-cell mediated, DHRs against a drug allergen whose antigenicity has been altered by exposure to ultraviolet radiation. Photoallergic reactions typically develop 24 to 48 hours after sunlight exposure, are eczematous, and may occur after days or months of drug exposure. Photoallergic reactions more frequently occur from topically applied agents such as sunscreens or fragrances but may also occur from systemically administered drugs including sulfonamides, quinolones, griseofulvin, ketoprofen, and quinine.[18]

SCARs often involve multiple organs. These syndromes include drug reaction with eosinophilia and systemic symptoms (DRESS) or drug-induced hypersensitivity syndrome (DiHS), acute generalized exanthematous pustulosis, and Stevens-Johnson syndrome (SJS)/toxic epidermal necrolysis (TEN) **(Table 2)**.

Other organ/organ system manifestations of delayed DHRs include renal (interstitial nephritis, nephrotic syndrome), liver (hepatitis), cardiovascular (myocarditis, vasculitis), pulmonary Loffler syndrome (cough, chest discomfort migratory infiltrates with or without peripheral eosinophilia), and/or hematologic systems (anemia, leukopenia, thrombocytopenia, lymphadenopathy). These manifestations are often times isolated and not associated with skin manifestations. Aseptic meningitis has been reported from NSAIDs, radiocontrast media, intravenous immunoglobulin replacement, and other agents.

Drug fever may occur in isolation or with other allergic manifestations. Drug fever usually occurs 7 to 10 days into a treatment course, with prompt defervescence within 48 hours of discontinuation of the responsible agent.

Table 2
Severe cutaneous adverse reactions

Type	Rash Features	Latent Period	Systemic Features	Laboratory Findings
AGEP	Pustules on erythematous background, flexural accentuation	Usually <3 d	High fever, edema	Neutrophilia, eosinophilia
DRESS/ DiHS	Itchy exanthem or urticarial papules/ plaques, erythroderma, nonerosive mucositis, >50% body surface area	2–8 wks[a]	Fever, edema, lymphadenopathy	Eosinophilia, atypical lymphocytes, hepatitis, renal impairment. Skin biopsy: interface dermatitis, apoptotic keratinocytes, scattered eosinophils
SJS/TEN	Painful dusky macular erythema, blisters, Nikolsky sign, erosive mucositis in ≥2 surfaces, palmoplantar tender erythema	4–21 d	Prodrome of flu-like symptoms, high fever, malaise, rarely pneumonitis	Skin biopsy: full-thickness epidermal necrosis
SS and SSLR	Itchy urticarial or serpiginous plaques, may start at injection site, predisposition for hands and feet	1–2 wks[a]	High fever, malaise, polyarthralgia or polyarthritis	Neutropenia, mild Eosinophilia, mild Proteinuria, low complement levels in severe cases. Histology nonspecific

Latent period from onset of drug administration.

Abbreviations: AGEP, acute generalized exanthematous pustulosis; d, days; SS, serum sickness; SSLR, serum sickness–like reactions.

[a] May be shorter latent period in sensitized patients.

Adapted from Peter JG, Lehloenya R, Diamini S, et al. Severe delayed cutaneous and systemic reactions to drugs: A global perspective on the science and art of current practice. J Allergy Clin Immunol Pract 2017;5(3):555; with permission.

Immunologic mechanisms

Most drugs are simple, small molecules (<1000 kD) that, by themselves, are poorly recognized by the immune system. However, drugs may become immunogenic when their native form or reactive metabolites bind to serum or tissue proteins and form hapten-protein carrier conjugates. These conjugates can act as complete antigens that are then recognized by the immune system and stimulate an immune response resulting in a DHR.

In contrast, large, complex drug molecules (eg, proteins) may directly stimulate immune responses through concentration-dependent interactions with immune receptors (eg, pharmacological interaction (p-i) model; see type IV reaction discussed later).

Immunologic reactions may be divided broadly into 4 categories according to the Gell and Coombs classification. Type I, II, and III are antibody mediated, whereas type IV reactions are T-cell mediated.[2,19] Although the Gell and Coombs framework is useful for recognizing patterns of clinical presentations, DHRs in a patient are sometimes complex and may be caused by combinations of immune responses and multiple effector mechanisms.

Type I reactions have an acute onset and involve drug-specific IgE antibody-mediated activation of mast cells and basophils. On initial exposure, a drug or its hapten-protein conjugate stimulates generation of drug-specific IgE by plasma cells of B-cell lineage, which then bind to high-affinity IgE receptors on the surfaces of mast cells and basophils. This results in a sensitized, asymptomatic state. On reexposure to the drug or one with a structurally similar antigenic region (cross-reacting agent), the drug binds to the IgE molecules, cross-linking them and activating mast cells and basophils. This results in the immediate release of histamine and tryptase as well as the rapid generation of leukotrienes and prostaglandins, resulting in anaphylaxis or any symptoms thereof (see earlier section on Immediate Reactions). Antibiotics are a common cause of type I DHRs.

Type II reactions have delayed onset (usually at least 5–8 days after exposure) and involve IgG or IgM antibody-mediated cell destruction by complement activation or cell clearance by macrophages.[20] Although type II reactions often occur after high-dose, prolonged, or frequent exposure to a drug, they may also occur during a treatment course.[19] Clinical sequelae include granulocytopenia, hemolytic anemia, and thrombocytopenia. Common causes include antibiotics, anticonvulsants, sulfonamides, and heparin. In heparin-induced thrombocytopenia, antibodies form against a conjugate of heparin and platelet factor 4 on platelets, triggering platelet destruction.

Type III reactions have delayed onset and result from formation of antibody-drug complexes (IgG > IgM) that are deposited in tissues. These complexes activate complement and other immune cells, causing tissue damage. Signs and symptoms typically occur one or more weeks after drug exposure and may manifest as serum sickness, vasculitis, or drug fever.[19]

Serum sickness presents with fever, urticarial or pruritic rash, arthralgia, and/or acute hepatitis glomerulonephritis. Causes may include antitoxins (rabies, botulism, venom) and rituximab. Serum sickness may occur sooner than 1 week in patients with a previous serum sickness reaction.

Antibiotics may also cause serum sickness-like reactions, with amoxicillin being the most common.[21]

Drug-induced antineutrophil cytoplasmic antibodies (ANCA) + vasculitis usually presents with palpable purpura and/or petechiae, fever, arthralgia, and lymphadenopathy. Hydralazine, minocycline, propylthiouracil, and levamisole-adulterated cocaine are the most commonly reported causes.[22]

Drug-induced lupus is principally a type III reaction, but lupus from different drugs may vary in both clinical presentation and associated autoantibodies. Hydralazine, procainamide, and minocycline typically cause serositis and less commonly rash. Drug-induced lupus from these agents is more typically associated with antihistone antinuclear antibodies and only rarely anti-double-stranded DNA, except pANCA occurs with minocycline. Drug-induced subacute cutaneous lupus (eg, from hydrochlorothiazide, calcium channel blockers, angiotensin converting enzyme [ACE] inhibitors and statins) is associated with a photosensitive rash as well as SS-A and SS-B antibodies; it is an atypical DHR in that rather than occurring shortly after drug introduction, it can often develop more than 6 months after drug introduction.[23]

Type IV reactions have delayed onset and are mediated by activated T cells (4 possible different subtypes) and may involve eosinophils, monocytes, and neutrophils. Type IV reactions typically occur at least 48 to 72 hours and sometimes days to weeks after exposure.[19] Most reactions involving T cells occur in the skin, a large T-cell reservoir.[24]

Clinical presentation is driven by the T-cell subset activated and may present with severe cutaneous reactions with or without organ involvement or may involve only a single organ (eg, drug-induced liver injury). Type IV reactions may also be accompanied by fever or present as drug fever only. Drugs or their metabolites may activate T cells (1) when hapten-protein conjugates or drug fragments are presented to T cells by antigen-presenting cells (APCs, eg, dendritic, Langerhans or B cells, or macrophages) or (2) by pharmacologic interaction with immune receptors (the p-i concept) in which drugs in their native state (*not* acting as haptens to form conjugates with proteins) noncovalently bind directly with T-cell receptors on T cells or with HLA molecules on APCs and then activate T cells. Abacavir is an example of a drug that acts through p-i interaction.[20] Allergic contact dermatitis and photoallergic reactions also occur through type IV mechanisms.

Nonimmunologic mechanisms

Nonallergic (nonimmunologic) mechanisms include but are not limited to direct stimulation of mast cell and/or basophils, complement activation, and alterations in metabolic pathways.

Drugs may directly (without IgE cross-linking) activate mast cells or basophils. Human G protein-coupled receptor MRGPRX2 has been identified as a mast cell receptor capable of causing histamine release in response to the following drugs/drug classes: quinolones (ciprofloxacin and levofloxacin), neuromuscular blocking agents (rocuronium), icatibant, vancomycin, and opioids.[13,25,26]

Complement activation and generation of anaphylatoxins C3a and C5a can activate mast cells through complement receptors. This can occur in reactions to Cremophor and oversulfated chondroitin sulfate–contaminated heparin.[27]

Examples of DHRs that occur because of alterations in metabolic pathways include (1) COX-1 inhibition by NSAIDs, which leads to overproduction of leukotrienes in sensitive individuals resulting in respiratory distress (aspirin-exacerbated respiratory disease [AERD]) and (2) ACE inhibition by ACE-inhibitors, leading to overproduction of bradykinin and other vasomediators.

MANAGEMENT
Acute Management

Acute treatment of DHRs involves immediate discontinuation of suspected drugs and treatment of signs and symptoms.

In anaphylaxis, epinephrine is lifesaving and the only drug proven effective and should be administered immediately. Adjunctive measures include antihistamines and glucocorticoids. Other cardiopulmonary resuscitative measures may also be required.

Itching from isolated, mild maculopapular/morbilliform rashes may respond to antihistamines, although the course of the rash is not altered. Progressive rashes or those associated with fever, nausea, or arthralgia should be treated with systemic steroids. Similarly, those with severe, prolonged drug reactions should be treated with systemic steroids and may require a slow taper over several weeks. DiHS/DRESS may require many months of treatment with systemic steroids.

Diagnostic Evaluations

Diagnosis of drug hypersensitivity requires a thorough history and identification of physical findings and symptoms that are compatible with characteristics and timing of drug-induced reactions. Thus, understanding the chronology, clinical manifestation, and mechanisms mentioned previously is essential. In selected cases, clinical diagnosis could be confirmed with demonstration of an elevated tryptase level obtained shortly after anaphylaxis, identification of IgE (in vitro or immediate-type skin testing) to a drug suspected to have caused anaphylaxis, or in very limited cases, delayed patch testing (to identify sensitized T cells) to a drug suspected to have caused a delayed reaction. Graded drug challenges can also be considered (see later discussion). Overall, objective testing for the diagnosis of drug allergy is limited (**Box 1**).[28]

Testing for Tryptase

Serum tryptase levels can aid in diagnosing anaphylaxis when the diagnosis is not clear by history and physical alone. Serum tryptase increases ~30 minutes after onset of anaphylaxis, peaks 1 to 2 hour after onset of reaction, and remains increased for up to 6 to 8 hours.[29] Commercial assays measure total tryptase, which is the sum of tryptase continuously secreted at baseline and released during activation of mast cells and basophils.[29] Tryptase level greater than 11.4 ng/mL or greater than $\geq 2 + 1.2 \times$ baseline tryptase levels supports anaphylaxis.[29] However, a negative tryptase level does not rule out anaphylaxis in part because tryptase is released from different mast cell and basophils subsets, depending on the trigger and severity of the reaction.[29]

Box 1
General considerations in evaluation of drug hypersensitivity reactions (DHRs)

Identify drugs that have a history of causing problems in the patient.

Determine whether there are cross-reactive agents and avoid them.

If the patient has a late reaction (eg, drug rash), take a careful history of all drugs used in the past month because the possible causative drug may have been discontinued.

Reactions are more likely to result from drugs introduced more recently.

Drugs administered with impunity for prolonged periods (eg, months to years) are rarely responsible for DHRs (notable exceptions are ACE inhibitors and drugs suspected to cause subacute cutaneous lupus erythematosus).

Have a high index of suspicion for drug reactions whenever a patient experiences adverse clinical manifestation.

Be mindful that drug reactions can involve internal organs (eg, nephritis, hepatitis, isolated lymphadenopathy), often in the absence of eosinophilia.

If an immunologic drug reaction is suspected, stop all nonessential drugs and substitute non–cross-reactive drugs (if possible).

Further evaluation may be needed
- When there is a history of prior DHR and the drug is essential (ie, there is no equally effective, structurally unrelated alternative) and the risk/possible benefit ratio for the suspect drug is positive.
- When there is a history of prior severe DHRs for other drugs; the best way to protect the patient is to find the culprit agents.

Further evaluation may not be needed if history does not suggest DHR
- Noncompatible symptomatology
- Noncompatible chronology
- Drug taken since with no reaction
- Same reaction without having taken the drug
- There are alternative diagnoses (eg, herpes virus eruption, chronic urticaria)

Adapted from Dykewicz MS. Drug allergy. In: Slavin R, Reisman R, editors. An Expert Guide to Allergy and Immunology. Philadelphia: American College of Physicians; 1999; p. 155. with permission.

Testing for Allergen-Specific Immunoglobulin E

Diagnosis of an IgE-mediated immediate reaction requires demonstration of allergen-specific IgE (by skin testing or in vitro testing) and clinical reactivity (either by history or supervised challenge). Allergen-specific IgE indicates sensitization, but not all patients with positive skin or in vitro testing will have a clinical reaction on challenge.

Skin and Patch Testing

Immediate-type skin testing (prick-puncture and intradermal) is a bioassay used to detect the presence of allergen-specific IgE on patient's mast cells and is only helpful for identifying risk for immediate reactions. Skin testing for most antibiotics (except penicillin [PCN]) lack negative predictive values. In a patient with history of an immediate drug reaction, a positive test with a nonirritating concentration of the medication suggests the presence of drug-specific IgE. However, a negative test does *not* rule out drug allergy due to the lack of negative predictive value.

Immediate-type skin testing requires knowledgeable personnel to avoid false-negative and false-positives results leading to under- or overdiagnosis of drug allergy, respectively. Skin test reactivity results can be repressed by antihistamines, topical steroids, and omalizumab.

Delayed-type patch testing involves application of drug, mixed into petrolatum or 0.9% saline, to a small area of skin under occlusion for 48 hours and then removed. The application site is then examined at 48 and 96 hours after placement. Conceptually, delayed patch testing might be used to evaluate risk for DHRs (type IV) to drugs. However, it currently has limited established utility for most drug allergens. Standardized and validated test concentrations and vehicles have not been fully studied or are disputed in the literature.

In Vitro Testing

Although a limited number of in vitro tests are available to identify risk for DHRs, most are not adequately standardized and their predictive value is not established. Immunoassays are marketed to assess hypersensitivity to neuromuscular blocking agents (NMBA) and some biological agents.[30] An in vitro test offered is the basophil activation test (BAT), which measures histamine release from human peripheral blood incubated with drug allergens. BAT is not standardized and few laboratories perform it.

TREATMENT OPTIONS

Future management of patients with a confirmed allergy to a drug includes administration of a non–cross-reactive alternative agent or desensitization to the culprit drug.

Graded Drug Challenges

Graded challenge testing (drug provocation testing) is used to exclude allergy to a medication in patients with a low probability of having an IgE-mediated drug allergy. Patients are given a test dose at a dose lower than that would cause a serious reaction followed by several escalating doses under continuous observation. Graded challenge does not modify or prevent allergic response to the drug; it is not a desensitization but a method used to confirm or deny drug allergy. Therefore, patients who tolerate a graded challenge are not allergic to the drug at the dose given. Graded challenges should be performed in a setting equipped to recognize and treat reactions. Graded challenge should not be performed in patients with history of SCARs (eg, DRESS/DiHS) to a drug in question because it could be potentially fatal.

Desensitization

Drug desensitization may be considered in patients with confirmed or high probability of an immediate (and in some cases type IV) DHR when the drug is essential.

Desensitization induces a temporary tolerance to allow patients with DHRs to receive an uninterrupted course of medication safely. Drug hypersensitivity returns once the medication is discontinued. Desensitization has been completed successfully for many drugs. However, because of the high risk of adverse reactions, particularly anaphylaxis, desensitization should only be performed by experienced physicians and only when the drug is essential (no alternatives available). Desensitization should never be attempted in patients with history of SCARs (eg, SJS/TEN) because even small doses of the drug may induce irreversible and potentially fatal reactions.

Drug desensitization involves administration of a drug in increasing doses until the therapeutic dose is reached. Temporary tolerance is maintained if the drug is given normally at its usual interval (eg, at least daily). Temporary tolerance is likely lost if 48 hours has elapsed since the last dose and thus, repeat desensitization is required before readministration.[31]

When patients have a history of an immediate reaction thought to be non–IgE mediated (eg, from many chemotherapy agents, most radiocontrast media reactions), premedication protocols that include antihistamines and systemic corticosteroids may be useful.

Rare immunologic complications may occur following desensitization in patients who require high dose or extended duration. Complications include serum sickness, hemolytic anemia, nephritis, and thrombocytopenia.[31]

REACTIONS TO SPECIFIC DRUGS
Penicillin and Other Beta-Lactam

IgE-mediated allergic responses are directed toward the drug-protein complex (antigenic determinants) that forms after penicillin (PCN) and/or its metabolites bind to tissue/serum proteins.

The allergic components of PCN are either the beta-lactam core ring structure (common to all PCNs, cephalosporins, and carbapenems) or less commonly, the R-group side chains that distinguish different PCNs from each other.[32] PCN cross-reactivity to cephalosporin is primarily due to R1 side chain group.[33] Risk of cross-reactivity to cephalosporin has been estimated to ~2%.[34] There is thought to be a lower incidence of immediate-type reactions to third- and fourth-generation cephalosporins than to the first- and second-generation compounds.

Most of the patients with IgE-mediated PCN reactions lose their sensitivity over time. After 5 and 10 years, approximately 50% and 80% of patients lose their sensitivity to PCN.

PCN skin testing is a safe and reliable way to assess for IgE-mediated reactions. Using both major and minor PCN determinants, PCN skin testing has a negative predictive value of 97% to 99%. Following negative skin testing, the absence of an allergy is usually confirmed by graded challenge under 1 to 2 doses to ensure an immediate reaction does not occur. PCN skin testing is contraindicated in patients with history of SCARs. Skin testing is *not* indicated in patients with a family history but no personal history of PCN allergy, because there is no increased risk of reaction.

If PCN testing is positive or cannot be completed in patients with suspected IgE-mediated reaction to PCN, the 2010 Joint Task Force on Practice Parameters for Drug Allergy recommends the following options:

1. Rapid desensitization if PCN is essential (eg, neurosyphilis).[7]
2. Use an alternative, non-beta-lactam drug.[7] An exception is aztreonam, a monobactam that has no cross-reactivity and can be safely given in PCN-allergic patients.[34]
3. Give a cephalosporin in graded challenge or via rapid desensitization.[7]
4. Administer a carbapenem via graded challenge.[7] Cross-reactivity of PCNs with carbapenems is less than 1%.[34]

In patients with a vague and/or distant history of PCN allergy, a graded challenge to PCN may be performed.[7] More recent guidelines have proposed that in patients with nonallergic symptoms or family history of PCN allergy, amoxicillin or PCN may be prescribed.[34] In patients with pruritis without rash or remote history (>10 years) *without* features of an IgE-mediated reaction to PCN class antibiotics, direct oral challenge to amoxicillin may be performed.[34]

Nonimmunologic reactions typically present as nonpruritic rash and are frequently seen with ampicillin and amoxicillin in patients with concomitant viral infections, allopurinol use, chronic lymphocytic leukemia, and hyperuricemia. These rashes are not associated with an increased risk of future intolerance to PCN antibiotics.

Cephalosporins

Cross-reactivity among cephalosporins as well as between cephalosporins and PCNs commonly arises from structural similarities in side chain groups (R1 > R2) or, rarely, from sensitization to the core beta-lactam ring present in both PCNs and cephalosporins or to metabolites of this ring. See PCN and other beta-lactams for more information about cross-reactivity.

Skin and in vitro testing for cephalosporin allergy are not validated and are not often used in clinical management. A safe and commonly used approach is selecting an alternative cephalosporin with a different side chain group from the implicated cephalosporin[35] (**Table 3**). However, patients with past immediate reactions to ceftazidime should avoid aztreonam because the two share identical side chains and cross-reactivity between the 2 drugs is reported.[35] Nonimmunologic disulfiram reaction may occur if cefoperazone is taken after alcohol ingestion.

Sulfonamides

Sulfonamides are divided into 2 distinct groups: antibiotics and nonantibiotics. Hypersensitivity to sulfonamide antibiotics is primarily mediated by immune responses to metabolites of the cyclic arylamine group common to all sulfonamide antibiotics. Notably, nonantibiotic sulfonamides do not contain this arylamine group.[36] Sulfonamide antibiotics include sulfamethoxazole, sulfadiazine, sulfadoxine, sulfisoxazole, and sulfapyridine (in sulfasalazine).[36]

Hypersensitivity reactions to sulfonamide antibiotics occur in ~2% to 4% of healthy patients and up to 50% to 60% of patients with HIV.[37] Immediate-type reactions are uncommon, with most hypersensitivity reactions presenting 1 to 2 weeks after start of therapy as a morbilliform rash with fever, with the fever sometimes preceding the rash. This can be accompanied by other organ involvement such as elevated liver enzymes and kidney dysfunction and can progress to SJS. Sulfonamide antimicrobials are highly associated with blistering dermatitis (SJS/TEN). Allergic reactions such as these, with systemic organ involvement such as DRESS and early stages of SJS, should be treated with systemic steroids and may require high doses (1–2 mg/kg q 6–8 hours) with a slow taper over many weeks, although other immunomodulators have been used. The rash may take several days to improve but the fever and malaise usually resolve in 24 to 48 hours. Topical steroids in addition often help speed the recovery

Table 3
Beta-lactam antibiotics with identical R-1 and R-2 side chains

Groups of B-lactam Antibiotics with Identical R-1 Side Chains

1	2	3	4	5	6	7	8
Amoxicillin	Ampicillin	Cefazolin	Cefoxitin	Cefdaloxime	Cefditoren	Aztreonam	Cefamandole
Cefadroxil	Cefaclor	Ceftezole	Cephaloridine	Cefdinir	Cefepime	Cefiderocol	Cefonicid
Cefatrizine	Cephalexin		Cephalothin	Cefixime	Cefodizime	Ceftazidime	
Cefprozil	Cephaloglycin				Cefotaxime		
	Cephradine				Cefpirome		
	Loracarbef				Cefpodoxime		
					Ceftriaxone		

Groups of B-lactam Antibiotics with Identical R-2 Side Chains

1	2	3	4	5	6
Cephalexin	Cefotaxime	Cefuroxime	Cefotetan	Cefaclor	Ceftibuten
Cefadroxil	Cephalothin	Cefoxitin	Cefamandole	Loracarbef	Ceftizoxime
Cephradine	Cephapirin		Cefoperazone		
	Cephaloglycin		Cefmetazole		
			Cefpiramide		

Adapted from Joint Task Force on Practice Parameters; American Academy of Allergy, Asthma and Immunology; American College of Allergy, Asthma and Immunology; Joint Council of Allergy, Asthma and Immunology. Drug allergy: An updated practice parameter. Ann Allergy Asthma Immunol 2010;105(4):273; with permission.

time of the rash. Tapering is guided by response to therapy and usually can start after 3 to 4 days. Underdosing may result in an incomplete response, and rapid tapering of steroids often results in rebound. Although there has been controversy in the past, most agree that SJS should be treated as such but corticosteroids are not indicated in TEN. In patients with severe cutaneous reactions but no fever or other organ involvement, a short course of systemic steroids (eg, prednisone 1–2 mg/kg/d for 5–7 days) may be beneficial.

Sulfonamide antibiotic allergy is diagnosed clinically based on a detailed history. No testing is available to assist in diagnosis. Patients with history of SCARs or blistering dermatitis should strictly avoid sulfonamides within the same group because reexposure could be fatal.

Cross-reactivity between sulfonamide antibiotics is variable.[38] In contrast, there is no convincing evidence of cross-reactivity between the antibiotic sulfonamides (that contain arylamine cyclic structures that generate target antigens through oxidative metabolism) and nonantibiotic sulfonamides (eg, diuretics, which do not contain an arylamine moiety).[39] However, sulfasalazine (a nonantimicrobial) should be avoided in patients allergic to sulfonamide antibiotics because sulfasalazine releases sulfapyridine (an antimicrobial) on exposure to gut bacteria.[39]

Desensitization protocols have been published for trimethoprim-sulfamethoxazole and nonantibiotic sulfonamides including sulfasalazine, torsemide, and furosemide.

Vancomycin

The most common vancomycin reaction is Red Man syndrome (RMS), which results from non–IgE-mediated histamine release from mast cells and basophils. This results in flushing, warmth, erythema, pruritus, and urticaria, affecting the face, neck, and torso. RMS usually occurs with rapid parenteral administration (>10 mg/min). Acute management involves stopping the infusion, treatment with H1 blockers (eg, diphenhydramine), and resuming at a slower infusion rate. Tolerance of future readministration is promoted by pretreatment with H1 blockers and a slower infusion rate. Rarely, IgE-mediated anaphylaxis can occur and is usually accompanied by angioedema and respiratory distress. Desensitization can be completed in cases of IgE-mediated anaphylaxis. Other rare severe cutaneous reactions from vancomycin include linear IgA bullous dermatitis, SJS/TEN, and DRESS/DiHS.

Angiotensin-Converting Enzyme Inhibitors

Cough and angioedema from ACE inhibitors are thought to be related to accumulation of bradykinin and other mediators. Cough may occur within hours of the first dose or months after therapy. Cough typically resolves within 1 to 4 weeks after discontinuation of the medication but may linger for up to 3 months. Angiotensin receptor blocker (ARB) agents are generally better tolerated, with a reported rate of cough of 3.3% compared with 9.9% with ACE inhibitors.[40]

ACE inhibitor–induced angioedema occurs in less than 1% of all patients treated, with higher occurrence in women and blacks.[41] More than 50% of episodes occur within the first week but some may occur even years after treatment.[42] Patients with a history of idiopathic/spontaneous angioedema or hereditary angioedema are at increased risk of developing angioedema from ACE inhibitors,[43] and therefore alternative agents (eg, ARBs, generally well tolerated in such patients) should be used, if indicated, in place of ACE inhibitors.

ACE inhibitor–induced angioedema is not associated with urticaria or pruritus and most commonly involves the lips, tongue, face, and upper airway. Angioedema could result in life-threatening airway obstruction and typically presents with throat hoarseness and inspiratory stridor. Visceral angioedema has been described in case reports and typically presents with diffuse abdominal pain with diarrhea. Acute episodes of ACE inhibitor angioedema will typically resolve over 2 to 5 days even if the ACE inhibitor is not discontinued but may then recur at highly variable intervals.[42] Alogliptin, an inhibitor of the bradykinin-degrading enzyme DPPIV used in patients with type 2 diabetes, is associated with increased risk of angioedema when taken concomitantly with ACE inhibitors.[41]

Management involves discontinuation of ACE inhibitors and if needed, airway support. In a retrospective study, 88% of patients had recurrence of angioedema 1 month after discontinuation of ACE inhibitors.[44] Intolerance to one ACE inhibitor usually predicts intolerance to the class. In patients unresponsive to usual measures, fresh frozen plasma and purified C1 inhibitor concentrate (if given early) have been beneficial in cases reports.[42,45] Icatibant has not been effective in trials.[46]

ARBs are generally well tolerated in patients with ACE-inhibitor angioedema. Systematic reviews reported a rate of 3.5% to 10% of recurrent angioedema in patients with a history of ACE-inhibitor angioedema.[47,48] This rate of recurrence may be contributed by recurrence of ACE-induced inhibitor angioedema.

Aspirin and Other Nonsteroidal Antiinflammatory Drugs

Drug hypersensitivity to NSAIDs may be categorized as pseudoallergic or less commonly, allergic reactions against structural moieties (**Table 4**). Reactions may manifest as cutaneous (urticaria/angioedema) and/or upper and lower respiratory symptoms (rhinoconjunctivitis, bronchospasm) or anaphylaxis. Skin testing is not helpful and in vitro testing is not available to assess patients with any type of suspected aspirin (acetylsalicylic acid [ASA]) or NSAID hypersensitivity.

Allergic reactions to nonsteroidal antiinflammatory drugs

Allergic NSAID reactions are either IgE (eg, generally anaphylaxis) or T-cell–mediated cutaneous reactions specific to one NSAID or a group of NSAIDs that have similar structural moieties (eg, propionic acid derivatives naproxen and ibuprofen but not ASA)[49,50] (see **Table 4**). In contrast to pseudoallergic reactions, patients with anaphylaxis to a particular NSAID structure may be able to tolerate other COX-1 inhibitors that have different chemical structures.

Pseudoallergic reactions to aspirin and nonsteroidal antiinflammatory drugs

Pseudoallergic reactions are thought to be related to drug-induced inhibition of COX-1, which leads to diminished production of prostaglandins (some that have a constitutive inhibitory effect on 5-lipoxygenase that produces proinflammatory leukotrienes). In sensitive individuals, this results in overproduction of leukotrienes. In patients with pseudoallergic reactions, patients may react to ASA or any NSAID that have notable COX-1 inhibition. Patients with pseudoallergic reactions to ASA/NSAIDs generally tolerate drugs that are weak COX-1 inhibitors (eg, salsalate, acetaminophen up to a dose of 1000 mg, or sodium or magnesium salicylate) or COX-2 inhibitors.[51] With exceptions, patient with pseudoallergic reactions tend to segregate into 2 different patient subgroups who have predominantly either respiratory reactions or cutaneous reactions (urticaria and/or angioedema).

Respiratory reactors include those with AERD (formerly termed Samter's Triad), a disorder classically characterized by asthma, chronic rhinosinusitis (CRS) with recurrent nasal polyps, and respiratory reactions induced by ASA and all COX-1 inhibitors. AERD usually presents in early adulthood with a prevalence rate of 7% to

Table 4
Classification of nonsteroidal antiinflammatory drug–induced hypersensitivity reactions

Reaction Timing	Clinical Symptoms	Cross-Reactivity Among COX-1 Inhibitors	Presence of Underlying Disease	Putative Mechanism
AERD				
Acute	Rhinitis, nasal congestion, bronchoconstriction, asthma exacerbation	Cross-reactive	Asthma/rhinosinusitis/nasal polyps	Pseudoallergic COX-1 inhibition
Multiple NSAID-exacerbated urticaria/angioedema in patients with underlying cutaneous disease				
Acute	Urticaria/angioedema	Cross-reactive	Chronic urticaria	Pseudoallergic COX-1 inhibition
Multiple NSAID-induced urticaria/angioedema in otherwise asymptomatic patients				
Acute	Urticaria/angioedema	Cross-reactive	None	Likely pseudoallergic, COX-1 inhibition
Single NSAID-induced anaphylactic reactions				
Acute	Anaphylaxis, urticaria/angioedema	Single-drug–induced, no COX-1–associated cross reactivity. May cross-react with an NSAID in same structural class (eg, propionic acid NSAIDs: ibuprofen and naproxen)	Atopy is common	IgE-mediated (presumed)
Delayed reactions to NSAIDs				
Delayed	Varied: fixed drug eruptions, severe bullous skin reactions, maculopapular drug eruptions	Can be single-drug–induced or cross-reactive	None	Varied: T-cell–mediated, cytotoxic T cells, natural killer cells, other

Abbreviations: AERD, Aspirin Exacerbated Respiratory Disease; NSAID, Non-steroidal Anti-Inflammatory Drug.
Adapted from Laidlaw TM, Cahill KN. Current knowledge and management of hypersensitivity to aspirin and NSAIDs. J Allergy Clin Immunol Pract 2017;5(3):539; with permission.

14% in patients with asthma and in 8% to 9% of patients with chronic nasal polyps with CRS.[52]

ASA desensitization and subsequent daily ASA therapy is an important option for chronic management of AERD, as this may reduce risk for recurrent nasal polyps, improve control of asthma or CRS, and decrease the need for frequent systemic corticosteroids to these symptoms.[51]

Cutaneous reactors develop urticaria and/or angioedema to COX-1 inhibitors. Many of these also have chronic spontaneous urticaria. Approximately 20% to 40% of patients with underlying chronic spontaneous urticaria will have worsening of their hives or swelling (angioedema) when they take either ASA or NSAIDs.

Management for pseudoallergic reactions includes avoidance of all significant COX-1 inhibitors, desensitization in selected patients followed by daily ASA/NSAID (to maintain desensitized state), and use of selective COX-2 inhibitors (eg, celecoxib) as needed for pain.[51] Oral challenges to confirm sensitivity may be completed under supervision of an experienced clinician.

ANESTHETIC AGENTS
Local Anesthetics

Most adverse reactions to local anesthetics (LA) are nonallergic. Clinical symptoms are often related to anxiety and pain including psychosomatic responses (hyperventilation and paresthesia), vasovagal symptoms (eg, sweating, nausea, bradycardia, pallor), or to the pharmacologic effects of LA or concomitantly administered epinephrine as a result of overdosing or accidental intravenous administration.[53]

Allergic reactions to LA are rare and manifest as immediate (eg, urticaria, anaphylaxis) or delayed (eg, allergic contact dermatitis) reaction. IgE-mediated LA was found to be responsible for 0.5% of patients in a retrospective study involving 402 patients.[54]

Evaluation for immediate reactions may involve immediate skin testing and subcutaneous graded challenge, whereas evaluation of delayed reactions (allergic contact dermatitis) involves patch testing.

LA are classified into benzoic acid esters (Group I: eg, benzocaine, procaine) or amides (Group II: eg, lidocaine, bupivacaine, mepivacaine).[53] Based on patch testing to assess delayed-type hypersensitivity, Group I LA cross-react with each other, but Group II agents do not cross-react within the group or with Group I agents. For immediate LA reactions, findings regarding cross-reactivity have been conflicting and some investigators feel the best approach is to choose an LA from a different group than that reported to cause a past reaction.[53] If the LA that caused the previous reaction is not known and skin testing cannot be completed, lidocaine is preferred due to rare reports of allergic reaction.[53] In patients with a delayed reaction, some investigators suggest delayed patch testing to other LA to help identify an agent the patient may tolerate.

Anesthesia-Related Agents

Perioperative anaphylaxis may be caused by antibiotics (PCN, cephalosporin), NMBAs (succinylcholine, alcuronium, pancuronium), induction agents (eg, thiopental), chlorhexidine, sugammadex, opioids, latex, and gelatin (in plasma substitute and sponges).[55] Anaphylaxis may be immunologically mediated or nonimmunologically mediated (eg, direct mast cell activation by NMBAs, opioids). Although in the United States, there are commercially available in vitro studies to assess hypersensitivity for some NMBAs, and skin testing can be performed for many agents, the predictive value of these tests is not validated.

RADIOGRAPHIC CONTRAST MEDIA

Radiocontrast media (RCM) immediate hypersensitivity reactions are believed to be primarily nonimmunologic (eg, direct mast cell activation, complement activation). However, IgE-mediated reactions to RCM may occur, and there is concern that these reactions to RCM are underreported and underrecognized. Skin testing is controversial but a recent panel proposed that skin testing to RCM may identify an alternative RCM agent when a skin test is positive to an RCM agent suspected to have caused a reaction.[56]

A previous reaction to RCM is the strongest indicator of a future reaction to RCM. The risk persists even if a patient has tolerated RCM without a reaction in the interim. Other risk factors include asthma, severe cardiovascular disease, and atopy.[56]

There is a common misconception that RCM reactions are cross-reactions because of shellfish allergy or povidone-iodine dermatitis. Shellfish allergy is due to IgE to shellfish proteins (eg, tropomyosin), which is structurally unrelated to iodine. Patients with shellfish allergy are not at significantly higher risk for RCM reaction and vice versa.[57] Moreover, patients with contact dermatitis to povidone-iodine do not have increased risk of RCM reactions and vice versa.[57]

For patients with history of RCM reactions, the use of nonionic, low-osmolar contrast with premedications significantly reduces the risk of reaction.[57] A commonly used pretreatment regimen involves systemic steroids (prednisone, 50 mg, 13 hours, 7 hours, and 1 hour before RCM administration) and H1-antihistamines (diphenhydramine, 50 mg, 1 hour before contrast administration).[58] In emergent cases, methylprednisolone, 40 mg, intravenously (IV) or hydrocortisone, 200 mg, IV immediately and every 4 hours until contrast given plus diphenhydramine, 50 mg, IV 1 hour before contrast may be helpful.[58] However, premedication with systemic steroids administered less than 4 hours before RCM exposure may not be reliably effective.[58]

CHEMOTHERAPEUTIC AGENTS

Chemotherapeutic agents may cause severe immediate reactions. Although most are nonimmune mediated, most infusion reactions from platinum agents are IgE mediated. Taxane agents may be IgE mediated (to the drug) or non–IgE-mediated (to chemotherapeutic solvents such as Cremophor and Polysorbate).[59] Skin testing may be useful in identifying sensitivities to platinum drugs and taxanes.

Anaphylactic-type reactions to first or second exposure are not generally IgE mediated. An exception is cetuximab, which may cause anaphylaxis on first initial exposure due to cross-reactivity to the carbohydrate determinant, alpha-gal, which is also present on red mammalian meat. Sensitization to carbohydrate alpha-gal is thought to be primarily due to multiple tick bites.[60]

For immediate DHRs to chemotherapeutic agents, a rapid 12-step desensitization protocol may be completed to induce temporary tolerance in nearly all patients who require chemotherapy. However, non–life-threatening reactions may still occur in ~6% of patients.[61]

DISCLOSURE

The authors have nothing to disclose.

REFERENCES

1. Thong B, Vervloet D. Drug allergies. World Allergy Organization; 2014. Available at: https://www.worldallergy.org/education-and-programs/education/allergic-disease-resource-center/professionals/drug-allergies.

2. Demoly P, Adkinson NF, Brockow K, et al. International consensus on drug allergy. Allergy 2014;69(4):420–37.
3. Thong BYH, Tan TC. Epidemiology and risk factors for drug allergy. Br J Clin Pharmacol 2011;71(5):684–700.
4. Gomes ER, Demoly P. Epidemiology of hypersensitivity drug reactions. Eur Ann Allergy Clin Immunol 2010;42(2):46.
5. Moss RB, Babin S, Yao-Pi H, et al. Allergy to semisynthetic penicillins in cystic fibrosis. J Pediatr 1984;104:460–6.
6. Paret G, Chovel-Sella A, Reif S, et al. Incidence of rash after amoxicillin treatment in children with infectious mononucleosis. Pediatrics 2013;131(5):e1424–7.
7. Solensky R, Khan DA, Weiss ME, et al. Drug allergy: an updated practice parameter. Ann Allergy Asthma Immunol 2010;105(4):259–73.
8. Caubet JC, Kaiser L, Lemaître B, et al. The role of penicillin in benign skin rashes in childhood: a prospective study based on drug rechallenge. J Allergy Clin Immunol 2011;127(1):218–22.
9. Davis CM, Shearer WT. Diagnosis and management of HIV drug hypersensitivity. J Allergy Clin Immunol 2008;121(4).
10. Khan DA. Pharmacogenomics and adverse drug reactions: Primetime and not ready for primetime tests. J Allergy Clin Immunol 2016;138(4):943–55.
11. Rieder MJ, Kanee A, Spielberg SP, et al. Prominence of slow acetylator phenotype among patients with sulfonamide hypersensitivity reactions. Clin Pharmacol Ther 2010;49(1):13–7.
12. Pichler WJ. An approach to the patient with drug allergy. In: Adkinson NF, editor UpToDate. Waltham (MA): UptoDate Inc. Available at: www.UptoDate.com. Accessed February 2, 2019.
13. Muraro A, Lemanske RF, Castells M, et al. Precision medicine in allergic disease—food allergy, drug allergy, and anaphylaxis—PRACTALL document of the European Academy of Allergy and Clinical Immunology and the American Academy of Allergy, Asthma and Immunology. Allergy 2017;72(7):1006–21.
14. Motala C, Dahl R, Ring J, et al. Revised nomenclature for allergy for global use: Report of the Nomenclature Review Committee of the World Allergy Organization, October 2003. J Allergy Clin Immunol 2004;113(5):832–6.
15. Bircher AJ. Exanthematous (maculopapular) drug eruption. In: Mockenhaupt M, editor. UpToDate. Waltham (MA): UptoDate Inc. Available at: www.uptodate.com. Accessed February 2, 2019.
16. Khan DA. Cutaneous drug reactions. J Allergy Clin Immunol 1994;6(3):83–122.
17. Ardern-Jones MR, Friedmann PS. Skin manifestations of drug allergy. Br J Clin Pharmacol 2011;71(5):672–83.
18. Vandergriff TW, Bergstresser PR. Chapter 91. Abnormal responses to ultraviolet radiation: idiopathic, probably immunologic, and photoexacerbated. In: Goldsmith LA, Katz SI, Gilchrest BA, et al, editors. Fitzpatrick's dermatology in general medicine. 8th edition. New York, NY: McGraw-Hill; 2012. Available at: http://accessmedicine.mhmedical.com/content.aspx?bookid=392&sectionid=41138800. Accessed October 21, 2019.
19. Pichler WJ. Drug allergy: classification and clinical features. In: Adkinson NF, editor. UpToDate. Waltham, MA: UpToDate Inc.
20. Pichler WJ. Drug allergy: pathogenesis. In: Adkinson NF, editor. UpToDate. Waltham (MA): UptoDate Inc. Available at: www.UptoDate.com. Accessed February 2, 2019.
21. Tatum AJ, Ditto AM, Patterson R. Severe serum sickness-like reaction to oral penicillin drugs: Three case reports. Ann Allergy Asthma Immunol 2001;86(3):330–4.

22. Pendergraft WF, Niles JL. Trojan horses: drug culprits associated with antineutrophil cytoplasmic autoantibody (ANCA) vasculitis. Curr Opin Rheumatol 2014; 26(1):42–9.

23. Srivastava M, Rencic A, Diglio G, et al. Drug-induced, Ro/SSA-positive cutaneous lupus erythematosus. Arch Dermatol 2003;139(1):45–9.

24. Brinster NK, Yamanaka K -i, Dowgiert RK, et al. The vast majority of CLA+ T cells are resident in normal skin. J Immunol 2014;176(7):4431–9.

25. Lansu K, Karpiak J, Liu J, et al. In silico design of novel probes for the atypical opioid receptor MRGPRX2. Nat Chem Biol 2017;13(5):529–36.

26. Serrano-Candelas E, Lafuente A, Navinés-Ferrer A, et al. MRGPRX2-mediated mast cell response to drugs used in perioperative procedures and anaesthesia. Sci Rep 2018;8(1):1–11.

27. Viswanathan K, Sasisekharan R, Nasr M, et al. Contaminated heparin associated with adverse clinical events and activation of the contact system. N Engl J Med 2008;358(23):2457–67.

28. Dykewicz MS. Drug allergy. In: Slavin R, Reisman R, editors. An expert guide to allergy and immunology. Philadelphia: American College of Physicians; 1999. p. 127–60.

29. Castells M. Diagnosis and management of anaphylaxis in precision medicine. J Allergy Clin Immunol 2017;140(2):321–33.

30. Kowal K, Dubuske L. Overview of in vitro allergy tests. In: Bochner BS, editor. UpToDate. Waltham (MA): UptoDate Inc. Available at: www.uptodate.com. Accessed February 2, 2019.

31. Castells MC, Solenksy R. Rapid drug desensitization for immediate hypersensitivity reactions. In: Adkinson NF, editor. UpToDate. Waltham (MA): UpToDate Inc. Accessed February 2, 2019.

32. Zagursky RJ, Pichichero ME. Cross-reactivity in β-lactam Allergy. J Allergy Clin Immunol Pract 2018;6(1):72–81.e1.

33. Macy E, Romano A, Khan D. Practical management of antibiotic hypersensitivity in 2017. J Allergy Clin Immunol Pract 2017;5(3):577–86.

34. Shenoy ES, Macy E, Rowe T, et al. Evaluation and management of penicillin allergy: a review. JAMA 2019;321(2):188–99.

35. Romano A, Valluzzi RL, Caruso C, et al. Cross-reactivity and tolerability of cephalosporins in patients with IgE-mediated hypersensitivity to penicillins. J Allergy Clin Immunol Pract 2018;6(5):1662–72.

36. Schnyder B, Pichler WJ. Allergy to sulfonamides. J Allergy Clin Immunol 2013; 131(1):256–7.e5.

37. Gruchalla RS. 10. Drug allergy. J Allergy Clin Immunol 2003;111(2 SUPPL. 2):548–59.

38. Tornero P, De Barrio M, Baeza ML, et al. Cross-reactivity among p-amino group compounds in sulfonamide fixed drug eruption: diagnostic value of patch testing. Contact Dermatitis 2004;51(2):57–62.

39. Wulf NR, Matuszewski KA. Sulfonamide cross-reactivity: is there evidence to support broad cross-allergenicity? Am J Health Syst Pharm 2013;70(17):1483–94.

40. McCrory DC, Samsa GP, Orlando LA, et al. Systematic review: comparative effectiveness of angiotensin-converting enzyme inhibitors and angiotensin ii receptor blockers for treating essential hypertension. Ann Intern Med 2013;148(1):16.

41. Cicardi M, Zuraw BL. Angioedema due to bradykinin dysregulation. J Allergy Clin Immunol Pract 2018;6(4):1132–41.

42. Banerji A. ACE inhibitor-induced angioedema. In: Saini S, editor. UpToDate. Waltham (MA): UptoDate Inc. Available at: www.UptoDate.com. Accessed February 2, 2019.

43. Orfan N, Patterson R, Dykewicz MS. Severe angioedema related to ACE inhibitors in patients with a history of idiopathic angioedema. JAMA 1990;264(10):1287–9.

44. Zanichelli A, Beltrami L, Vacchini R, et al. Long-term follow-up of 111 patients with angiotensin-converting enzyme inhibitor-related angioedema. J Hypertens 2011; 29(11):2273–7.

45. Warrier MR, Copilevitz CA, Dykewicz MS, et al. Fresh frozen plasma in the treatment of resistant angiotensin-converting enzyme inhibitor angioedema. Ann Allergy Asthma Immunol 2004;92(5):573–5.

46. Straka BT, Ramirez CE, Byrd JB, et al. Effect of bradykinin receptor antagonism on ACE inhibitor-associated angioedema. J Allergy Clin Immunol 2017;140(1):242–8.e2.

47. Haymore BR, Yoon J, Mikita CP, et al. Risk of angioedema with angiotensin receptor blockers in patients with prior angioedema associated with angiotensin-converting enzyme inhibitors: a meta-analysis. Ann Allergy Asthma Immunol 2008;101(5):495–9.

48. Beavers CJ, Dunn SP, Macaulay TE. The role of angiotensin receptor blockers in patients with angiotensin-converting enzyme inhibitor-induced angioedema. Ann Pharmacother 2011;45(4):520–4.

49. Kowalski ML, Makowska JS, Blanca M, et al. Hypersensitivity to nonsteroidal anti-inflammatory drugs (NSAIDs) - classification, diagnosis and management: review of the EAACI/ENDA and GA2LEN/HANNA. Allergy 2011;66(7):818–29.

50. Kowalski ML, Makowska JS. Seven steps to the diagnosis of NSAIDs hypersensitivity: How to apply a new classification in real practice? Allergy Asthma Immunol Res 2015;7(4):312–20.

51. Laidlaw TM, Cahill KN. Current knowledge and management of hypersensitivity to aspirin and NSAIDs. J Allergy Clin Immunol Pract 2017;5(3):537–45.

52. Rajan JP, Wineinger NE, Stevenson DD, et al. Prevalence of aspirin-exacerbated respiratory disease among asthmatic patients: a meta-analysis of the literature. J Allergy Clin Immunol 2015;135(3):676–81.e1.

53. Schatz M. Allergic reactions to local anesthetics. In: Adkinson NF, editor. UpToDate. Waltham (MA): UptoDate Inc. Available at: www.UptoDate.com. Accessed February 2, 2019.

54. Trautmann A, Goebeler M, Stoevesandt J. Twenty years' experience with anaphylaxis-like reactions to local anesthetics: genuine allergy is rare. J Allergy Clin Immunol Pract 2018;6(6):2051–8.e1.

55. Ebo DG, Faber M, Elst J, et al. In vitro diagnosis of immediate drug hypersensitivity during anesthesia: a review of the literature. J Allergy Clin Immunol Pract 2018;6(4):1176–84.

56. Sánchez-Borges M, Aberer W, Brockow K, et al. Controversies in drug allergy: radiographic contrast media. J Allergy Clin Immunol Pract 2019;7(1):61–5.

57. Hong SJ, Cochran ST. Immediate hypersensitivity reactions to radiocontrast media: Prevention of recurrent reactions. In: Adkinson NF, editor. UpToDate. Waltham (MA): UpToDate Inc. Accessed February 2, 2019.

58. ACR Committee on Drugs and Contrast Media. ACR Manual on Contrast Media. Version 10.3. Reston, Virginia: American College of Radiology; 2018. p. 22–8.

59. Castells MC, Matulonis UA, Horton TM. Infusion reactions to systemic chemotherapy. In: Drews RE, Adkinson F, editors. UpToDate. Waltham (MA): UptoDate Inc. Available at: www.UptoDate.com. Accessed February 2, 2019.

60. Gold D, Chan E, Satinover SM, et al. Cetuximab-Induced Anaphylaxis and IgE Specific for Galactose-α-1,3-Galactose. N Engl J Med 2008;358(11):1109–17.

61. Castells MC, Tennant NM, Sloane DE, et al. Hypersensitivity reactions to chemotherapy: Outcomes and safety of rapid desensitization in 413 cases. J Allergy Clin Immunol 2008;122(3):574–80.

Approach to Patients with Stinging Insect Allergy

Elissa M. Abrams, MD[a], David B.K. Golden, MD[b],*

KEYWORDS

- Stinging insect • Anaphylaxis • Venom immunotherapy • Large local reaction

KEY POINTS

- Large local and systemic cutaneous reactions to stinging insects are benign, and can be treated with supportive measures.
- Anaphylaxis to a stinging insect requires allergy evaluation for skin prick testing and consideration of venom immunotherapy.
- Venom immunotherapy is safe and effective, and is considered the gold standard in treatment of anaphylaxis to stinging insects.

INTRODUCTION

Although insect stings usually cause localized inflammation, both large local reactions (LLRs) and systemic reactions (SRs) can occur. Systemic allergic reactions to insect stings affect about 3% of adults and up to 0.8% of children.[1,2] In the United States there are at least 40 fatal stings per year.[3] LLRs to stinging insects are also common, affecting up to 10% of adults, but rarely progress to SRs.[4–6] This article reviews the diagnosis, acute and long-term management, and prognosis of stinging insect reactions. The focus is on stinging insects found in North America (hornets, wasps, yellow jackets, honeybees) and the endemic threat of imported fire ant stings in the southeastern United States.

INSECT DESCRIPTION

There are 3 common stinging families of the Hymenoptera order: bees (honeybee, rarely bumblebee), vespids (yellow jacket, yellow hornet, white faced hornet, and wasp), and stinging ants (in particular the imported fire ant).

Disclosure: Neither author has any conflicts to disclose.
[a] Department of Pediatrics, Section of Allergy and Clinical Immunology, University of Manitoba, FE125-685 William Avenue, Winnipeg, Manitoba R2A 5L9, Canada; [b] Department of Medicine, Johns Hopkins University School of Medicine, 20 Crossroads Drive Suite 16, Owings Mills, MD 21117, USA
* Corresponding author.
E-mail address: Dgolden1@jhmi.edu

Knowledge of the nesting patterns and life cycles of stinging insects can help identify which insect was involved in the reaction, can aid in recommending avoidance measures, and can also provide some prognostic information.

Yellow jackets (Vespid family, genus *Vespula*) cause the most frequent insect-sting reactions in North America (**Table 1**). They live in large in-ground or above-ground nests and are aggressive; some species occasionally leave a stinger embedded at the site of the sting. Stings from yellow jackets often occur during yard work or gardening, and at outdoor activities and events (especially in locations near food such as picnics and trash cans).[7] Wasps (Vespid family, genus *Polistes*) live in exposed honeycomb-patterned nests in shrubs and under eaves of barns or houses.[7] They are moderately aggressive, do not leave a stinger, and can also nest in fencing and playground equipment.[7] Hornets (Vespid family, genus *Dolichovespula*) live in large enclosed nests in trees or shrubs, are highly aggressive, and do not leave a stinger.[7] Yellow jackets, wasps, and hornets are all scavengers attracted by food and drinks. Honeybees live in commercial hives or in the wild, are generally nonaggressive, and routinely leave a stinger after they sting.[7] Africanized honeybees (found in several states, including Texas, California, and Arizona) are more prone to swarming and aggressive behavior than native honeybees.

Imported fire ants (IFAs) are an endemic threat, particularly in the southern United States.[8,9] They are black or red and live in nests of soil most commonly in open areas, such as along roadways, fields, and playgrounds.[8] They are highly aggressive, and often sting multiple times by grasping the skin with their mandible and stinging with their abdomen in a radial pattern causing a sterile pseudopustule in the area of the sting.[8] This is a clinical presentation that is specific for IFAs stings.

SRs from other insect or spider bites are rare. LLRs from multiple mosquito bites, termed skeeter syndrome, can resemble hives and require symptomatic management only.[10]

CLINICAL MANIFESTATIONS

Normal reactions to insect stings and bites are localized to the area of the sting and include erythema, burning, pruritus, and mild swelling (**Table 2**).[7] These reactions usually resolve within hours to days with few or no supportive measures.[7]

Table 1
Characteristics of common stinging insects of the Hymenoptera order

Insect	Dwelling	Aggression Level	Stinger Left in Place
Honeybee	Commercial hives or in the wild	Nonaggressive	Routinely
Yellow jacket	Large in-ground or above-ground nests	Highly aggressive	Occasionally
Wasp	Exposed honeycomb-patterned nests in shrubs and under eaves of barns or houses	Moderately aggressive	No
Hornets	Large enclosed nests in trees or shrubs	Highly aggressive	No
Imported fire ants	Nests of soil particularly in open areas	Highly aggressive	No; do cause a pathognomonic sterile pustule

Table 2
Clinical manifestations of stinging insect reactions

Reaction	Clinical Manifestations	Resolution
Normal	Erythema, burning, pruritus, mild swelling localized to area of sting	Hours to days
LLR	Swelling contiguous with the site of the sting and increases in size over 1–2 d	3–10 d
Cutaneous SR	Urticaria, angioedema, pruritus, or flushing, within minutes to hours, systemic (distant from the site of the sting)	24 h
Anaphylaxis	Combination of cutaneous, respiratory, gastrointestinal, or cardiovascular symptoms within hours of sting	24 h

Adapted from Golden DB, Demain J, Freeman T, et al. Stinging insect hypersensitivity: A practice parameter update 2016. Ann Allergy Asthma Immunol 2017;118(1):28-54; with permission.

Immunoglobulin (Ig) E–mediated allergic reactions to stinging insects present in 2 forms: LLRs and SRs. LLRs involve swelling contiguous with the site of the sting that begins within several hours of the sting, increases in size for 1 to 2 days, and then resolves over 3 to 10 days.[7] These reactions can cause lymphangitic streaks, but can be differentiated from cellulitis by their early presence after only 24 to 48 hours, and by the absence of systemic symptoms such as fever or neutrophilia.[7] The risk of a future SR in patients with a history of LLR is low, with studies documenting the risk to be less than 10% for all SRs, and less than 3% for severe anaphylaxis.[5–7]

IgE-mediated SRs can be divided into cutaneous SRs and anaphylaxis. Cutaneous SRs cause only generalized urticaria, angioedema, pruritus, or flushing. Cutaneous SRs are the most common type of systemic SR in children (60% of all SRs), but are uncommon in adults (15% of all SRs).[11] Anaphylaxis involves a wide range of possible cutaneous, respiratory (cough, wheeze, dyspnea, stridor, throat tightness), gastrointestinal (abdominal pain, nausea, vomiting, diarrhea), and cardiovascular symptoms (arrhythmias, infarction, hypotonia, syncope, light-headedness, incontinence).[12–14] Cutaneous symptoms are absent in about 20% of cases of anaphylaxis.[12] In addition, anaphylaxis presents differently in adults and children with stinging insect allergy; in particular, vascular symptoms such as hypotension are more common in adults and cutaneous SRs are more common in children.[12,15] The most common symptoms contributing to anaphylaxis fatality are laryngeal edema and vascular collapse.[12,16]

Systemic symptoms usually occur within minutes to hours after a sting.[7,12] The onset of reaction is within 20 minutes in 75%, and within 40 minutes in 87% of cases of sting anaphylaxis, although reactions have been reported to begin 5 hours or more after the sting.[15] More severe reactions may occur if there are multiple stings at once, or if there are repeated stings in a short period of time (such as less than a 2-month duration).[17] In general, there is a correlation between immediacy of reaction onset and severity of symptoms, with more rapid onset of symptoms associated with more severe reactions.[18] Half of all fatal reactions occur in people with no history of a prior reaction to a stinging insect.[1,19]

Cutaneous SRs carry a very low risk for a more severe anaphylaxis in the future. Studies have shown a less than 10% risk of a future SR (and <3% chance of a more severe anaphylaxis) in people with cutaneous SRs.[7,20,21] In contrast, those with anaphylaxis to a stinging insect have a high risk of future anaphylactic reactions (30%–60%).[7,22,23]

Serum sickness–like reactions[24] and cold urticaria[25] have been reported after insect stings. In addition, there are rare reports of non–IgE-mediated reactions to stinging insects, including nephropathy,[26] neuropathy,[27] rhabdomyolysis,[28] and immune thrombocytopenic purpura.[29]

CLINICAL DIAGNOSIS

Clinical history should include information to help determine which insect was the possible cause, including the location and activity at the time of the sting, visual identification of the insect if possible, and whether the insect left a stinger embedded in the skin. The clinical history should include details about the earliest symptoms of the reaction, its progression, findings of any physicians involved in the care of the reaction, treatments for the reaction, and time to resolution. Subtle indicators can have prognostic implications, such as the presence/or absence of cutaneous symptoms (absence of cutaneous symptoms usually indicates a more severe reaction), and whether the patient had to sit or lie down (this can indicate hypotension or cardiovascular involvement, which is also a poor prognostic indicator). Any history of previous stings and/or episodes of anaphylaxis should be included.

A review of pertinent medical history, and in particular other atopic conditions such as asthma (which, if poorly controlled, can be a risk factor for more severe anaphylaxis),[12] should be included. All medications should be reviewed, especially antihypertensives (such as β-blockers and angiotensin-converting enzyme inhibitors [ACEIs]) because antihypertensives can potentially make anaphylaxis more severe or refractory to standard management.[12]

ACUTE MANAGEMENT

For LLRs, conservative measures may be considered for symptomatic control, such as nonsedating antihistamines, oral analgesics, and cold compresses (**Fig. 1**).[6,7,30] A short course of oral corticosteroids could be considered if swelling is extreme, progressive, or localized to certain areas, such as the head and neck. Antibiotics are not indicated.

Cutaneous SRs also require only symptomatic measures, such as nonsedating antihistamines. Oral steroids have no role in the management of systemic urticaria, which resolves quickly and spontaneously.

For anaphylaxis, first-line therapy is intramuscular epinephrine (0.01 mg/kg of a 1:1000 solution to a maximum of 0.3 mg in children and 0.5 mg in adults), followed by observation in the emergency department (ED) for a minimum of 4 to 6 hours.[12,14,31–33] Epinephrine is the only definitive medical intervention available for stinging insect anaphylaxis. Beneficial mechanisms include vasoconstriction

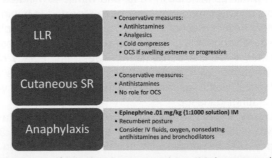

Fig. 1. Acute management of stinging insect reactions. IM, intramuscular; IV, intravenous; OCS, oral corticosteroids.

(alleviating hypotension and laryngeal edema), increased force/rate of cardiac contractions, and bronchodilation.[12] Delayed use of epinephrine is associated with increased risk of anaphylaxis fatality,[16,34,35] and increased risk of biphasic anaphylaxis.[36–38] There is no contraindication to epinephrine use in anaphylaxis, including concurrent cardiac disease.[12,13]

In addition, recumbent posture is essential in an SR because while lying down there is improved venous return in the context of reduced circulation.[39] Increased risk of anaphylaxis fatality has been shown in patients with a change to upright posture, and has been postulated to occur because, with standing up or sitting, venous return decreases (empty ventricle syndrome), resulting in no cardiac flow and ultimately pulseless electrical activity.[39]

Adjunct therapies in anaphylaxis include nonsedating antihistamines, bronchodilators, intravenous fluids, and supplemental oxygen.[13,33] Antihistamines are not first-line therapy and should not be used in place of epinephrine. Although oral corticosteroids are often prescribed to prevent a biphasic reaction, evidence to support their efficacy is lacking.[40,41]

Observation in the ED for anaphylaxis should be a minimum of 4 to 6 hours and may be longer in patients at risk of a biphasic reaction, such as individuals with delayed epinephrine administration, as well as those who require more than 1 dose of epinephrine, those to whom a beta-agonist is administered in the ED, and/or those who present with a wide pulse pressure.[42]

Before discharge from the ED, self-injectable epinephrine (SIE) should be prescribed to patients with an anaphylactic reaction. In general, SIEs are not required in those with a history of a cutaneous SR or those with an LLR to a stinging insect, because the risk of a future SR is less than 10%, and the risk of severe anaphylaxis is less than 3%.[7] However, individual preference and physician/patient comfort level may guide this decision as well as other extraneous factors (such as occupational proximity to stinging insects). Carrying SIE does not improve health-related quality of life in patients with a prior reaction to a stinging insect.[43,44] A study examining the possible negative aspects of SIE prescription found it to be inconvenient and burdensome to most people with stinging insect allergy.[44]

It should be reiterated to patients that there is no contraindication to use of SIE with a future anaphylactic reaction, and that delays in epinephrine use are associated with poorer outcomes in anaphylaxis. It should also be explained that antihistamines should never be used in place of epinephrine.

LONG-TERM MANAGEMENT

All patients with a history of a reaction to a stinging insect, whether it be an LLR or an SR, benefit from a discussion of stinging insect avoidance measures (**Fig. 2**). Avoidance measures include removing all known nests by a trained professional, avoiding walking barefoot outside and covering arms/legs when outdoors for long periods, staying away from areas with exposed outdoor food (such as garbage bins), and avoidance of eating/drinking outdoors when possible. Insect-allergic persons should ensure that everything consumed outdoors is visible, because stinging insects can crawl inside the food or drink (eg, sandwiches, salads, beverage containers, straws). In the mouth or throat, even an LLR can prove life threatening.[7] Insect repellants do not deter stinging insects but insecticides are effective if available.

Most patients with severe reactions (and all patients with anaphylaxis) benefit from an allergy referral to discuss the relative risk of a future SR, perform diagnostic testing, and review whether or not venom immunotherapy (VIT) is indicated.

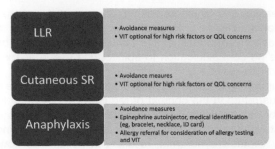

Fig. 2. Long-term management of stinging insect reactions. ID, identity; QOL, quality of life.

In patients with low risk of a future SR, such as those with LLRs or cutaneous SRs, SIE is not required.

In patients with a history of anaphylaxis to a stinging insect allergy, SIE should be prescribed and proper technique and use should be reviewed. A medical identification item (eg, bracelet, necklace, or identification card) should be discussed and an anaphylaxis action plan provided. All this should be done pending allergy evaluation and attention should be given to optimizing risk factors for more severe/refractory anaphylaxis, such as controlling asthma, and discussing early intervention with SIE.[12]

DIAGNOSTIC TESTS

In general, diagnostic testing is only required in patients with a history of anaphylaxis to stinging insects, because the risk of a more severe SR is low (<10%) in patients with LLRs or cutaneous SRs.[7] Diagnostic testing is not indicated for preemptive screening in patients without a history of reactivity because there is a high rate of asymptomatic sensitization; up to 20% of the general population have positive testing but only 5% to 15% of those have future reactions.[2,45,46] Diagnostic testing is not indicated in people with a family history of stinging insect allergy; it is generally not heritable and asymptomatic sensitization is possible.[1]

One exception to preemptive testing is in patients with mastocytosis, a systemic mast cell disorder.[47] In these patients, insect stings are the most common cause of anaphylaxis, and reactions, if they occur, are more severe and potentially fatal.[48] In patients with mastocytosis, stinging insect testing is indicated even if there is no history of a prior reaction.[7]

Skin testing is, in general, the preferred method of testing to stinging insects because it is highly sensitive and safe.[49] Skin testing is performed intradermally with commercial venom protein extracts (yellow jacket, yellow hornet, white faced hornet, wasp, honeybee) that are supplied as lyophilized venom protein extracts, to be reconstituted before testing. It is recommended to include all 5 common stinging insects in testing (sensitization can occur to multiple venoms even in the context of a single reaction). Skin testing should always include positive (histamine) and negative (diluent) controls.[7] Although guidelines recommend starting intradermal testing at a low concentration,[7] recent studies suggest that testing at a target concentration of 1 μg/mL can be done safely.[50]

There are differing criteria for defining a positive skin test, but all involve a wheal and flare response. The most recent North American stinging insect guideline recommends defining a positive test if there is at least a 5 to 10-mm wheal and 11 to 20 mm of surrounding erythema.[7] Skin test size does not correlate reliably with reaction severity.[7]

Negative skin tests can occur despite a consistent clinical history (this can occur in up to 30% of patients with a history of a reaction),[51–54] and can occur for a variety of reasons: an anergic period that may last a few weeks after a recent reaction, loss of sensitivity many years after a reaction, and variability in skin testing over time. If skin testing is negative, consideration could be given to serum allergen-specific IgE antibodies to the stinging insect venoms. However, this test is less sensitive than skin testing and is not usually first line. Repeat skin testing could also be considered 3 to 6 months later.[51,55] Allergen-specific IgE antibodies are also useful in situations in which skin testing cannot be performed, such as with dermatographism, severe atopic dermatitis, or use of antihistamines and other medications that block the cutaneous response to histamine.

For fire ant reactions, whole-body extract is available and used for skin testing, which often starts as a screening skin prick testing, and then serial intradermal skin testing (increasing concentrations to a maximum concentration of 1:1000 weight/volume).[7,8] IFA does not cross-react with other venoms, such as vespid or honeybee. As a result, if clinical history is compatible with IFA reaction (ie, the insect was visualized, or there was the presence of a sterile pustule at the sting site), testing for other venoms is not usually necessary.

Serum tryptase level is typically increased during the first hours after onset of anaphylaxis, but should be normal at baseline unless there is an underlying mast cell disorder. A baseline serum tryptase measurement is recommended in patients with a history of a severe SR to a stinging insect (in particular with hypotension or absence of urticaria), because it is abnormal in up to 25% of patients. Baseline serum tryptase level is also abnormal in many patients with a history of sting anaphylaxis but negative venom skin tests and specific IgE.[7] It should also be considered in all patients with a history of anaphylaxis to a stinging insect.[47,56–58] In addition to screening for the presence of mastocytosis, serum tryptase levels stratify risk: people with a high serum tryptase level have a higher risk of severe (and even fatal) reactions to future stings, and a less reliable response to VIT.[59,60]

Sting challenges are considered the gold standard in research settings. Studies have shown that none of the commonly used criteria for insect-sting hypersensitivity (such as skin testing or serum-specific IgE) correlate consistently with the reaction severity after a sting. As a result, this is the ultimate measure of risk (and potentially of VIT efficacy) in patients with stinging insect reactions. However, there are concerns about the risk of the procedure (anaphylaxis can occur, including severe anaphylaxis, such as hypotension).[61] In addition, they are not consistently reproducible, with up to 21% of patients reacting on a second sting challenge but not on the first.[61] Some investigators have expressed ethical concerns about the use of sting challenges,[62] and they are used primarily as a research tool.[7,58,63]

VENOM IMMUNOTHERAPY

VIT is an established and highly effective disease-modifying therapy that can dramatically reduce the risk of future SRs to a stinging insect in people with a history of anaphylaxis. VIT involves subcutaneous injections of Hymenoptera venom, in gradually increasing doses up to a maintenance dose that is antigenically equivalent to 2 to 10 stings. Immunotherapy modulates the immune system in many ways, including increased production of IgG-blocking antibodies, increased production of interleukin-10, and induction of regulatory T lymphocytes.

VIT is indicated in people with a history of anaphylaxis to a stinging insect and positive venom allergy tests (either skin tests or venom-specific IgE).[7,11] It is not routinely indicated in those with LLRs or cutaneous SRs,[5,21] but may be considered because of other factors, including occupation (high risk of stings), quality of life, and perception of risk.[7]

The most significant side effect to VIT is the potential for anaphylaxis, which occurs in less than 5% of patients.[7] LLRs occur in up to 50% of patients on VIT, but rarely interfere with treatment.[7] Premedication with antihistamines and/or leukotriene receptor antagonists, such as montelukast, helps to reduce LLRs to VIT.[11,64] There is also some evidence that antihistamine before treatment, during the initial dose buildup phase of VIT, may improve its efficacy.[64,65] If there is an SR while on VIT, the dosing schedule is usually adjusted. Almost all patients can complete VIT with schedule adjustment, even if there has been an SR.[49]

Some medications, such as ACEIs and β-blockers, have been thought to increase the risk of anaphylaxis to VIT, and potentially make anaphylaxis more difficult to treat. However, the evidence on this is inconsistent and it is recommended that the benefits of VIT outweigh any risk associated with these medications in patients with cardiovascular disease.[7] Several recent studies have refuted the notion that use of β-blockers or ACEIs makes anaphylaxis more refractory to therapy, or increases the risk of SRs to VIT.[18,66–69]

Guidelines recommend to include in VIT all venoms to which there is known sensitization (ie, positive allergy tests), although some experts choose to include only the insect that was known to, or most likely to, have caused the reaction.[7] There is a high degree of cross-reactivity among vespids (people sensitized to yellow jacket are also sensitized to hornets 95% of the time), although this cross-reactivity is less with wasps (50%). There is minimal cross-reactivity between vespids and honeybee.[70–72]

VIT reduces the risk of a future SR to a sting in people with a history of anaphylaxis from 40% to 70% to approximately 2% in most patients.[73–76] This risk reduction is less for single-vespid venom (5%–10% risk of an SR if stung while on VIT) and honeybee (15%–25% risk of an SR if stung while on VIT).[73–76] However, there is an almost universal reduction in the severity of SR to a sting while on VIT.

There are different schedules available that vary based on how quickly the patient achieves the maintenance dose, including traditional (4–6 months), semirush (6–8 weeks), rush (2–3 days), and ultrarush (3–6 hours) protocols. There is no evidence that there is increased risk of adverse reactions with any specific protocol (other than ultrarush protocols, which can increase the risk of anaphylaxis during buildup dosing).[77–80]

The maintenance dose is 100 μg of each venom, although in young children there is some evidence that a dose of 50 μg of each venom may be as protective.[81–83] Once patients reach maintenance dosing, they usually receive subcutaneous injections every 4 weeks for at least 1 year, then every 6 to 8 weeks for 2 to 3 years, and then every 12 weeks.

The recommended duration of VIT is at least 3 years and usually 5 years.[7] There is some evidence that 5 years of VIT provides more persistent protection than 3 years, although a mean duration of 3.5 years was reported to have been sufficient in children.[84–87] It is recommended that some patients at higher risk remain on VIT for longer than 5 years, such as those with honeybee anaphylaxis, mastocytosis, a severe anaphylactic reaction, or an SR during VIT.[7]

During VIT, repeat skin testing and/or serum-specific IgE may be considered every 2 to 3 years, although they do not reliably predict successful protection or sustained unresponsiveness. If both venom skin tests and serum IgE become negative, then VIT could presumably be discontinued, but this occurs very infrequently in less than

5 years. Even when venom skin tests become negative, there is usually still some detectable venom-specific IgE.

Once at maintenance VIT, most patients no longer require SIE because their risk of a future anaphylactic reaction to a stinging insect is very low.[7] Patients with frequent exposure or in remote locations may warrant having an epinephrine injector. In addition, patients who discontinue VIT after more than 5 years of treatment also no longer require SIE. Exceptions include patients who should not discontinue VIT because of higher risk, such as those with mastocytosis, honeybee anaphylaxis, severe reactions while on VIT, or underlying medical conditions such as uncontrolled asthma.

IMPORTED FIRE ANT IMMUNOTHERAPY

Immunotherapy is also available for IFA, and is recommended in people with a history of anaphylaxis to IFA and positive skin test/allergen-specific IgE to IFA whole-body extract (although there is no venom extract for IFA, the whole-body extract does contain a significant amount of venom allergens).[7] In contrast with venom reactions, it is also recommended in people with cutaneous reactions to IFA because the natural history of these reactions is less well described.[7] Studies have shown that stings with IFA are difficult to avoid in endemic areas, increasing the salience of immunotherapy.[88]

The buildup schedule for fire ant usually follows the traditional (4–6 months) schedule. As with venom, rush immunotherapy for fire ant has been reported to be as safe as the slower schedules.[89] The maintenance dose is usually 0.5 mL of a 1:100 weight/volume vaccine/extract, although there is wide variability in commonly prescribed maintenance dosing patterns.[7,90]

Although there are no controlled trials, studies have shown IFA immunotherapy to be safe and effective, with less than 2% risk of anaphylaxis in sting challenges after immunotherapy.[89,91] In studies to date, SRs with IFA immunotherapy are in the range of 5% to 9%, although in general these are milder than initial reactions.[89,92] Studies have shown similar safety with various protocols, including rush protocols (which achieve maintenance dosing in 2 days),[89] with the exception of increased SRs during ultrarush (1 day) protocols, especially in the absence of premedication.[93] The duration of immunotherapy for IFA is also less well defined, with recommendations extrapolated from those for VIT.[7]

PROGNOSIS

Patients with a history of anaphylaxis to a stinging insect have up to a 50% to 60% risk of future anaphylaxis (25%–40% risk in children) to stinging insects, which may decrease over time (**Table 3**).[20,45,73,94] The best predictor of future reaction severity is previous reaction severity: 25% to 40% of moderate reactors, 40% to 75% of severe reactors, and 95% of patients with mastocytosis have a future anaphylactic reaction when stung. The subsequent reactions are rarely more severe than previous reactions. In addition, the risk remains present for decades.[7,22,23]

This risk is reduced significantly with VIT: during VIT the risk is approximately 2% (if mixed vespid) and, after completion of VIT, the risk of a future reaction is 10% (although only about 2% require epinephrine).[85,95,96] There is some degree of risk stratification. After 5 years of VIT, two-thirds of patients have a less than 3% risk of relapse, whereas one-third of patients have a 30% to 50% chance of relapse. In patients with a cutaneous SR, or LLR, the risk of future anaphylaxis is less than 5%.[4,5,30,97]

Table 3
Prognosis of stinging insect reactions

Reaction Type	Risk of SR with Future Sting (%)
LLR	<10 (<3 for severe anaphylaxis)
Cutaneous SR	<10 (<3 risk of severe anaphylaxis)
Anaphylaxis	50–60 (25–40 in children)
On maintenance VIT	2 (mixed vespid venom); 5 (single vespid venom); 15 (honeybee venom)
After completing ≥5 y of VIT	10 per sting; only 2 require epinephrine (>40 in high-risk patients; <3 in low-risk patients)

There are several factors related to long-term prognosis. In general, prognosis is less favorable in men, with elderly age, and with increasing number of prior stings.[60] Future SRs are more common with honeybee stings than vespid stings (and, within vespids, more common with hornets than yellow jackets).[11] However, even within a single species, reactivity can vary from sting to sting and may be related to differences in amount of venom protein from sting to sting.[98] Prognosis is worse if there is concurrent mastocytosis (or increased basal serum tryptase level),[47,56,57,59,60] reactions while on VIT,[7] previous severe SRs,[22,96] and concurrent medical comorbidities. In these circumstances, VIT may be prolonged and ongoing SIE is recommended.

SUMMARY

Although stinging insect allergy is uncommon, it can be life threatening and is treatable. Diagnosis involves a clinical history and confirmative testing, including first-line skin testing, and sometimes supplemental serum-specific IgE. Serum tryptase levels can be used to stratify risk. Immediate management includes treatment of anaphylaxis with intramuscular epinephrine; for LLRs and cutaneous SRs, treatment is supportive. Long-term management includes VIT in patients with a history of anaphylaxis, and avoidance measures for any patient with a history of a reaction to a stinging insect of any type. SIE should be on hand for any patient with a history of a SR to a stinging insect, and counseling around its use and indications, and carrying it on the person, is recommended. Immunotherapy is effective and safe in reducing the risk of a future SR to a stinging insect, with sustained unresponsiveness to stings for many years after VIT in most cases.

REFERENCES

1. Bilo BM, Bonifazi F. Epidemiology of insect-venom anaphylaxis. Curr Opin Allergy Clin Immunol 2008;8(4):330–7.
2. Golden DB, Marsh DG, Kagey-Sobotka A, et al. Epidemiology of insect venom sensitivity. JAMA 1989;262(2):240–4.
3. Graft DF. Insect sting allergy. Med Clin North Am 2006;90(1):211–32.
4. Pucci S, D'Alo S, De Pasquale T, et al. Risk of anaphylaxis in patients with large local reactions to hymenoptera stings: a retrospective and prospective study. Clin Mol Allergy 2015;13:21.
5. Graft DF, Schuberth KC, Kagey-Sobotka A, et al. A prospective study of the natural history of large local reactions after Hymenoptera stings in children. J Pediatr 1984;104(5):664–8.

6. Severino M, Bonadonna P, Passalacqua G. Large local reactions from stinging insects: from epidemiology to management. Curr Opin Allergy Clin Immunol 2009; 9(4):334–7.
7. Golden DBK, Demain J, Freeman T, et al. Stinging insect hypersensitivity: a practice parameter update 2016. Ann Allergy Asthma Immunol 2017;118(1):28–54.
8. Steigelman DA, Freeman TM. Imported fire ant allergy: case presentation and review of incidence, prevalence, diagnosis, and current treatment. Ann Allergy Asthma Immunol 2013;111(4):242–5.
9. Kemp SF, deShazo RD, Moffitt JE, et al. Expanding habitat of the imported fire ant (Solenopsis invicta): a public health concern. J Allergy Clin Immunol 2000;105(4): 683–91.
10. Simons FE, Peng Z. Skeeter syndrome. J Allergy Clin Immunol 1999;104(3 Pt 1): 705–7.
11. Golden DBK. Insect sting anaphylaxis. Immunol Allergy Clin North Am 2007; 27(2):261–72, vii.
12. Simons FER. Anaphylaxis. J Allergy Clin Immunol 2010;125(2 Suppl 2):S161–81.
13. Simons FER, Ardusso LRF, Bilo MB, et al. 2012 update: World Allergy Organization Guidelines for the assessment and management of anaphylaxis. Curr Opin Allergy Clin Immunol 2012;12(4):389–99.
14. Simons FER, Ardusso LRF, Bilo MB, et al. World allergy organization guidelines for the assessment and management of anaphylaxis. World Allergy Organ J 2011;4(2):13–37.
15. Lockey RF, Turkeltaub PC, Baird-Warren IA, et al. The Hymenoptera venom study I, 1979-1982: demographics and history-sting data. J Allergy Clin Immunol 1988; 82(3 Pt 1):370–81.
16. Pumphrey RSH, Gowland MH. Further fatal allergic reactions to food in the United Kingdom, 1999-2006. J Allergy Clin Immunol 2007;119(4):1018–9.
17. Pucci S, Antonicelli L, Bilo MB, et al. Shortness of interval between two stings as risk factor for developing Hymenoptera venom allergy. Allergy 1994;49(10): 894–6.
18. Stoevesandt J, Hain J, Kerstan A, et al. Over- and underestimated parameters in severe Hymenoptera venom-induced anaphylaxis: cardiovascular medication and absence of urticaria/angioedema. J Allergy Clin Immunol 2012;130(3): 698–704.e1.
19. Mosbech H. Death caused by wasp and bee stings in Denmark 1960-1980. Allergy 1983;38(3):195–200.
20. Reisman RE, Dvorin DJ, Randolph CC, et al. Stinging insect allergy: natural history and modification with venom immunotherapy. J Allergy Clin Immunol 1985; 75(6):735–40.
21. Valentine MD, Schuberth KC, Kagey-Sobotka A, et al. The value of immunotherapy with venom in children with allergy to insect stings. N Engl J Med 1990;323(23):1601–3.
22. Reisman RE. Natural history of insect sting allergy: relationship of severity of symptoms of initial sting anaphylaxis to re-sting reactions. J Allergy Clin Immunol 1992;90(3 Pt 1):335–9.
23. Golden DBK, Breisch NL, Hamilton RG, et al. Clinical and entomological factors influence the outcome of sting challenge studies. J Allergy Clin Immunol 2006; 117(3):670–5.
24. Reisman RE, Livingston A. Late-onset allergic reactions, including serum sickness, after insect stings. J Allergy Clin Immunol 1989;84(3):331–7.

25. Wong CG, Borici-Mazi R. Delayed-onset cold anaphylaxis after hymenoptera sting. Ann Allergy Asthma Immunol 2012;109(1):77–8.
26. Dhanapriya J, Dineshkumar T, Sakthirajan R, et al. Wasp sting-induced acute kidney injury. Clin Kidney J 2016;9(2):201–4.
27. Goldstein N, Rucker W, Woltman H. Neuritis occurring after insect sting. JAMA 1960;173(15):1727–30.
28. Akdur O, Can S, Afacan G. Rhabdomyolysis secondary to bee sting. Case Rep Emerg Med 2013;2013:258421.
29. Akbayram S, Akgun C, Dogan M, et al. Acute ITP due to insect bite: report of 2 cases. Clin Appl Thromb Hemost 2011;17(4):408–9.
30. Golden DBK. Large local reactions to insect stings. J Allergy Clin Immunol Pract 2015;3(3):331–4.
31. Boyce JA, Assa'ad A, Burks AW, et al. Guidelines for the diagnosis and management of food allergy in the United States: report of the NIAID-Sponsored Expert Panel. J Allergy Clin Immunol 2010;126(6 0):S1–58.
32. Cheng A. Emergency treatment of anaphylaxis in infants and children. Paediatr Child Health 2011;16(1):35–40.
33. Sicherer SH, Simons FER. Epinephrine for first-aid management of anaphylaxis. Pediatrics 2017;139(3). https://doi.org/10.1542/peds.2016-4006.
34. Sampson HA, Mendelson L, Rosen JP. Fatal and near-fatal anaphylactic reactions to food in children and adolescents. N Engl J Med 1992;327(6):380 4.
35. Bock SA, Munoz-Furlong A, Sampson HA. Further fatalities caused by anaphylactic reactions to food, 2001-2006. J Allergy Clin Immunol 2007;119(4):1016–8.
36. Tole JW, Lieberman P. Biphasic anaphylaxis: review of incidence, clinical predictors, and observation recommendations. Immunol Allergy Clin North Am 2007; 27(2):309–26, viii.
37. Ellis AK, Day JH. Incidence and characteristics of biphasic anaphylaxis: a prospective evaluation of 103 patients. Ann Allergy Asthma Immunol 2007; 98(1):64–9.
38. Lee JM, Greenes DS. Biphasic anaphylactic reactions in pediatrics. Pediatrics 2000;106(4):762–6.
39. Pumphrey RSH. Fatal posture in anaphylactic shock. J Allergy Clin Immunol 2003;112(2):451–2.
40. Choo KJL, Simons FER, Sheikh A. Glucocorticoids for the treatment of anaphylaxis. Evid Based Child Health 2013;8(4):1276–94.
41. Alqurashi W, Ellis AK, Ottawa F. Do corticosteroids prevent biphasic anaphylaxis? J Allergy Clin Immunol Pract 2017;5(5):1194–205.
42. Alqurashi W, Stiell I, Chan K, et al. Epidemiology and clinical predictors of biphasic reactions in children with anaphylaxis. Ann Allergy Asthma Immunol 2015;115(3):217–23.e2.
43. Oude Elberink JNG, De Monchy JGR, Van Der Heide S, et al. Venom immunotherapy improves health-related quality of life in patients allergic to yellow jacket venom. J Allergy Clin Immunol 2002;110(1):174–82.
44. Oude Elberink JNG, van der Heide S, Guyatt GH, et al. Analysis of the burden of treatment in patients receiving an EpiPen for yellow jacket anaphylaxis. J Allergy Clin Immunol 2006;118(3):699–704.
45. Golden DB, Marsh DG, Freidhoff LR, et al. Natural history of Hymenoptera venom sensitivity in adults. J Allergy Clin Immunol 1997;100(6 Pt 1):760–6.
46. Sturm GJ, Kranzelbinder B, Schuster C, et al. Sensitization to Hymenoptera venoms is common, but systemic sting reactions are rare. J Allergy Clin Immunol 2014;133(6):1635–43.e1.

47. Vos BJPR, van Anrooij B, van Doormaal JJ, et al. Fatal anaphylaxis to yellow jacket stings in mastocytosis: options for identification and treatment of at-risk patients. J Allergy Clin Immunol Pract 2017;5(5):1264–71.
48. Bonadonna P, Zanotti R, Muller U. Mastocytosis and insect venom allergy. Curr Opin Allergy Clin Immunol 2010;10(4):347–53.
49. Golden DBK. Anaphylaxis to insect stings. Immunol Allergy Clin North Am 2015; 35(2):287–302.
50. Quirt JA, Wen X, Kim J, et al. Venom allergy testing: is a graded approach necessary? Ann Allergy Asthma Immunol 2016;116(1):49–51.
51. Clayton WF, Georgitis JW, Reisman RE. Insect sting anaphylaxis in patients without detectable serum venom-specific IgE. Clin Allergy 1985;15(4):329–33.
52. Golden DB, Kagey-Sobotka A, Norman PS, et al. Insect sting allergy with negative venom skin test responses. J Allergy Clin Immunol 2001;107(5):897–901.
53. Golden DBK, Tracy JM, Freeman TM, et al. Negative venom skin test results in patients with histories of systemic reaction to a sting. J Allergy Clin Immunol 2003;112(3):495–8.
54. Reisman RE. Guidelines for management of people with histories of insect sting anaphylaxis and subsequent negative venom skin tests. J Allergy Clin Immunol 2004;113(2):364 [author reply: 364–5].
55. Goldberg A, Confino-Cohen R. Timing of venom skin tests and IgE determinations after insect sting anaphylaxis. J Allergy Clin Immunol 1997;100(2):182–4.
56. Bonadonna P, Perbellini O, Passalacqua G, et al. Clonal mast cell disorders in patients with systemic reactions to Hymenoptera stings and increased serum tryptase levels. J Allergy Clin Immunol 2009;123(3):680–6.
57. Niedoszytko M, Bonadonna P, Oude Elberink JNG, et al. Epidemiology, diagnosis, and treatment of Hymenoptera venom allergy in mastocytosis patients. Immunol Allergy Clin North Am 2014;34(2):365–81.
58. Rueff F, Przybilla B, Muller U, et al. The sting challenge test in Hymenoptera venom allergy. Position paper of the Subcommittee on Insect Venom Allergy of the European Academy of Allergology and Clinical Immunology. Allergy 1996; 51(4):216–25.
59. Haeberli G, Bronnimann M, Hunziker T, et al. Elevated basal serum tryptase and hymenoptera venom allergy: relation to severity of sting reactions and to safety and efficacy of venom immunotherapy. Clin Exp Allergy 2003;33(9):1216–20.
60. Rueff F, Przybilla B, Bilo MB, et al. Predictors of severe systemic anaphylactic reactions in patients with Hymenoptera venom allergy: importance of baseline serum tryptase-a study of the European Academy of Allergology and Clinical Immunology Interest Group on Insect Venom Hypersensitivity. J Allergy Clin Immunol 2009;124(5):1047–54.
61. Franken HH, Dubois AE, Minkema HJ, et al. Lack of reproducibility of a single negative sting challenge response in the assessment of anaphylactic risk in patients with suspected yellow jacket hypersensitivity. J Allergy Clin Immunol 1994; 93(2):431–6.
62. Reisman RE. Insect sting challenges: do no harm. J Allergy Clin Immunol 1995; 96(5 Pt 1):702–3.
63. Franken HH, Dubois AE, Kauffman HF, et al. Hymenoptera sting challenge tests. Lancet 1991;338(8778):1344.
64. Brockow K, Kiehn M, Riethmuller C, et al. Efficacy of antihistamine pretreatment in the prevention of adverse reactions to Hymenoptera immunotherapy: a prospective, randomized, placebo-controlled trial. J Allergy Clin Immunol 1997;100(4): 458–63.

65. Muller UR, Jutel M, Reimers A, et al. Clinical and immunologic effects of H1 antihistamine preventive medication during honeybee venom immunotherapy. J Allergy Clin Immunol 2008;122(5):1001–7.e4.

66. White JL, Greger KC, Lee S, et al. Patients Taking beta-Blockers Do Not Require Increased Doses of Epinephrine for Anaphylaxis. J Allergy Clin Immunol Pract 2018;6(5):1553–8.e1.

67. White KM, England RW. Safety of angiotensin-converting enzyme inhibitors while receiving venom immunotherapy. Ann Allergy Asthma Immunol 2008;101(4): 426–30.

68. Muller UR, Haeberli G. Use of beta-blockers during immunotherapy for Hymenoptera venom allergy. J Allergy Clin Immunol 2005;115(3):606–10.

69. Tejedor-Alonso MA, Farias-Aquino E, Perez-Fernandez E, et al. Relationship between anaphylaxis and use of beta-blockers and angiotensin-converting enzyme inhibitors: a systematic review and meta-analysis of observational studies. J Allergy Clin Immunol Pract 2018. https://doi.org/10.1016/j.jaip.2018.10.042.

70. Reisman RE, Wypych JI, Mueller UR, et al. Comparison of the allergenicity and antigenicity of Polistes venom and other vespid venoms. J Allergy Clin Immunol 1982;70(4):281–7.

71. King TP, Joslyn A, Kochoumian L. Antigenic cross-reactivity of venom proteins from hornets, wasps, and yellow jackets. J Allergy Clin Immunol 1985;75(5): 621–8.

72. King TP, Spangfort MD. Structure and biology of stinging insect venom allergens. Int Arch Allergy Immunol 2000;123(2):99–106.

73. Hunt KJ, Valentine MD, Sobotka AK, et al. A controlled trial of immunotherapy in insect hypersensitivity. N Engl J Med 1978;299(4):157–61.

74. Muller U, Helbling A, Berchtold E. Immunotherapy with honeybee venom and yellow jacket venom is different regarding efficacy and safety. J Allergy Clin Immunol 1992;89(2):529–35.

75. Boyle RJ, Elremeli M, Hockenhull J, et al. Venom immunotherapy for preventing allergic reactions to insect stings. Cochrane Database Syst Rev 2012;(10):CD008838.

76. Lange J, Cichocka-Jarosz E, Marczak H, et al. Natural history of Hymenoptera venom allergy in children not treated with immunotherapy. Ann Allergy Asthma Immunol 2016;116(3):225–9.

77. Golden DBK. Rush venom immunotherapy: ready for prime time? J Allergy Clin Immunol Pract 2017;5(3):804–5.

78. Roll A, Hofbauer G, Ballmer-Weber BK, et al. Safety of specific immunotherapy using a four-hour ultra-rush induction scheme in bee and wasp allergy. J Investig Allergol Clin Immunol 2006;16(2):79–85.

79. Sturm G, Kranke B, Rudolph C, et al. Rush Hymenoptera venom immunotherapy: a safe and practical protocol for high-risk patients. J Allergy Clin Immunol 2002; 110(6):928–33.

80. Birnbaum J, Charpin D, Vervloet D. Rapid Hymenoptera venom immunotherapy: comparative safety of three protocols. Clin Exp Allergy 1993;23(3):226–30.

81. Reisman RE, Livingston A. Venom immunotherapy: 10 years of experience with administration of single venoms and 50 micrograms maintenance doses. J Allergy Clin Immunol 1992;89(6):1189–95.

82. Konstantinou GN, Manoussakis E, Douladiris N, et al. A 5-year venom immunotherapy protocol with 50 mug maintenance dose: safety and efficacy in school children. Pediatr Allergy Immunol 2011;22(4):393–7.

83. Golden DB, Kagey-Sobotka A, Valentine MD, et al. Dose dependence of Hymenoptera venom immunotherapy. J Allergy Clin Immunol 1981;67(5):370–4.

84. Keating MU, Kagey-Sobotka A, Hamilton RG, et al. Clinical and immunologic follow-up of patients who stop venom immunotherapy. J Allergy Clin Immunol 1991;88(3 Pt 1):339–48.

85. Lerch E, Muller UR. Long-term protection after stopping venom immunotherapy: results of re-stings in 200 patients. J Allergy Clin Immunol 1998;101(5):606–12.

86. Committee on Insects. The discontinuation of Hymenoptera venom immunotherapy. J Allergy Clin Immunol 1998;101(5):573–5.

87. Muller UR, Ring J. When can immunotherapy for insect sting allergy be stopped? J Allergy Clin Immunol Pract 2015;3(3):324–30.

88. Letz AG, Quinn JM. Frequency of imported fire ant stings in patients receiving immunotherapy. Ann Allergy Asthma Immunol 2009;102(4):303–7.

89. Tankersley MS, Walker RL, Butler WK, et al. Safety and efficacy of an imported fire ant rush immunotherapy protocol with and without prophylactic treatment. J Allergy Clin Immunol 2002;109(3):556–62.

90. Haymore BR, McCoy RL, Nelson MR. Imported fire ant immunotherapy prescribing patterns in a large health care system during a 17-year period. Ann Allergy Asthma Immunol 2009;102(5):422–5.

91. Freeman TM, Hylander R, Ortiz A, et al. Imported fire ant immunotherapy: effectiveness of whole body extracts. J Allergy Clin Immunol 1992;90(2):210–5.

92. La Shell MS, Calabria CW, Quinn JM. Imported fire ant field reaction and immunotherapy safety characteristics: the IFACS study. J Allergy Clin Immunol 2010; 125(6):1294–9.

93. Arseneau AM, Nesselroad TD, Dietrich JJ, et al. A 1-day imported fire ant rush immunotherapy schedule with and without premedication. Ann Allergy Asthma Immunol 2013;111(6):562–6.

94. van Halteren HK, van der Linden PW, Burgers JA, et al. Discontinuation of yellow jacket venom immunotherapy: follow-up of 75 patients by means of deliberate sting challenge. J Allergy Clin Immunol 1997;100(6 Pt 1):767–70.

95. Golden DB, Kagey-Sobotka A, Lichtenstein LM. Survey of patients after discontinuing venom immunotherapy. J Allergy Clin Immunol 2000;105(2 Pt 1):385–90.

96. Reisman RE. Duration of venom immunotherapy: relationship to the severity of symptoms of initial insect sting anaphylaxis. J Allergy Clin Immunol 1993;92(6): 831–6.

97. Carlson J, Golden DBK. Large local reactions to insect envenomation. Curr Opin Allergy Clin Immunol 2016;16(4):366–9.

98. Hoffman DR, Jacobson RS. Allergens in hymenoptera venom XII: how much protein is in a sting? Ann Allergy 1984;52(4):276–8.

Food Allergy in Adults
Presentations, Evaluation, and Treatment

Mahboobeh Mahdavinia, MD, PhD

KEYWORDS

- Food allergy • Prevalence • Adult • Severity

KEY POINTS

- Food allergy is on the rise globally, in all age groups, and across all continents.
- Food allergy in adults differs from children; adults are often allergic to foods less frequently seen in children and their presenting symptoms may differ.
- Providers need to recognize the various presentations of food allergy, including those that may be life threatening, and, in those cases, in particular, explicitly describe the condition and the associated danger to all patients.

INTRODUCTION

Food allergy (FA) is an important and concerning public health problem, which has been increasing in incidence.[1,2] FA reactions can be life threatening and are a common cause of anaphylaxis presenting to emergency departments (EDs).[3] The prevalence of FA has been rapidly increasing in children in the past couple decades.[4–7] As these children are growing into adults, this trend is being observed in adults as well. Data on adult FA, however, is more limited. In addition, there is an increased incidence of new-onset FA in adults. In fact, 40% to 60% of cases of fish or shellfish allergy start in adulthood.[8,9]

EPIDEMIOLOGY

The estimated North American population prevalence of reported FA is 3.9% to 8% in infants and children and 6.6% to 10% in adults. Although multiple studies have been investigating the epidemiology of FA, there is still a need for comprehensive, nationwide, population-based studies on FA prevalence and the risks associated with FA in the United States. Most reports have depended on self-reported symptoms of FA, resulting in inaccurate prevalence (possibly underestimated) in adults with unrecognized symptoms, such as abdominal pain.[4,8,10] Furthermore, relying on patients' reports of possible FA might result in overestimation of the prevalence.

Division of Allergy and Immunology, Department of Internal Medicine, Rush University Medical Center, Professional Building, 1725 West Harrison Street, Suite 117, Chicago, IL 60612, USA
E-mail address: Mahboobeh_Mahdavinia@rush.edu

Med Clin N Am 104 (2020) 145–155
https://doi.org/10.1016/j.mcna.2019.08.008
0025-7125/20/© 2019 Elsevier Inc. All rights reserved.

A recent article investigated the self-reported FA (srFA) prevalence data in adults by comparing the US Food and Drug Administration Food Safety Surveys at 3 time points: 2001, 2006, and 2010.[7] This study found an increase in srFA without an associated increase in physician diagnosis of FA in adults. This discrepancy is alarming and possibly indicates an overdiagnosis of FA, with multiple nutritional and psychosocial consequences, and a resulting negative impact on the individual's health and quality of life. Patients may be increasingly avoiding foods without seeking medical advice.[1,2] This can potentially result in social isolation or contribute to the development of eating disorders. Furthermore, unnecessary avoidance of foods and limited diets can result in malnutrition and failure to thrive, especially in children and the elderly. Therefore, a proper diagnosis is essential in all suspected patients. These data point to a need for educational programs for patients with this condition about seeking proper help from health care providers.

Diagnosis of FA is based on both food allergen sensitization and development of classical allergic symptoms with ingestion of the food. Elevated sIgE or a positive skin test to a food is an evidence for allergen sensitization but does not mean a person is allergic to the food, unless that person develops IgE-mediated symptoms with ingestion of that specific food. In other words, only a subset of individuals reporting food-related reactions are sensitized to those foods and only a subset of those who are sensitized have true FA. For these reasons, there are few data on the true prevalence of FA (IgE mediated) in the adult populations. Both self-reported reactions and sensitization, however, can be used as markers for trends in the prevalence of true FA. The rate of sensitization to at least 1 common food allergen among adults is as high as 14.9% in the United States.[11] These sensitization rates range from 11% to 24% among Europeans.[11] In agreement with reported FA, the rate of food sensitization is very high in the United States, with rates as high as 16.8% reported in 2010.[12] The highest prevalence of food sensitization is in children ages 1 year to 5 years (28%) and declines steadily with age.[12] In line with this, clinical FA prevalence declines with age, highest in 1-year-old to 5-year-old children (4.2%) and lowest in adults 60 years old and older (1.3%).[12]

srFA among adults is more common in women.[4,7] The rate of sensitization to food allergens, however, is similar in both men and women.[12] Food sensitization to peanut, shrimp, and milk is more prevalent in men.[12]

Previous studies have estimated the prevalence of FA to be different among individuals based on race, with the highest-risk group in the United States non-Hispanic African Americans.[4] This is true for both srFA[4] and objective sensitization to food allergens.[12]

srFA also is associated with higher household education level.[4] Food sensitization is more prevalent, however, in individuals living in poverty and least prevalent in higher-income households.[12]

REACTIONS

As the prevalence of FA increases, increased awareness is needed. Most child-care facilities and schools are developing protective policies and programs to provide a safe environment for children with FA, such as a separate table for younger food-allergic children and having children carry their own self-injectable epinephrine (SIE). There is a need for public awareness for protecting adults with the condition as well. Proper labeling of food with all hidden ingredients and keeping a detailed list of ingredients in all food services and restaurants can prevent accidental exposure and reactions. In a large study, adults reported that 8.4% of FA-related reactions were treated with an intramuscular epinephrine in an ED.[7] In this same survey, 34% of adults with srFA had gone more than 5 years without an FA-related reaction.[7] A longitudinal study investigating FA-related ED trends reported a decrease in the frequency of FA-related ED visits from 2001 to 2009 among US adults.[13] The relatively long period of time with no reactions reported by Verrill and colleagues[7] as well as the decreased rate of FA-related ED visits indicate a possible shift toward improved prevention of reactions in adults with FA.

FOODS

Among adults with srFA, 75%report reactions to at least 1 of the 8 major food allergens.[7] These allergens include milk, wheat, egg, soy (seen most commonly in children), peanut, tree nuts, fish, and shellfish. Milk is the most commonly reported allergen reported in 4.1% of US adults followed by shellfish reported in 3.6% of adults.[7] Milk and shellfish have been reported as the most common allergens in adults in another national study based on the National Health and Nutrition Examination Survey in 2007 to 2010.[4] Other common allergens reported among adults are peanut and tree nuts, together accounting for approximately 25% of the cases.[9] A majority of these cases of allergy to peanut and tree nuts are childhood onset. In addition to the 8 major food allergens, fruits and vegetables represent the largest reported food group to cause reactions, with 2.7% of adults in the United States reporting reacting to this large food group.[7] Reported reactions to raw fruits and vegetables could be due to another type of food-related allergy, known as pollen FA syndrome (PFAS), which results in symptoms mostly confined to the mouth and lips, such as oral pruritis or swelling of the lips. PFAS is to foods that cross-react with pollen or airborne allergens and is seen in patients who first develop the aeroallergen sensitivity. This syndrome is discussed in more detail later.

PRESENTATION

As discussed previously, not all patients who report symptoms with foods are clinically food allergic. FA can start at any age, however, and many adults do develop new FAs; therefore, a detailed oriented history is an essential key to this diagnosis, with special attention to the following: temporal association of symptoms in relation to food exposure; type and severity of reaction; response to treatment; and reproducibility of the reaction. The diagnosis is confirmed with evidence of sensitization to the culprit by skin prick test (SPT) or serologic testing measuring sIgE.

Temporal Relationship

IgE-mediated FA is characterized by almost immediate onset of symptoms (mostly within 2 hours). Delayed reactions hours after ingestion could be due to food intolerances or other rare types of FAs, such as food protein–induced enterocolitis (FPIES) or delayed anaphylaxis or hives to mammalian meats secondary to a galactose-α-1,3-galactose (α-gal) allergy. These are discussed in more detail later. Therefore, even patients who report a consistent, delayed reaction to a specific food need to be referred to an allergist for evaluation.

Symptoms

The typical FA symptoms indicating an IgE-mediated FA are characterized by almost immediate onset of symptoms (within 3 hours) and consist of urticaria, angioedema, bronchospasm, nausea, vomiting, occasionally diarrhea, and, in severe cases, dizziness due to hypotension, loss of consciousness, and shock (anaphylactic shock).[1]

Many adults presenting for evaluation for possible FA complain of nonspecific symptoms, such as bloating, changes in bowel movements, chronic abdominal pain, or tiredness. These nonspecific symptoms are not indicative of an IgE-mediated FA and fall mostly into other types of food intolerance. Some other types of food-related reactions, such as FPIES, can result in delayed abdominal pain and vomiting to the point of severe tiredness and even lethargy. These patients do not have other classical symptoms of FA, such as cutaneous or respiratory tract symptoms. Although FPIES was originally thought to be a pediatric disease, it is more commonly reported in adults now, especially to crustaceans. This condition is in the differential for patients presenting with delayed GI symptoms, especially with seafood, and should be referred to an allergist for evaluation. Because FPIES is not IgE mediated, serologic testing to foods are negative.

Response to Treatment

It is important to know whether symptoms were resolved or improved with treatments, such as antihistamines, and if epinephrine was needed/given. How severe was the reaction? Did it require treatment in the ED and, if so, what was given? It also is important to know how long the symptoms lasted after treatment. Patients who develop severe respiratory symptoms and anaphylaxis are at higher risk for development of severe reactions again.[1,2]

History of Re-exposure

FA symptoms are reproducible. It is not advised to ever try eating the food again if there is concern of allergy but often patients have eaten the food since the reaction and tolerated it before coming for evaluation. If patients have consumed the same food/foods since their reaction without developing any symptoms, they do not have classic IgE-mediated FA. There are a few exceptions to this. For example, some foods are tolerated after exposed to high heat. This is most commonly seen in individuals who are allergic to egg and milk but can tolerate egg and milk in baked goods.[14] These food-allergic patients are sensitized to a heat-sensitive protein in the milk or egg that is broken down with baking and only react to the raw and or lightly cooked products. Patients with PFAS react only to raw fruits or vegetables and tolerate these foods in cooked or canned forms. Also, some fish-allergic patients can tolerate canned fish, such as canned tuna.

Some other types of food sensitivity could be dependent on the amount of food consumed or related to co-occurrence of other factors, such as exercise in the case of food-dependent, exercise-induced anaphylaxis. This condition is thought to be due to IgE sensitization to the food, often wheat, that is tolerated alone, but causes anaphylaxis if combined with exercise or in some cases nonsteroidal anti-inflammatory drugs or aspirin.

EVALUATIONS

A diagnosis of FA needs to be confirmed with evidence of sensitization to the culprit food either by SPT or serologic testing measuring serum-specific IgE. These tests without a supporting clinical history are not useful and should not be used for diagnosis of FA.[1] A positive allergy test (SPT or serum-specific IgE) alone is only indicative of sensitization and not allergy.[1] In other words, the patient has developed antibodies but does not react. Larger SPT wheal size or higher concentration of sIgE levels do correlate with higher likelihood of clinical reaction due to IgE-mediated allergy.[15] None of these markers correlates with severity of food-related allergic reactions, however.[15] There is no role for SPT or food-specific IgE levels in the diagnosis of non–IgE-mediated FA.[1,15] In cases of diagnostic uncertainty, oral challenge to food/foods is needed. These challenges need to be done in a controlled setting usually as open food challenges. If patients consent, a blinded, placebo-controlled food challenge is preferred[16] but if the patient is thought to be not allergic, open challenge usually is done. Other laboratory tests, such as component-resolved diagnostics testing, can help in decision making and can increase the diagnostic accuracy.[17] Component-resolved diagnostics testing uses individual allergenic proteins within a food to identify reactivity to the specific food proteins rather than whole allergens used for standard allergy testing.[18] For some foods, specific food proteins are associated with anaphylaxis whereas others are associated with PFAS. Adjuvant use of this modality can provide a more accurate assessment in the diagnosis of FA and the risks involved in exposure. For example, peanut is a common food allergen in the United States, commonly causing life-threatening anaphylaxis. Peanut allergy also is seen in PFAS, however, because some proteins in peanut cross-react with allergy to birch tree. Component testing in the context of a patient's history/reaction can help delineate PFAS from primary peanut allergy, which causes anaphylaxis and is life threatening. In the former, Ara H 8 is the protein to which patients are sensitized whereas anaphylaxis is associated with sensitivity to Ara H 2. Serologic IgE testing may be positive in both cases, and diagnosing based on this can cause unnecessary food avoidance and the emotional burdens associated with this (fear of foods, fear of eating out, and need to carry SIE.)

TYPES OF FOOD ALLERGIES

There are 4 distinct syndromes that represent an IgE-mediated allergic reaction to foods (**Table 1**). The first and most common is a typical anaphylactic-type FA. These reactions are potentially life threatening and are detailed previously.

The second type of FA is a delayed anaphylactic reaction to mammalian meats. The allergenic epitope is α-gal, a carbohydrate commonly expressed on nonprimate mammalian proteins; this conditions is called α-gal allergy α-gal syndrome,[19] and patients with this allergy can have severe reactions to the anticancer drug cetuximab. The α-gal syndrome is an increasingly recognized condition and is secondary to tick bites by the lone star tick. This unique type of allergy was first described in the southern states of the United States,[19] where there is exposure to lone star ticks and chiggers, and it has increasingly been reported across the world. There is evidence from multiple regions of the world, including Australia, Europe, and the United States, that the primary cause of this allergic response is tick bites, which can itch for 10 days or more. Diagnosis of α-gal syndrome is complicated and is made by a detailed history of delayed hives or anaphylaxis after eating red meat, supported by the presence of specific IgE to beef, pork, and lamb and the lack of IgE to chicken, turkey, and fish. SPTs generally are negative, but intradermal testing could be positive.[20] Testing for the IgE to α-gal can be done at some academic centers. Management of this condition consists of detailed education based on avoidance of both ingestion of red meat and further tick bites because this allergy may wane in time if no further exposure to tick bites.

The third type of IgE-mediated food reactions is food-dependent, exercise-induced anaphylaxis, which occurs only in the context of food allergen ingestion and exercise within a short interval, usually vigorous exercise, such as running, but brisk walking can induce symptoms.[21] IgE to that food should be demonstrable. It is the combination of ingestion of the culprit food and exercise that precipitates reactions, whereas

Table 1
Types of food-related adverse reactions

Disorder	Mechanism	Clinical Features	Common Food Triggers
Classic FA	IgE	Cutaneous: hives, angioedema Respiratory: bronchospasm, laryngeal angioedema GI: nausea/vomiting, diarrhea, cramps Systemic: hypotension, loss of consciousness, anaphylactic shock	Most common: milk, fish, shellfish, egg, wheat, peanut, tree nuts, soy, and sesame But can occur with any food
Oral allergy syndrome or food pollen syndrome	IgE to cross-reactive allergens between aeroallergens and food	Itching and rarely mild swelling confined to the oropharyngeal area	Fresh fruits and vegetables
Food-dependent, exercise-induced anaphylaxis	IgE-mediated hypersensitivity in conjunction with exercise	Anaphylaxis in cases of consumption of the specific food along with exercise	Most common: wheat, shellfish, tree nuts, peanuts, fish, pork, beef, eggs, peaches, apples, milk
α-Gal allergy	IgE	Delayed anaphylactic reaction to mammalian meats	Red meat
EoE and EGIDs	Both IgE mediated and non-IgE mediated	GI symptoms Dysphagia and food impaction in EoE Diarrhea/constipation, abdominal pain, vomiting, and bloating in other forms of EGID Narrowing and fibrosis of the GI lumen in severe cases.	Milk, wheat, egg, and legumes Less commonly peanut, tree nuts, fish, and shellfish
FPIES	Non-IgE Immunologic	Delayed nausea, vomiting, diarrhea and abdominal cramps	Wheat, milk, soy, other grains
Food intolerance	Non-IgE Nonimmunologic	Variable symptoms Examples • Nonspecific GI symptoms • Migraine headaches • Flushing with scombroid fish poisoning	Any food Examples • Lactose intolerance with milk • Scombroid fish poisoning

the food and exercise are each tolerated separately. It has been recently shown that in some cases, exercise is not the only factor precipitating the attacks. In some patients, other augmentation factors, such as high alcohol or acetylsalicylic acid intake, along with ingestion of significant amount of the culprit food can result in IgE-mediated symptoms at rest.[21] Thus, food-dependent, exercise-induced anaphylaxis seems more correctly characterized as a type of FA in which symptoms develop in the presence of augmenting factors, with exercise, however, as the primary factor in all cases. Thus, diagnosis and management are made more complicated.

All these reactions also could be life threatening because they cause anaphylaxis. All these patients need to be evaluated by an allergy specialist and educated well about avoidance and treatment of accidental exposures, including the use of SIE. The fourth condition is oral allergy syndrome, also referred to as PFAS. PFAS is caused by cross-reactivity between aeroallergens and food. This type of allergy is also called FA type 2 and often manifests as immediate-onset symptoms of itching and rarely mild swelling confined to the oropharyngeal area after eating fresh fruits or vegetable.[22,23] The syndrome is believed to begin with sensitization to pollen allergens, such as birch tree pollen (Bet v1). Bet v1 (profilin) is a heat-labile protein abundantly found in birch pollen. It plays an important role in the selective polymerization of actin filaments in the required direction, an important element for successful pollen formation and dispersion that is shared by most plants.[24–26] This allergen cross-reacts with allergens found in multiple fruits, such as apples, pears, and peaches. Another example of PFAS is mugwort pollen cross-reacting with celery.[27] These proteins are sensitive to gastric enzymes, protecting the individual from systemic symptoms.[28] Similarly, these proteins are heat sensitive; therefore, patients can tolerate ingesting cooked fruits or vegetable with no symptoms. In a survey, PFAS was reported as the most prevalent new-onset FA in adults.[22] It is associated with significant decline in health-related quality of life.[29] At the molecular level, the most common allergens causing PFAS are PR10 proteins and profilins. PR10 are found in species belonging to the Rosaceae family, such as peach, apple, pear, and cherry. Although rare, allergy to fresh fruits, such as apples and peaches, also might be life threatening, causing anaphylaxis. This occurs when the cross-reactive protein is a lipid transfer protein, which is stable to heat and enzymes. Allergy to lipid transfer protein has been reported mostly in the Mediterranean region of Europe.[30] Diagnosis of PFAS is made by typical clinical presentation and can be confirmed by fresh food prick testing to the fruit or vegetables plus evidence of sensitization to the cross-reactive pollen.[31,32]

There is another group of food-related conditions that falls into the broad category of eosinophilic gastrointestinal disorders (EGIDs). These conditions are confined to the gastrointestinal (GI) tract (see **Table 1**).[33] EGID are characterized by increased eosinophils in GI tract mucosal biopsies. Eosinophilic esophagitis (EoE) is the best characterized EGID. The current body of literature suggests that the pathogenesis of EGID is based on an inflammatory response to foods manifested by type 2 helper T-cell inflammation and includes both IgE-mediated and non–IgE-mediated components. The exact pathophysiology, however, is still unknown. Patients with EoE commonly complain of long-standing progressive dysphagia and can suffer from food impactions. Current recommendations for diagnosis of EoE include the combination of esophageal dysfunction symptoms that do not respond to proton pump inhibitor therapy and evidence for increased eosinophils in esophageal biopsies. A large majority of EoE patients have other atopic diseases, such as allergic rhinitis, asthma, PFAS, and/or IgE-mediated FAs.[34] The most common food associated with EoE in adults is milk followed by wheat and egg. The treatment is based on identifying the triggering food.

This often requires repeated endoscopies and biopsies after food elimination of the most common foods and foods the patient suspects followed by reintroduction to the foods. Endoscopies and biopsies are needed because symptoms do not always correlate with pathology. In most cases, patients are also treated with orally taken topical steroids, such as swallowed budesonide or fluticasone.[35] Studies with biologics are ongoing.

DIFFERENTIAL DIAGNOSIS

Food intolerance is a nonimmune reaction after ingestion of a food and is often misinterpreted as FA by patients. Food intolerance may occur in cases of exposure to metabolic substances (eg, lactose intolerance), due to exposure to toxins in foods (eg, microbial contamination or scombroid fish poisoning) or other metabolically active components of foods, such as caffeine or tyramine (found in aged cheese), which can trigger migraine. These reactions might also be via undefined mechanisms. A detailed history, as described previously, can help distinguish food intolerance from FA; however, in many cases referral to an allergist and further testing is needed.

Two other types of reactions can mimic IgE-mediated classic FA to seafood. The first reaction is due to scombroid poisoning, which is a non–IgE-mediated reaction that mimics a classic allergic reaction. This reaction is typically due to mishandling of fish. Although the symptoms can be identical to a true allergic reaction, such as flushing, itching, and even shortness of breath, they are not reproducible, which is different from IgE-mediated reactions that occur on every ingestion of the culprit fish. Another type of reaction to seafood is due to sensitization to tropomyosins, which are major allergens in crustaceans.[36] Tropomyosins from shellfish and fish have a high degree of homology with house dust mite and cockroaches.[37] Shrimp tropomyosin (Pen a 1) has more than 80% amino acid sequence similarity to house dust mite (Der p 10)[37] and cockroach (Per a 7).[38] Shellfish tropomyosins widely cross-react with tropomyosins in dust mite and cockroach.[36] It has been hypothesized that, similar to the oral allergy syndrome reaction to fruit and vegetables that are cross-reacting plant allergens, shellfish allergy in adolescents and adults may be secondary to sensitization to inhalant allergens, including dust mite and cockroach, which contain a cross-reacting tropomyosin.[36] These reactions usually are only cutaneous, milder, and occur with ingestion of larger amounts of the cross-reactive food, which distinguishes them from classic IgE-mediated FA, wherein ingestion of a small amount of the food (a bite) can result in anaphylaxis. Recently, cases of delayed food related reactions to seafood that resemble adult FPIES have been reported. Although the mechanism of these reactions is not completely understood, it might be linked to sensitivity to these cross-reactive epitopes.

TREATMENT

Currently there is no cure for FA. The current recommended treatment includes strict avoidance of the food, education for recognition of an allergic reaction (especially to teachers, school staff, and caregivers), and providing management plans (action plans) in cases of accidental exposure and allergic reaction. These plans need to elaborate on the spectrum of symptoms and include instruction to use specific emergency medications, such as epinephrine autoinjectors and antihistamines.[16] Patients need to be instructed to read food labels, be attentive and diligent when eating out or eating prepared foods, and be careful about cross-contact of allergenic foods in buffets or during meal preparation (shared cutting boards, slicers, and mixers).

Epinephrine is the only proved treatment of anaphylaxis and for this reason patients should always carry SIE because accidental exposures can occur anywhere, even in the home. Steroids and antihistamines, although unproved, may help as well but are second line to epinephrine. Patients and family should be instructed on the use of SIE and this should be demonstrated in the office with a training device.

A majority of patients with IgE-mediated FA suffer from other atopic conditions and asthma is commonly seen in these individuals.[1,5] During an FA reaction, asthmatic patients tend to have severe asthma attacks. Therefore, proper management of asthma at baseline and treatment of acute asthma attacks in the context of FA is crucial. Risk factors identified with fatal or near-fatal reactions to food include asthma (especially if uncontrolled at baseline), no epinephrine given, and delay in giving epinephrine. Having had previously mild reactions is not a predictor of future reactions, and severe reactions, including anaphylactic shock, can happen with any exposure. A robust team, including the patient, family, primary care provider, and allergy specialist, is the best approach to avoid devastating outcomes.

SUMMARY

Adult FA, especially srFA indicative of perceived symptoms with food, is a common condition. In some cases, the history represents persistence of childhood FA into adulthood; however, in many cases, the symptoms have started in adulthood. An understanding of the underlying pathogenesis of FA can aid the health providers in deciding on appropriate testing and treatment plans. It needs to be determined especially whether the condition is potentially life threatening or not. It is of utmost importance for practitioners to pay attention to the timing and type of symptoms, specific allergens, and possible cofactors in order to make an accurate diagnosis. The most important role of the provider is to risk-stratify the patient, provide detailed action plans, and recommend appropriate avoidance measures. For example, exercise-induced anaphylaxis can be a confusing diagnosis because symptoms are not reproducible and require the exercise cofactor to be present. Definitive treatment of most FA syndromes are lacking, and avoidance is the main recommendation. Many trials are ongoing, however, and some have promising results for emerging treatment options for inducing tolerance in cases of accidental exposures to food allergens.

REFERENCES

1. Boyce JA, Assa'ad A, Burks AW, et al. Guidelines for the diagnosis and management of food allergy in the united states: summary of the NIAID-sponsored expert panel report. J Allergy Clin Immunol 2010;126(6):1105–18.
2. Flokstra-de Blok BM, Dubois AE, Vlieg-Boerstra BJ, et al. Health-related quality of life of food allergic patients: comparison with the general population and other diseases. Allergy 2010;65(2):238–44.
3. Atkins D, Bock SA. Fatal anaphylaxis to foods: epidemiology, recognition, and prevention. Curr Allergy Asthma Rep 2009;9(3):179–85.
4. McGowan EC, Keet CA. Prevalence of self-reported food allergy in the National Health and Nutrition Examination Survey (NHANES) 2007-2010. J Allergy Clin Immunol 2013;132(5):1216–9.e5.
5. Branum AM, Lukacs SL. Food allergy among children in the United States. Pediatrics 2009;124(6):1549–55.
6. Sampson HA. Anaphylaxis and emergency treatment. Pediatrics 2003;111(6 Pt 3):1601–8.

7. Verrill L, Bruns R, Luccioli S. Prevalence of self-reported food allergy in U.S. adults: 2001, 2006, and 2010. Allergy Asthma Proc 2015;36(6):458–67.
8. Sicherer SH, Munoz-Furlong A, Sampson HA. Prevalence of seafood allergy in the United States determined by a random telephone survey. J Allergy Clin Immunol 2004;114(1):159–65.
9. Kamdar TA, Peterson S, Lau CH, et al. Prevalence and characteristics of adult-onset food allergy. J Allergy Clin Immunol Pract 2015;3(1):114–5.e1.
10. Sicherer SH, Munoz-Furlong A, Godbold JH, et al. US prevalence of self-reported peanut, tree nut, and sesame allergy: 11-year follow-up. J Allergy Clin Immunol 2010;125(6):1322–6.
11. Burney P, Summers C, Chinn S, et al. Prevalence and distribution of sensitization to foods in the European Community Respiratory Health Survey: a EuroPrevall analysis. Allergy 2010;65(9):1182–8.
12. Liu AH, Jaramillo R, Sicherer SH, et al. National prevalence and risk factors for food allergy and relationship to asthma: results from the National Health and Nutrition Examination Survey 2005-2006. J Allergy Clin Immunol 2010;126(4):798–806.e13.
13. Clark S, Espinola JA, Rudders SA, et al. Favorable trends in the frequency of U.S. emergency department visits for food allergy, 2001-2009. Allergy Asthma Proc 2013;34(5):439–45.
14. Leonard SA, Nowak-Wegrzyn AH. Baked milk and egg diets for milk and egg allergy management. Immunol Allergy Clin North Am 2016;36(1):147–59.
15. Sampson HA. Utility of food-specific IgE concentrations in predicting symptomatic food allergy. J Allergy Clin Immunol 2001;107(5):891–6.
16. Anagnostou K, Stiefel G, Brough H, et al. Active management of food allergy: an emerging concept. Arch Dis Child 2015;100(4):386–90.
17. Schussler E, Kattan J. Allergen component testing in the diagnosis of food allergy. Curr Allergy Asthma Rep 2015;15(9):55.
18. Valenta R, Lidholm J, Niederberger V, et al. The recombinant allergen-based concept of component-resolved diagnostics and immunotherapy (CRD and CRIT). Clin Exp Allergy 1999;29(7):896–904.
19. Commins SP, Satinover SM, Hosen J, et al. Delayed anaphylaxis, angioedema, or urticaria after consumption of red meat in patients with IgE antibodies specific for galactose-alpha-1,3-galactose. J Allergy Clin Immunol 2009;123(2):426–33.
20. Steinke JW, Platts-Mills TA, Commins SP. The alpha-gal story: lessons learned from connecting the dots. J Allergy Clin Immunol 2015;135(3):589–96 [quiz: 597].
21. Feldweg AM. Food-dependent, exercise-induced anaphylaxis: diagnosis and management in the outpatient setting. J Allergy Clin Immunol Pract 2017;5(2):283–8.
22. Skypala IJ, Bull S, Deegan K, et al. The prevalence of PFS and prevalence and characteristics of reported food allergy; a survey of UK adults aged 18-75 incorporating a validated PFS diagnostic questionnaire. Clin Exp Allergy 2013;43(8):928–40.
23. Eriksson NE, Formgren H, Svenonius E. Food hypersensitivity in patients with pollen allergy. Allergy 1982;37(6):437–43.
24. Baek K, Liu X, Ferron F, et al. Modulation of actin structure and function by phosphorylation of Tyr-53 and profilin binding. Proc Natl Acad Sci U S A 2008;105(33):11748–53.
25. Breiteneder H, Radauer C. A classification of plant food allergens. J Allergy Clin Immunol 2004;113(5):821–30 [quiz: 831].

26. Haarer BK, Brown SS. Structure and function of profilin. Cell Motil Cytoskeleton 1990;17(2):71–4.
27. Egger M, Mutschlechner S, Wopfner N, et al. Pollen-food syndromes associated with weed pollinosis: an update from the molecular point of view. Allergy 2006; 61(4):461–76.
28. Rodriguez-Perez R, Crespo JF, Rodriguez J, et al. Profilin is a relevant melon allergen susceptible to pepsin digestion in patients with oral allergy syndrome. J Allergy Clin Immunol 2003;111(3):634–9.
29. Beyer S, Franke A, Simon JC, et al. Measurement of health-related quality of life in adult patients with birch pollen-associated food allergy. J Dtsch Dermatol Ges 2016;14(4):397–404.
30. Asero R, Pravettoni V. Anaphylaxis to plant-foods and pollen allergens in patients with lipid transfer protein syndrome. Curr Opin Allergy Clin Immunol 2013;13(4): 379–85.
31. Zuidmeer L, Goldhahn K, Rona RJ, et al. The prevalence of plant food allergies: a systematic review. J Allergy Clin Immunol 2008;121(5):1210–8.e4.
32. Anhoej C, Backer V, Nolte H. Diagnostic evaluation of grass- and birch-allergic patients with oral allergy syndrome. Allergy 2001;56(6):548–52.
33. Rothenberg ME. Eosinophilic gastrointestinal disorders (EGID). J Allergy Clin Immunol 2004;113(1):11–28 [quiz: 29].
34. Mahdavinia M, Bishehsari F, Hayat W, et al. Association of eosinophilic esophagitis and food pollen allergy syndrome. Ann Allergy Asthma Immunol 2017;118(1): 116–7.
35. Cianferoni A, Spergel J. Eosinophilic esophagitis: a comprehensive review. Clin Rev Allergy Immunol 2016;50(2):159–74.
36. Reese G, Ayuso R, Lehrer SB. Tropomyosin: an invertebrate pan-allergen. Int Arch Allergy Immunol 1999;119(4):247–58.
37. Wong L, Huang CH, Lee BW. Shellfish and house dust mite allergies: is the link tropomyosin? Allergy Asthma Immunol Res 2016;8(2):101–6.
38. Santos AB, Chapman MD, Aalberse RC, et al. Cockroach allergens and asthma in Brazil: identification of tropomyosin as a major allergen with potential cross-reactivity with mite and shrimp allergens. J Allergy Clin Immunol 1999;104(2 Pt 1):329–37.

Atopic Dermatitis in Adults

Jonathan I. Silverberg, MD, PhD, MPH[a,b,*]

KEYWORDS

- Atopic dermatitis • Eczema • Epidemiology • Treatment • Comorbidities • Burden

KEY POINTS

- Atopic dermatitis is common in adults in the United States and worldwide.
- Atopic dermatitis is associated with different genetic, immunologic, and epidemiologic risk factors in adults than in children.
- One in 4 adults with atopic dermatitis report adult onset of their disease.
- Atopic dermatitis is associated with major patient and societal burden.
- Atopic dermatitis is associated with multiple atopic and mental health comorbidities.

INTRODUCTION

Atopic dermatitis (AD) was once thought to be primarily a pediatric disease that remitted with increasing age. However, recent epidemiologic studies showed that AD is a common and burdensome disorder in adults. Moreover, emerging studies have shown that there are different genetic, immunologic, and epidemiologic risk factors for AD in adults than in children. This article examines the pathophysiology, epidemiology, heterogeneous clinical presentation, burden, diagnosis, and treatment of adult AD.

PATHOPHYSIOLOGY
Genetics

AD is thought to occur via a combination of genetic, environmental, immunologic, and behavioral factors.[1-3] Genetic inheritance plays an essential role in the predisposition for childhood AD. Monozygotic twins have a higher rate of AD concordance than dizygotic twins (~80% vs ~20%).[4,5] Filaggrin (FLG) gene null mutations are the most well-

Disclosure: Dr J.I. Silverberg served as a consultant and/or advisory board member for Abbvie, Asana, Arena, Dermavant, Dermira, Eli Lilly, Galderma, Glaxosmithkline, Glenmark, Kiniksa, Leo, Menlo, Pfizer, Regeneron-Sanofi, and Realm receiving honoraria; speaker for Regeneron-Sanofi; and received research grants from GlaxoSmithKline and Galderma. The author has nothing else to disclose.

[a] Northwestern University Feinberg School of Medicine, Chicago, IL, USA; [b] Northwestern Medicine Multidisciplinary Eczema Center, Chicago, IL, USA
* 676 North Saint Clair Street, Suite 1600, Chicago, IL 60611.
E-mail address: JONATHANISILVERBERG@GMAIL.COM
twitter: JONATHANMD (J.I.S.)

Med Clin N Am 104 (2020) 157–176
https://doi.org/10.1016/j.mcna.2019.08.009
0025-7125/20/© 2019 Elsevier Inc. All rights reserved.

studied genetic determinant of AD. FLG codes for the protein filaggrin, which is broken down into a natural moisturizing factor in the stratum corneum and plays an integral role in skin-barrier function.[6] FLG null mutations lead to a deficiency of natural moisturizing factor,[7] xerosis in AD,[8] and disrupted epidermal barrier function allowing increased penetration of allergens and development of a T-helper cell type 2 (Th-2)–predominant phenotype.[9] FLG loss-of-function mutations lead to AD with early childhood onset, greater severity,[10] and persistence into adulthood.[11,12]

However, FLG null mutations are not detected in most children with AD. FLG mutations were only identified in a large minority of European[13] and Asian[14] populations,[15] and not South African and Ethiopian[16,17] or African American populations.[15] Moreover, FLG mutations may not be responsible for adolescent-onset and adult-onset AD. A study of 241 patients with AD found that the 4 most common filaggrin loss-of-function mutations were only associated with early childhood-onset AD ($\leq$8 years), but not late childhood–onset (8–17 years) or adult-onset disease ($\geq$18 years).[10] In contrast, the −1903/A polymorphism of the mast-cell chymase (MCC) gene may play a role in adult-onset AD because it is associated with AD in adults, but not allergic rhinitis or asthma,[18,19] and is inversely associated with serum immunoglobulin (Ig) E levels in adult patients with AD.[19,20] Other important genetic factors linked to adult AD include polymorphisms of the interleukin (IL)-4 receptor[21] and the vitamin D receptor.[22] Future research is needed to understand the genetics of adult AD, particularly adult-onset AD.

Immunologic Factors

Th-2 and other T-cell subsets contribute to AD pathogenesis. In the acute and chronic phases of AD, a skewed Th-2 response is seen, leading to increased activity of IL-4, IL-5, IL-13, IL-31, and so forth. However, Th-1 responses are upregulated in the chronic phase of AD. A study of 28 adults with AD and 6 healthy controls found that IL-13 messenger RNA (mRNA) was expressed in 27 of 28 AD skin lesions examined, but only 3 of 6 controls; the level of expression of IL-13 mRNA was significantly higher in lesional skin compared with healthy controls.[23] However, IL-4 mRNA was expressed in only 3 of 28 AD lesions and 0 of 6 controls.[23] A study of 16 patients with AD and 12 healthy controls found significantly higher expression of IL-1b, IL-1RA, IL-5, IL-6, IL-8, IL-13, IL-18, thymus and activation regulated chemokine (TARC), tumor necrosis factor alpha, Monokine induced by gamma interferon (MIG), and interferon γ-induced protein 10 kDa (IP-10) in AD skin lesions compared with non-lesional AD skin and/or healthy skin.[24] Furthermore, interstitial fluid levels of IL-13 and IP-10 but not IL-4 in AD skin lesions strongly correlated with AD severity as judged by the SCORAD Scoring Atopic Dermatitis) total and objective scores.[24]

Few studies have compared the immune differences of AD in children versus adults. A recent study of 19 children aged less than 5 years with new-onset AD compared the immune phenotype in skin with 15 adults with AD.[25] Children compared with adults with AD showed comparable or greater epidermal hyperplasia and immune infiltration, and decreased filaggrin expression on histology and immunohistochemistry as well as activation of Th-2, Th-22, and Th-1 axes on quantitative real-time polymerase chain reaction. However, children showed higher induction of Th-17–related cytokines, antimicrobials, Th-9, IL-33, and innate markers than adults. These results suggest that the immune mechanisms of AD may differ between children and adults.

EPIDEMIOLOGY OF ADULT ATOPIC DERMATITIS

A study of 27,157 adults (aged 18–85 years) from a US population-based study (2010 National Health Interview Survey) found the prevalence of "dermatitis, eczema, or any other red, inflamed skin rash" in the past year with or without a personal history of asthma and/or hay fever was 3.2% and 10.2%, respectively.[26] The former definition likely underestimates the true prevalence by excluding patients without atopic disease. The latter likely overestimates the true prevalence by including other dermatoses. The true prevalence of AD is likely between 3% and 10%. A study of 34,613 adults (2012 National Health Interview Survey) found the prevalence of "eczema or skin allergy" in the past year to be 7.2%.[27] The question used was similar to one previously validated for self-report of AD, but did not include health care diagnosis.[28] A study of 4972 adults (2005–2006 National Health and Nutrition Examination Survey) found that the lifetime prevalence of health care–diagnosed eczema in adults was 7.4%.[29] A study of 2893 adults from a US population-based study (AD in America) found the prevalence of AD to be 7.3% using adapted United Kingdom Working Party criteria. Together, these studies suggest that the prevalence of AD in US adults is ~7%.

The prevalence of adult AD ranged from 2% to 17% in previous international studies.[30] A recent international, Web-based survey found the prevalence of previously diagnosed and active AD ranged from 2.1% to 4.9%.[31] Similar to the results of the National Health Interview Survey in the United States, AD prevalence was found to decrease from childhood to adolescence but remained stable into adulthood.[30,32] Together, it seems that the prevalence of AD in adults is similar to that in adolescents and is stable throughout adulthood. Globally, AD prevalence is often highest in high-income countries.[32,33]

It has been widely observed that AD shows a female preponderance, particularly in adolescence and adulthood.[32,34,35] This increased prevalence in female patients from puberty onward is also observed in other atopic disorders.[36]

HETEROGENEITY OF ATOPIC DERMATITIS
Morphology

AD is a heterogeneous disease with a broad spectrum of clinical manifestations. AD is highly polymorphic with a wide spectrum of lesions including acute oozing and crusting, subacute lesions with dryness and scaling, and chronic lesions with lichenification and/or prurigo nodules; erythema, excoriations, and dryness can occur at all stages of disease. In addition, there are myriad lesional morphologies that are present in AD, including nummular, psoriasiform, papular lichenoid lesions, and follicular eczema.

There are also several distinguishing clinical features that occur more commonly in some racial and ethnic groups than others. Erythema in skin of color often appears hyperpigmented or violaceous. A previous study of Nigerian patients with AD found that 54.1% had lichenoid lesions and 70.3% had a perifollicular, micropapular rash on the extensor aspects of the joints.[37]

A recent systematic review and meta-analysis of 101 studies identified 78 different clinical signs and characteristics of AD, with considerable variability by global region and patient age.[38] The review included 38 pediatric and 36 adult studies that reported a proportion of at least 1 AD feature with sufficient data for meta-analysis. Adults studies reported 2-fold or higher rates of erythroderma, Hertoghe sign (thinning or loss of outer third of eyebrows), hand eczema, papular lichenoid lesions, course influenced by emotions and/or environment, prurigo nodules, lichenification, nail involvement, nipple eczema, and nummular lesions. Thus, it seems that AD manifests differently in adults than in children, and in different races/ethnicities and regions.

Distribution

The distribution of lesions is also heterogeneous. In early childhood, lesions have a predilection for the face and extensor areas, whereas older children and adults tend to have flexural eczema. Adults, particularly those with adult onset or recurrence, seem to have a lesional predilection on the head/neck and hands.[39,40]

A recent US population-based study of 602 adults with AD found that the most common sites of skin lesions were reported to be the popliteal fossae, lower legs, dorsal feet, and antecubital fossae.[41] Other commonly reported sites include the face, scalp, hands, and genitals. Most persons with AD reported symmetry of lesions on the extremities. Most persons with active lesions in the antecubital or popliteal areas reported lesions elsewhere. There were no significant differences of lesional distribution by sex. Lesions on the trunk were significantly more common in black and Hispanic people. Age greater than or equal to 60 years was associated with a significantly higher proportion of lesions on the buttocks or genitals.

A statistical approach called latent class analysis was used to identify the dominant patterns of AD lesion distribution and revealed 5 different subsets. The most common subset (35.3% of adults with AD) consisted of lower probabilities of lesions affecting any sites, consistent with milder and less extensive disease. The second most common subset (26.9%) consisted of higher probabilities of lesions involving the anterior and posterior neck and trunk. The third most common subset (19.0%) consisted of higher probabilities of lesions involving the antecubital fossae and upper extremities. The fourth most common subset (9.7%) consisted of lesions involving the arms, posterior hands, genitals, and buttocks, and to a lesser extent face, palms, and legs. The least common subset (9.1%) consisted of higher probabilities of lesions affecting all sites, consistent with severe and more extensive disease.

Atopic Dermatitis Symptoms

There is a complex constellation of symptoms in AD, including pruritus, xerosis, pain, and sleep disturbance, which leads to a large impairment in quality of life.[27,42,43] A US population-based survey (AD in America study) found that pruritus was reported to be the most burdensome symptom by more than half of adults with AD (54.4%), followed by excessive dryness or scaling (19.6%) and red or inflamed skin (7.2%).[42] However, adults with moderate to severe AD in particular were less likely to report itch or excessive dryness and scaling as their most burdensome symptoms. Adults with moderate to severe AD were more likely to report that other symptoms were most burdensome, such as blisters or bumps, red or inflamed skin, sleep disturbance, pain, open sores, or oozing.

Pain

Skin pain has recently been recognized as an important symptom in AD. A prospective dermatology practice–based study of 305 adolescents and adults found that 42.7% of patients reported skin pain in the past week, with 13.8% reporting severe or very severe pain.[44] Skin pain was heterogeneous, with patients regarding pain as part of their itch (16.8%), secondary to scratching (11.2%), or both (72.0%). Patients with skin pain were more likely to describe their itch using descriptors similar to those used in neuropathic pain; for example, sharp, tingling, and pinpricklike. Patients with both severe itch and skin pain had even poorer quality of life and mental health symptoms than patients with either or neither being severe.

Pain from AD was reported in 61% of adults with AD from the AD in America study, of whom 33% experienced pain at least weekly and 22% reported severe pain (intensity ≥ 7).[45] AD pain was heterogeneous, with 27% reporting pain from open areas caused by scratching, 27% from fissures, 25% from inflamed red skin, and only 10% from burning secondary to creams or ointments. AD severity and pain were correlated overall. However, pain from scratching was more likely in mild AD; constant pain and pain from inflamed skin were more likely in severe AD. Overall, 3.8% and 8.2% of adults with AD from the AD in America study reported that pain was the most or second most burdensome symptom of their AD; the proportion increased in those with moderate-severe AD.[42] Optimal treatment approaches for pain in AD have not yet been examined.

Sleep disturbance

Patients with AD have sleep disturbances secondary to severe itch and secondary itch-scratch cycle,[46] poor sleep hygiene, circadian rhythm–induced modification of itch,[47] and potentially secondary effects of inflammatory cytokines on sleep regulation.[48] Adults with AD were found to have poor sleep quality with less sleep, more frequent and prolonged awakening, overall lower sleep efficiency, and increased daytime dysfunction.[49–53] A US population-based study of 34,613 adults (2012 National Health Interview Survey) found that adults with self-reported AD were more likely to report fatigue, regular daytime sleepiness and regular insomnia (25%–33%), and either short or long sleep duration.[27] Adults with AD and sleep disturbances reported poorer overall health status, and a higher number of sick days and doctor visits.[27] Another US population-based study of 5563 adults (2005–2006 National Health and Nutrition Examination Survey) found that adults with AD were more likely to report short sleep duration, trouble falling asleep, nighttime awakenings, early morning awakenings, leg jerks, and leg cramps during sleep. They were more likely to feel unrested, being overly sleepy during the day and feeling as if they did not get enough sleep.[43] Sleep disturbances are well recognized to have detrimental effects throughout all fields of medicine, including poor school and work performance; impaired health-related quality of life[49,54–57]; increased direct and indirect costs for patients, payers, and society[49,54,56–58]; psychological distress[59,60]; motor vehicle accidents; and workplace injury.[61–63] Together, sleep disturbances seem to be both common and burdensome in children and adults with AD. In addition, sleep disturbances may be an important mediator of poor outcomes and the development of comorbid health conditions in adults with AD.

Profound sleep disturbances despite optimized topical therapy for AD should prompt consideration for stepping up treatment using oral systemic therapy, biologics, or phototherapy. Patients with AD can develop poor sleep hygiene over many years of being unable to fall or stay asleep at night; for example, watching late night movies or infomercials, or consumption of large amounts of caffeine or other stimulants to overcome fatigue. Efforts should also be made to improve the sleep hygiene of patients with AD. Adjunctive treatments should be considered to improve the sleep of adults with AD. Sedating antihistamines may improve patients' sleep, even though there is insufficient evidence to support their efficacy as a treatment of itch or inflammation in AD.[64] A recent randomized controlled trial of 48 Taiwanese children with AD found high-dose melatonin (3 g/d) was well tolerated and resulted in modest improvements of AD severity and decreased sleep-onset latency.[65] In addition, referral to a sleep medicine specialist may be warranted when sleep disturbances do not improve with optimal control of AD and/or adjunctive treatments for sleep.

Age of Onset

AD is typically reported to begin in the first year of life in 50% of cases and by age 5 years in 85%.[66–68] However, the cited studies included cohorts of children, but did not assess adolescents or adults. As such, it is impossible to extrapolate about how commonly AD starts in adolescents or adults. Recent studies suggest there is considerable heterogeneity with respect to the course of AD in adults, including adult-onset AD.

A few studies examined whether adult-onset AD presents with distinct phenotypes compared with childhood-onset AD. Wang and colleagues[69] found that adult-onset AD (n = 407) versus pediatric-onset AD (n = 275) was associated with higher rates of dermatitis affecting the feet, with lower rates of dermatitis affecting the conjunctiva/eyelids (7.1% vs 21.8%), ears (9.6% vs 18.9%), and face (16.7% vs 51.3%). The study also found that adult-onset AD was more associated with the presence of vesicles and nodules (19.7% vs 9.8%; 13.8% vs 4%, respectively), and less associated with xerosis (55% vs 60.7%). Son and colleagues[70] found that adult-onset AD (n = 48) versus pediatric-onset AD (n = 232) was associated with higher rates of dermatitis affecting the head/neck (22.9% vs 16.4%), and possibly lower rates of dermatitis of the flexor surfaces of the extremities (29.2% vs 51.3%). The study also found that adult-onset AD was more associated with white dermatographism (4.2% vs 2.6%) and sign of Hertoghe (thinning or loss of outer third of eyebrows; 8.3% vs 3.9%), but less associated with xerosis (56.3% vs 63.8%) and pruritus after sweating (37.5% vs 51.3%). A recent study also examined phenotypical differences, and found that adult-onset AD (n = 149) versus pediatric-onset AD (n = 207) was associated with lower rates of dermatitis affecting the conjunctiva (24.2% vs 53.6%) and face (28.2% vs 57%); possibly more likely to present morphologically with nummular eczema (14.1% vs 5.8%); and was less associated with pruritus after sweating (60.4% vs 66.7%) and Dennie-Morgan fold (extra infraorbital crease; 10.7% vs 36.2%).[71] However, a US population-based study found no significant differences of lesional distribution by age of onset.

Patients with adult-onset AD were consistently found to have lower rates of conjunctivitis or any allergic disease in multiple studies, although higher rates of allergic rhinitis in some studies, lower rates of family history of allergic disease, but no differences in asthma.[72]

A systematic review and meta-analysis of 17 studies examining AD onset later than 10 years of age found that 26.1% of adults with AD reported adult onset of their disease overall, with all studies reporting substantial proportions of adult-onset AD.[72] AD onset was found to commonly occur even at middle and mature age. Most of the studies that found high proportions of childhood-onset AD only studied patients into early adulthood. Five studies retrospectively examined medical records and confirmed that patients with adult-onset AD did not have childhood AD.[39,40,73–75] Three studies followed patients prospectively and verified that the AD diagnosis was correct and did not change over time.[76–78] Thus, AD seems to commonly begin at all ages. Pediatric and adolescent studies may have missed this observation because they did not examine cohorts with older adults.

BURDEN OF ATOPIC DERMATITIS

AD is associated with a substantial patient burden and poor health-related quality of life secondary to its heterogeneous and often severe signs and symptoms.[79,80] The high prevalence and patient burden of AD made it one of the most burdensome skin disorders globally in 2013 in both children and adults.[81] A recent cross-sectional study of 2893 adults found significantly decreased short-form 6D health utility scores in adults with mild AD and even lower scores in moderate and severe AD.[82] AD was associated with higher total loss of quality of life–adjusted years than autoimmune disorders, diabetes, food allergy, and heart disease in both men and women, indicating a major population or societal burden.[82]

In the United States, adults with AD reported significantly limited access to care with inability to afford prescription medications and inability to get a timely medical appointment, both contributing to delay of care or inadequate treatment.[83]

AD may also affect performance at school and/or work. Roughly one-third of patients with AD thought that their disease affected their occupational performance; 14% thought that AD negatively influenced their career trajectory.[51] Previous studies found that adults with AD are more likely to take sick leave,[84,85] retire early,[84] and change occupation.[85,86] In the United States, adults with AD were more likely to have greater than or equal to 6 half-days in bed and greater than or equal to 6 lost workdays from all causes, with approximately 6 million lost workdays from their eczema.[83]

Health care Use for Adult Atopic Dermatitis

A US population-based survey (AD in America study) found that outpatient use for AD was low in adults with mild AD (29.3%–34.7%) and increased in those with moderate (36.2%–49.8%) and severe (50.6%–86.6%) AD. AD severity was the major predictor of outpatient use, followed by timeliness of appointments, expenses, and insurance coverage. One in 10 adults with AD reported having greater than or equal to 1 urgent care, emergency department or hospital visit in the past year. Urgent care or emergency department visits were more common among adults with black and Hispanic race/ethnicity, lower household income, lower education level, and AD prescriptions being denied by their insurance companies. Similarly, US adults with AD (2010 and 2012 National Health Interview Survey) had more visits to doctors, urgent/emergency care, and hospitalizations.[83]

A study of the patterns and predictors of outpatient use (1993–2015 National Ambulatory Medical Care Survey) found that AD visits occurred predominantly at primary care providers (PCPs), followed by dermatologists, and far less commonly allergists.[87] The frequency of AD visits increased from 1996 to 2015 overall and particularly among PCPs. However, the frequency of AD visits to dermatologists decreased over time.[87] Adults with self-pay were more likely to see a dermatologist, whereas adults with comorbid allergic rhinitis or food allergies were more likely to see an allergist.[87] AD visits were more likely to be acute visits among PCPs, and chronic visits among dermatologists.[87]

A study of emergency department use in the United States (2006–2012 National Emergency Department Sample) estimated that the incidence of emergency department visits for AD or eczema significantly increased between 2006 and 2012. Emergency department visits with versus without a primary diagnosis of AD were associated with Medicaid or no insurance and lower household income quartiles, and were more likely to occur during weekends and summer months. These results suggest there are socioeconomic and health care disparities with respect to emergency department use and access to care in general for AD. The total costs of emergency department visits for AD significantly increased, from $127,275,080 in 2006 to $265,541,084 in 2012. In addition, hospitalizations for AD or eczema were estimated to have $8,288,083 and $3,333,868 total annual costs per year for US adults and children (2002–2012 National Inpatient Sample).[88] Further, adults with AD were estimated to have $371 to $489 higher out-of-pocket costs per person-year compared with those without AD (2010 and 2012 National Health Interview Survey).[83] Together, the outpatient, emergency department and inpatient direct costs and indirect costs of AD are estimated to be approximately $5.2 billion annually in the United States.[89]

COMORBIDITIES OF ATOPIC DERMATITIS

Emerging research has shown that AD is associated with numerous medical and mental health comorbidities in adults. However, much of the research into these comorbidities is nascent. There is strong evidence to support the association of AD with atopic disease, as well as depression, anxiety, and suicidality.

Atopic Disease

Several US population-based studies examined the prevalence of atopic comorbidities in adults with AD. The lifetime and 1-year prevalences of self-reported asthma were 25.5% and 18.7%; 1-year prevalence of allergic rhinitis was 28.4%; and 1-year history of food allergy was 13.2% (2012 National Health Interview Survey).[90] The lifetime prevalence of asthma and allergic rhinitis and 1-year prevalence of food allergy were increased in adults with more severe AD.[91] Eosinophilic esophagitis has more recently been recognized as a comorbidity of AD and atopic disease.[92] Patients with AD, particularly those with severe AD, warrant increased screening for the presence and control of comorbid atopic disease. There is an enormous body of literature examining the relationship of AD with atopic comorbidities that is beyond the scope of this review. Of note, AD can present in the context of systemic atopy, and exposure to allergens may exacerbate the AD or make it difficult to control. Aeroallergens (eg, dust mite) can contribute to allergic asthma and rhinoconjunctivitis, and in some patients may contribute to AD. Inhalation of house dust mite has been shown to exacerbate AD in sensitized patients. Patients with allergic rhinoconjunctivitis may rub their eyes and face, thereby worsening their AD on the eyelids and face. Screening for systemic atopy, treatment such as nasal steroids, and aeroallergen avoidance might therefore result in improved skin disease in some individuals, in addition to improving allergic airway disease. However, recent systematic reviews and meta-analyses found no consistent evidence of efficacy for dust mite reduction and avoidance measures alone[93] or specific allergen immunotherapy[94] in treating AD. Moreover, dust mite avoidance was not found to be effective for primary prevention of AD.[95] For patients with a history of worsening or difficult-to-control AD, or those with signs or symptoms on exposure to 1 or more potential allergens, referral to an allergist should be considered. AD can also be exacerbated by food exposures in a small subset of patients with AD, particularly in infants and young children with severe AD.[96] However, a systematic review of 9 studies found no benefit for unselected egg and cow's milk elimination diets in AD.[97] In addition, foods as a cause of AD exacerbation in adults is extremely rare. Thus, patients with AD should not be advised to empirically eliminate different foods from their diet. Rather, appropriate food allergy testing by an allergist should be considered in patients with persistent AD in spite of optimized management and topical therapy and/or a reliable history of an immediate allergic reaction after ingestion of foods, with careful interpretation of test results.[98]

Depression, Anxiety, and Suicidality

Two systematic reviews and meta-analyses examined the relationship of AD with depression, suicidal ideation, and/or anxiety. The first performed a meta-analyses of depression (n = 23 studies), anxiety (n = 13 studies), and suicidality (n = 6 studies), and found significant higher odds ratio of depression and anxiety in adults with AD, depression in children with AD, and suicidality in adults and adolescents with AD.[99] The second performed a meta-analysis of 36 studies and found that 1 in 5 persons with AD had depression[100] and patients with AD had higher rates of clinical depression, antidepressant use, and suicidality in adults.[100] Depression occurred particularly in patients with moderate-severe AD.[100] AD was also associated with higher rates of depressive symptoms overall,[100] including having little interest in doing things, feeling down, feeling hopeless, feeling tired or having little energy, having a poor appetite, feeling bad about themselves, having difficulty concentrating, moving or speaking slowly or too fast, and having thoughts of being better off dead.[101]

Adults with AD had higher prevalences of abnormal (≥11) Hospital Anxiety and Depression Scale anxiety and depression subscores, particularly in more severe AD (AD in America study).[102] Importantly, 100% of respondents with severe scores for AD and itch had borderline or abnormal anxiety and depression scores. However, 13% to 55% of adults with AD who had borderline and/or abnormal anxiety or depression scores reported not being diagnosed with anxiety or depression. These results suggest that many patients with AD have undiagnosed anxiety and depression, and underscore the important of increased mental health screening in primary care and specialty practice settings.

Symptoms of anxiety and depression may be secondary to AD; that is, Diagnostic and Statistical Manual of Mental Disorders (DSM) IV Axis III disorders (secondary to a medical condition). In many (if not most) instances, these symptoms resolve with improved control of AD signs and symptoms. However, symptoms of anxiety and depression may be indicators of DSM-IV Axis I diagnoses, such as major depressive disorder or generalized anxiety disorder. It is important that clinicians managing patients with AD screen for anxiety and/or depression and treat or refer appropriately.

Other Comorbidities

Patients with AD were also found to have increased body mass index and/or obesity,[103,104] poor cardiovascular outcomes,[105] type II diabetes mellitus,[105] ocular complications such as atopic keratoconjunctivitis and keratoconus,[106–108] osteoporosis and fracture of bone or joint disease,[29,109] dental complications,[110] warts, and extracutaneous infections.[111] Many of these comorbidities are related to AD severity and poor long-term disease control. Future research is needed to determine the mechanisms of association between AD and comorbidities and optimize screening and treatment approaches for comorbidities.

DIAGNOSIS
Diagnostic Criteria

AD is diagnosed clinically based on a combination of history, physical examination, and ruling out other entities in the differential diagnosis. There are no specific diagnostic criteria for AD in adults. The diagnostic criteria of Hanifin and Rajka[112] (H-R) were developed for AD in children and adults in 1980 (**Box 1**) and are the most commonly used criteria in clinical trials of AD in both children and adults.[113] H-R criteria include flexural eczematous lesions as a major criterion. Early age of onset is a minor (but not major) criterion in H-R. Thus, a patient can meet the H-R criteria if they have adult-onset disease with flexural involvement. Further research is warranted to determine the optimal criteria for diagnosing adult-onset or adult-recurrent AD in clinical practice and trials. Formal diagnostic criteria are rarely used in clinical practice. However, they can be helpful in guiding clinicians toward the diagnosis of AD, particularly in adult-onset cases of eczema. However, all criteria for AD are imperfect. Other disorders, such as allergic contact dermatitis or cutaneous T-cell lymphoma, occasionally fulfill the clinical criteria for AD. Therefore, it is imperative that clinicians consider the broader differential diagnosis of AD in adults (**Box 2**). Of note, many disorders in the differential diagnosis of AD can mimic AD (eg, allergic

---

Box 1
Hanifin and Rajka diagnostic criteria for atopic dermatitis

- At least 3 major criteria:
  - Pruritus
  - Typical morphology and distribution (flexural lichenification/linearity in adults)
  - Chronic or chronically relapsing dermatitis
  - Personal or family history of atopy

- At least 3 of 23 minor criteria:
  - Xerosis
  - Ichthyosis, palmar hyperlinearity, or keratosis pilaris
  - Immediate skin-test reactivity
  - Increased serum IgE level
  - Early age of onset
  - Tendency toward cutaneous infections
  - Tendency toward nonspecific hand or foot dermatitis
  - Nipple eczema
  - Cheilitis
  - Recurrent conjunctivitis
  - Dennie-Morgan infraorbital fold
  - Keratoconus
  - Anterior subcapsular cataracts
  - Orbital darkening
  - Facial pallor or erythema
  - Pityriasis alba
  - Anterior neck folds
  - Itch when sweating
  - Intolerance to wool and lipid solvents
  - Perifollicular accentuation
  - Food intolerance
  - Course influenced by environmental or emotional factors
  - White dermatographism

From Hanifin J, Rajka G. Diagnostic features of atopic dermatitis. Acta Derm Venereol (Stockh) 1980;92(Suppl):44-47; with permission.

---

contact dermatitis or cutaneous T-cell lymphoma) or develop as comorbid diagnoses in patients with long-standing AD (eg, allergic or irritant contact dermatitis).

Biopsy

Diagnostic testing is not required but can support the diagnosis of AD and exclude alternate diagnoses. Biopsy should be considered for lesions that are atypical appearing and/or refractory to conventional therapy. A punch biopsy with standard hematoxylin-eosin staining can be helpful to exclude other disorders that have distinct histologic patterns; for example, cutaneous T-cell lymphoma, psoriasis, and cutaneous lupus. Acute eczematous lesions are characterized by epidermal spongiosis and dermal perivascular mononuclear infiltrates with eosinophils and a predominance of T cells and presence of eosinophils. Chronic eczematous lesions are characterized hyperkeratosis, epidermal hyperplasia, irregular elongation of the rete ridges, and variable amounts of spongiosis and dermal eosinophils. These histologic patterns are found in other eczematous disorders and cannot distinguish AD from other eczematous disorders, such as allergic contact dermatitis, irritant contact dermatitis, or nummular dermatitis. An additional punch biopsy of perilesional skin and examination using direct immunofluorescence may help exclude autoimmune blistering disorders, such as bullous pemphigoid and dermatitis herpetiformis. Biopsies and

Box 2
Differential diagnosis of adult-onset atopic dermatitis
Allergic contact dermatitis
Irritant contact dermatitis
Cutaneous T-cell lymphoma/Sezary syndrome
Psoriasis
Nummular dermatitis
Cutaneous lupus
Eczematous drug eruption
Dermatomyositis
Urticarial bullous pemphigoid
Dermatitis herpetiformis
Transient acantholytic dermatosis
Seborrheic dermatitis
Asteatotic eczema
Skin infection (ie, impetigo)
Molluscum dermatitis
Langerhans cell histiocytosis
Scabies
Zinc deficiency
Immunodeficiency (Wiskott-Aldrich syndrome, hyper-IgE syndrome)

histopathology have low reliability to distinguish between inflammatory skin diseases.[114] They cannot and should not substitute for a thorough history and physical examination.

Patch Testing

A multidisciplinary consensus guideline recommended that patch testing be performed in all patients with adolescent-onset or adult-onset AD, because allergic contact dermatitis can mimic AD.[115] Patients with AD that has worsened or become more generalized should also be patch tested, because there may be an allergenic trigger of their underlying AD. Patch testing is indicated in patients with a lesional distribution that is changing or atypical for AD, or one that is localized and suggestive of contact dermatitis, such as dermatitis of the head and neck, eyelids, hands, and feet. Nummular eczematous lesions can occur in patients with AD without evidence of allergic contact dermatitis,[71] but may be a sign of allergic contact dermatitis and warrant patch testing.[116,117]

Patients with AD have higher rates of positive patch test reactions to ingredients in their topical medications, including corticosteroids and antibiotics, and personal care products, including emollients, salves, and cleansers.[118–120] An expanded patch-testing screening series is recommended in order to assess these allergens, such as American Contact Dermatitis Society Core Allergen Series or North American Contact Dermatitis Group standard series, with supplemental allergen series as indicated.[120] The Thin-Layer Rapid Use Epicutaneous test lacks many of the allergens previously found to be relevant in patients with AD and is generally inadequate in patients with AD.[120]

Other Laboratory Tests

Skin scrapings with in-office microscopic evaluation may be warranted to exclude scabies or fungal infections, which are important clinical disorders to exclude in patients presenting for a new-onset pruritic dermatitis.

Skin prick testing, total serum IgE, allergen-specific IgE, and peripheral eosinophil levels are not required to diagnose AD. These tests are not useful in patients with suspected adult-onset AD, which has been shown to be associated with lower rates of atopy and atopic disease than child-onset AD.[72] Moreover, food allergy testing is not routinely recommended for the assessment of AD in children or adults.

A white blood cell count may reveal abnormalities secondary to lymphoma. Severe pruritus in general and even classic-appearing AD can develop in patients as a paraneoplastic disorder in non-Hodgkin lymphoma. Anecdotally, I have observed multiple cases of severe pruritus and/or AD appearing as early as 1 to 2 years before the diagnosis of lymphoma. All patients with elderly onset of AD should have close clinical follow-up and be up to date with all age-appropriate malignancy screenings. This scenario can also occur in younger patients and should be considered in the differential diagnosis of severe generalized pruritus.

Genetic testing may help exclude immunodeficiencies that manifest with AD, such as Job syndrome. Of note, extreme increases of total serum IgE level (>10,000 IU/mL) are commonly found in patients with AD, particularly in those with moderate to severe disease. However, such extreme increases are typically not associated with recurrent infections, skeletal abnormalities, or other stigmata of Job syndrome or other immunodeficiencies. Work-up for immunodeficiencies should be prompted by a relevant clinical history, and not only by very high IgE levels.

Other laboratory tests are rarely needed and the clinical scenario should guide their use. Antineutrophil cytoplasmic antibody may help exclude Churg-Strauss syndrome, which can manifest with a classic presentation of AD and/or asthma.[121] Antinuclear antibody, complement levels, erythrocyte sedimentation rate, and other laboratory testing may help exclude systemic lupus erythematosus or other autoimmune disorders. Indirect immunofluorescence may be helpful to exclude autoimmune blistering disease. Testing for human immunodeficiency virus (HIV) may be indicated to rule out atopiclike dermatitis in HIV in patients with specific risk factors and/or other stigmata of HIV (eg, increased infections).[122] Testing may be indicated for syphilis, which rarely can present with an eczematous pattern.[123]

TREATMENT

There are no treatment guidelines specifically for adult AD. Current AD treatment guidelines for adults and children recommend a step-care approach.[124,125] Patient education should encourage gentle skincare, bathing practices, trigger avoidance, and appropriate use of moisturizers and emollients. Regular tap water baths have been shown to be effective at reducing AD severity. A recent meta-analysis found that bleach baths were no more effective than water baths.[126] Patients should be encouraged to shower or bath daily using gentle nonsoap cleansers, avoid excessively prolonged water-exposure time or use of scalding hot water, and apply moisturizers immediately after drying off.[126] Patients may require additional application of moisturizers throughout the day to offset severe xerosis, particularly during colder weather months. The choice of emollients should be based on patient preference, with ointments generally being more effective and creams and lotions being more patient friendly. Moisturizers and emollients have shown good efficacy in AD and may have adequate efficacy as a monotherapy in the mildest forms of AD. However, they have inadequate efficacy as a monotherapy in many cases of mild AD and virtually all cases of moderate or severe AD. The next treatment step includes adding antiin-flammatory agents, such as topical corticosteroids (TCSs), calcineurin inhibitors (TCIs), and/or phosphodiesterase E4 (PDE4) inhibitors. Midpotency TCSs (eg, triam-cinolone and mometasone) can be applied to most body sites with AD lesions. Super-potent TCSs (eg, betamethasone and clobetasol) should be reserved for refractory lesions. Mild-potency TCS (eg, desonide or hydrocortisone) and steroid-sparing agents (eg, TCI and PDE4 inhibitors) can be used in sensitive areas, such as face, axillae, and groin. Once-daily application of TCS, TCI, or PDE4 inhibitors can be effec-tive to treat active lesions, although twice-daily is more effective than once-daily appli-cation. TCS should not be applied to the same skin areas daily for more than 3 to 4 consecutive weeks owing to concern about skin atrophy. TCS and TCI can also be applied proactively 1 to 2 times a week to clear skin in areas prone to flaring in order to prevent recurrent flares. When optimal use of topical therapy is inadequate, the next treatment step includes adding oral systemic therapy, biologic therapy, and/or photo-therapy. Patients with inadequate response to topical therapy in the primary care setting should be referred to an appropriate AD specialist for advanced treatment. Topical and/or oral antibiotics should only be used for frank skin infections, and are not recommended for the treatment of AD.[127]

SUMMARY

AD is common in adulthood, and is associated with a large patient-based and population-based burden. Adult AD shares many common features with childhood AD, although it has different epidemiology, immune phenotypes, and clinical manifes-tations in adults than in children. AD has a very negative effect on quality of life in both children and adults so referral to a specialist should be considered in patients whose AD is difficult to control or refractory to therapy. Newer, more targeted therapies, including biologics, are available but further research is necessary to better under-stand the pathogenesis and optimal treatment approaches in adult AD.

REFERENCES

1. Guttman-Yassky E, Nograles KE, Krueger JG. Contrasting pathogenesis of atopic dermatitis and psoriasis–part II: immune cell subsets and therapeutic concepts. J Allergy Clin Immunol 2011;127(6):1420–32.

2. Proksch E, Brasch J. Abnormal epidermal barrier in the pathogenesis of contact dermatitis. Clin Dermatol 2012;30(3):335–44.

3. Leung DY, Boguniewicz M, Howell MD, et al. New insights into atopic dermatitis. J Clin Invest 2004;113(5):651–7.

4. Larsen FS, Holm NV, Henningsen K. Atopic dermatitis. A genetic-epidemiologic study in a population-based twin sample. J Am Acad Dermatol 1986;15(3):487–94.

5. Schultz Larsen F. Atopic dermatitis: a genetic-epidemiologic study in a population-based twin sample. J Am Acad Dermatol 1993;28(5 Pt 1):719–23.

6. Rawlings AV, Harding CR. Moisturization and skin barrier function. Dermatol Ther 2004;17(Suppl 1):43–8.

7. Kezic S, Kemperman PM, Koster ES, et al. Loss-of-function mutations in the filaggrin gene lead to reduced level of natural moisturizing factor in the stratum corneum. J Invest Dermatol 2008;128(8):2117–9.
8. O'Regan GM, Sandilands A, McLean WH, et al. Filaggrin in atopic dermatitis. J Allergy Clin Immunol 2009;124(3 Suppl 2):R2–6.
9. Scharschmidt TC, Man MQ, Hatano Y, et al. Filaggrin deficiency confers a paracellular barrier abnormality that reduces inflammatory thresholds to irritants and haptens. J Allergy Clin Immunol 2009;124(3):496–506, 506.e1-6.
10. Rupnik H, Rijavec M, Korosec P. Filaggrin loss-of-function mutations are not associated with atopic dermatitis that develops in late childhood or adulthood. Br J Dermatol 2015;172(2):455–61.
11. Heede NG, Thyssen JP, Thuesen BH, et al. Anatomical patterns of dermatitis in adult filaggrin mutation carriers. J Am Acad Dermatol 2015;72(3):440–8.
12. Barker JN, Palmer CN, Zhao Y, et al. Null mutations in the filaggrin gene (FLG) determine major susceptibility to early-onset atopic dermatitis that persists into adulthood. J Invest Dermatol 2007;127(3):564–7.
13. Palmer CN, Irvine AD, Terron-Kwiatkowski A, et al. Common loss-of-function variants of the epidermal barrier protein filaggrin are a major predisposing factor for atopic dermatitis. Nat Genet 2006;38(4):441–6.
14. Chen H, Common JE, Haines RL, et al. Wide spectrum of filaggrin-null mutations in atopic dermatitis highlights differences between Singaporean Chinese and European populations. Br J Dermatol 2011;165(1):106–14.
15. Margolis DJ, Apter AJ, Gupta J, et al. The persistence of atopic dermatitis and filaggrin (FLG) mutations in a US longitudinal cohort. J Allergy Clin Immunol 2012;130(4):912–7.
16. Thawer-Esmail F, Jakasa I, Todd G, et al. South African amaXhosa patients with atopic dermatitis have decreased levels of filaggrin breakdown products but no loss-of-function mutations in filaggrin. J Allergy Clin Immunol 2014;133(1):280–2.e1-2.
17. Winge MC, Bilcha KD, Lieden A, et al. Novel filaggrin mutation but no other loss-of-function variants found in Ethiopian patients with atopic dermatitis. Br J Dermatol 2011;165(5):1074–80.
18. Mao XQ, Shirakawa T, Yoshikawa T, et al. Association between genetic variants of mast-cell chymase and eczema. Lancet 1996;348(9027):581–3.
19. Iwanaga T, McEuen A, Walls AF, et al. Polymorphism of the mast cell chymase gene (CMA1) promoter region: lack of association with asthma but association with serum total immunoglobulin E levels in adult atopic dermatitis. Clin Exp Allergy 2004;34(7):1037–42.
20. Tanaka K, Sugiura H, Uehara M, et al. Association between mast cell chymase genotype and atopic eczema: comparison between patients with atopic eczema alone and those with atopic eczema and atopic respiratory disease. Clin Exp Allergy 1999;29(6):800–3.
21. Oiso N, Fukai K, Ishii M. Interleukin 4 receptor alpha chain polymorphism Gln551Arg is associated with adult atopic dermatitis in Japan. Br J Dermatol 2000;142(5):1003–6.
22. Heine G, Hoefer N, Franke A, et al. Association of vitamin D receptor gene polymorphisms with severe atopic dermatitis in adults. Br J Dermatol 2013;168(4):855–8.
23. Tazawa T, Sugiura H, Sugiura Y, et al. Relative importance of IL-4 and IL-13 in lesional skin of atopic dermatitis. Arch Dermatol Res 2004;295(11):459–64.

24. Szegedi K, Lutter R, Res PC, et al. Cytokine profiles in interstitial fluid from chronic atopic dermatitis skin. J Eur Acad Dermatol Venereol 2015;29(11): 2136–44.
25. Esaki H, Brunner PM, Renert-Yuval Y, et al. Early-onset pediatric atopic dermatitis is TH2 but also TH17 polarized in skin. J Allergy Clin Immunol 2016;138(6): 1639–51.
26. Silverberg JI, Hanifin JM. Adult eczema prevalence and associations with asthma and other health and demographic factors: a US population-based study. J Allergy Clin Immunol 2013;132(5):1132–8.
27. Silverberg JI, Garg NK, Paller AS, et al. Sleep disturbances in adults with eczema are associated with impaired overall health: a US population-based study. J Invest Dermatol 2015;135(1):56–66.
28. Silverberg JI, Patel N, Immaneni S, et al. Assessment of atopic dermatitis using self-report and caregiver report: a multicentre validation study. Br J Dermatol 2015;173(6):1400–4.
29. Garg NK, Silverberg JI. Eczema is associated with osteoporosis and fractures in adults: a US population-based study. J Allergy Clin Immunol 2015;135(4): 1085–7.e2.
30. Harrop J, Chinn S, Verlato G, et al. Eczema, atopy and allergen exposure in adults: a population-based study. Clin Exp Allergy 2007;37(4):526–35.
31. Barbarot S, Auziere S, Gadkari A, et al. Epidemiology of atopic dermatitis in adults: Results from an international survey. Allergy 2018;73(6):1284–93.
32. Odhiambo JA, Williams HC, Clayton TO, et al. Global variations in prevalence of eczema symptoms in children from ISAAC Phase Three. J Allergy Clin Immunol 2009;124(6):1251–8.e23.
33. Shaw TE, Currie GP, Koudelka CW, et al. Eczema prevalence in the United States: data from the 2003 National Survey of Children's Health. J Invest Dermatol 2011;131(1):67–73.
34. Pesce G, Marcon A, Carosso A, et al. Adult eczema in Italy: prevalence and associations with environmental factors. J Eur Acad Dermatol Venereol 2015;29(6): 1180–7.
35. Sandstrom MH, Faergemann J. Prognosis and prognostic factors in adult patients with atopic dermatitis: a long-term follow-up questionnaire study. Br J Dermatol 2004;150(1):103–10.
36. Osman M. Therapeutic implications of sex differences in asthma and atopy. Arch Dis Child 2003;88(7):587–90.
37. Nnoruka EN. Current epidemiology of atopic dermatitis in south-eastern Nigeria. Int J Dermatol 2004;43(10):739–44.
38. Yew YW, Thyssen JP, Silverberg JI. A systematic review and meta-analysis of the regional and age-related differences in atopic dermatitis clinical characteristics. J Am Acad Dermatol 2019;80(2):390–401.
39. Ozkaya E. Adult-onset atopic dermatitis. J Am Acad Dermatol 2005;52(4): 579–82.
40. Bannister MJ, Freeman S. Adult-onset atopic dermatitis. Australas J Dermatol 2000;41(4):225–8.
41. Silverberg JI, Margolis DJ, Boguniewicz M, et al. Distribution of atopic dermatitis lesions in United States adults. J Eur Acad Dermatol Venereol 2019;33(7): 1341–8.
42. Silverberg JI, Gelfand JM, Margolis DJ, et al. Patient burden and quality of life in atopic dermatitis in US adults: A population-based cross-sectional study. Ann Allergy Asthma Immunol 2018;121(3):340–7.

43. Yu SH, Attarian H, Zee P, et al. Burden of sleep and fatigue in US adults with atopic dermatitis. Dermatitis 2016;27(2):50–8.

44. Vakharia PP, Chopra R, Sacotte R, et al. Burden of skin pain in atopic dermatitis. Ann Allergy Asthma Immunol 2017;119(6):548–52.e3.

45. Silverberg JI, Gelfand JM, Margolis DJ, et al. Pain is a common and burdensome symptom of atopic dermatitis in United States adults. J Allergy Clin Immunol Pract 2019. [Epub ahead of print].

46. Camfferman D, Kennedy JD, Gold M, et al. Eczema and sleep and its relationship to daytime functioning in children. Sleep Med Rev 2010;14(6):359–69.

47. Gupta AK, Cooper EA, Paquet M. Recurrences of dermatophyte toenail onychomycosis during long-term follow-up after successful treatments with mono- and combined therapy of terbinafine and itraconazole. J Cutan Med Surg 2013; 17(3):201–6.

48. Bender BG, Leung DY. Sleep disorders in patients with asthma, atopic dermatitis, and allergic rhinitis. J Allergy Clin Immunol 2005;116(6):1200–1.

49. Bender BG, Leung SB, Leung DY. Actigraphy assessment of sleep disturbance in patients with atopic dermatitis: an objective life quality measure. J Allergy Clin Immunol 2003;111(3):598–602.

50. Bender BG, Ballard R, Canono B, et al. Disease severity, scratching, and sleep quality in patients with atopic dermatitis. J Am Acad Dermatol 2008;58(3): 415–20.

51. Zuberbier T, Orlow SJ, Paller AS, et al. Patient perspectives on the management of atopic dermatitis. J Allergy Clin Immunol 2006;118(1):226–32.

52. Hanifin JM, Reed ML, Eczema P, et al. A population-based survey of eczema prevalence in the United States. Dermatitis 2007;18(2):82–91.

53. Torrelo A, Ortiz J, Alomar A, et al. Atopic dermatitis: impact on quality of life and patients' attitudes toward its management. Eur J Dermatol 2012;22(1):97–105.

54. Beikert FC, Langenbruch AK, Radtke MA, et al. Willingness to pay and quality of life in patients with atopic dermatitis. Arch Dermatol Res 2014;306(3):279–86.

55. Hon KL, Leung TF, Wong KY, et al. Does age or gender influence quality of life in children with atopic dermatitis? Clin Exp Dermatol 2008;33(6):705–9.

56. Ricci G, Bendandi B, Bellini F, et al. Atopic dermatitis: quality of life of young Italian children and their families and correlation with severity score. Pediatr Allergy Immunol 2007;18(3):245–9.

57. Beattie PE, Lewis-Jones MS. An audit of the impact of a consultation with a paediatric dermatology team on quality of life in infants with atopic eczema and their families: further validation of the Infants' Dermatitis Quality of Life Index and Dermatitis Family Impact score. Br J Dermatol 2006;155(6):1249–55.

58. Skaer TL, Sclar DA. Economic implications of sleep disorders. Pharmacoeconomics 2010;28(11):1015–23.

59. Schmitt J, Chen CM, Apfelbacher C, et al. Infant eczema, infant sleeping problems, and mental health at 10 years of age: the prospective birth cohort study LISAplus. Allergy 2011;66(3):404–11.

60. Romanos M, Gerlach M, Warnke A, et al. Association of attention-deficit/ hyperactivity disorder and atopic eczema modified by sleep disturbance in a large population-based sample. J Epidemiol Community Health 2010;64(3): 269–73.

61. Gander PH, Marshall NS, Harris RB, et al. Sleep, sleepiness and motor vehicle accidents: a national survey. Aust N Z J Public Health 2005;29(1):16–21.

62. Young T, Blustein J, Finn L, et al. Sleep-disordered breathing and motor vehicle accidents in a population-based sample of employed adults. Sleep 1997;20(8): 608–13.

63. Akerstedt T, Fredlund P, Gillberg M, et al. A prospective study of fatal occupational accidents – relationship to sleeping difficulties and occupational factors. J Sleep Res 2002;11(1):69–71.

64. Hoare C, Li Wan Po A, Williams H. Systematic review of treatments for atopic eczema. Health Technol Assess 2000;4(37):1–191.

65. Chang YS, Chou YT, Lee JH, et al. Atopic dermatitis, melatonin, and sleep disturbance. Pediatrics 2014;134(2):e397–405.

66. Kay J, Gawkrodger DJ, Mortimer MJ, et al. The prevalence of childhood atopic eczema in a general population. J Am Acad Dermatol 1994;30(1):35–9.

67. Nutten S. Atopic dermatitis: global epidemiology and risk factors. Ann Nutr Metab 2015;66(Suppl 1):8–16.

68. Spergel JM, Paller AS. Atopic dermatitis and the atopic march. J Allergy Clin Immunol 2003;112(6 Suppl):S118–27.

69. Wang X, Shi XD, Li LF, et al. Prevalence and clinical features of adult atopic dermatitis in tertiary hospitals of China. Medicine 2017;96(11):e6317.

70. Son JH, Chung BY, Kim HO, et al. Clinical features of atopic dermatitis in adults are different according to onset. J Korean Med Sci 2017;32(8):1360–6.

71. Silverberg JI, Vakharia PP, Chopra R, et al. Phenotypical differences of childhood- and adult-onset atopic dermatitis. J Allergy Clin Immunol Pract 2018; 6(4):1306–12.

72. Lee HH, Patel KR, Singam V, et al. A systematic review and meta-analysis of the prevalence and phenotype of adult-onset atopic dermatitis. J Am Acad Dermatol 2019;80(6):1526–32.e7.

73. Garmhausen D, Hagemann T, Bieber T, et al. Characterization of different courses of atopic dermatitis in adolescent and adult patients. Allergy 2013; 68(4):498–506.

74. Jaafar RB, Pettit JH. Atopic eczema in a multiracial country (Malaysia). Clin Exp Dermatol 1993;18(6):496–9.

75. Tay YK, Khoo BP, Goh CL. The profile of atopic dermatitis in a tertiary dermatology outpatient clinic in Singapore. Int J Dermatol 1999;38(9):689–92.

76. Johansson EK, Ballardini N, Bergstrom A, et al. Atopic and nonatopic eczema in adolescence: is there a difference? Br J Dermatol 2015;173(4):962–8.

77. Mortz CG, Andersen KE, Dellgren C, et al. Atopic dermatitis from adolescence to adulthood in the TOACS cohort: prevalence, persistence and comorbidities. Allergy 2015;70(7):836–45.

78. Punekar YS, Sheikh A. Establishing the sequential progression of multiple allergic diagnoses in a UK birth cohort using the General Practice Research Database. Clin Exp Allergy 2009;39(12):1889–95.

79. Weidinger S, Novak N. Atopic dermatitis. Lancet 2016;387(10023):1109–22.

80. Kim DH, Li K, Seo SJ, et al. Quality of life and disease severity are correlated in patients with atopic dermatitis. J Korean Med Sci 2012;27(11):1327–32.

81. Murray CJ, Vos T, Lozano R, et al. Disability-adjusted life years (DALYs) for 291 diseases and injuries in 21 regions, 1990-2010: a systematic analysis for the Global Burden of Disease Study 2010. Lancet 2012;380(9859):2197–223.

82. Silverberg JI, Gelfand JM, Margolis DJ, et al. Health Utility Scores of Atopic Dermatitis in US Adults. J Allergy Clin Immunol Pract 2019;7(4):1246–52.e1.

83. Silverberg JI. Health care utilization, patient costs, and access to care in US adults with eczema: a population-based study. JAMA Dermatol 2015;151(7):743–52.

84. Holm EA, Esmann S, Jemec GB. The handicap caused by atopic dermatitis–sick leave and job avoidance. J Eur Acad Dermatol Venereol 2006;20(3):255–9.

85. Nyren M, Lindberg M, Stenberg B, et al. Influence of childhood atopic dermatitis on future worklife. Scand J Work Environ Health 2005;31(6):474–8.

86. Drucker AM, Wang AR, Li WQ, et al. The burden of atopic dermatitis: summary of a report for the National Eczema Association. J Invest Dermatol 2017;137(1):26–30.

87. Singh P, Silverberg JI. Outpatient utilization patterns for atopic dermatitis in the United States. J Am Acad Dermatol 2019 Mar 15. https://doi.org/10.1016/j.jaad.2019.03.021 [Epub ahead of print]. [pii:S0190-9622(19)30435-30439].

88. Narla S, Hsu DY, Thyssen JP, et al. Inpatient financial burden of atopic dermatitis in the United States. J Invest Dermatol 2017 Jul;137(7):1461–7.

89. Lim HW, Collins SAB, Resneck JS Jr, et al. The burden of skin disease in the United States. J Am Acad Dermatol 2017;76(5):958–72.e2.

90. Hua T, Silverberg JI. Atopic dermatitis in US adults: epidemiology, association with marital status, and atopy. Ann Allergy Asthma Immunol 2018;121(5):622–4.

91. Silverberg JI, Gelfand JM, Margolis DJ, et al. Association of atopic dermatitis with allergic, autoimmune, and cardiovascular comorbidities in US adults. Ann Allergy Asthma Immunol 2018;121(5):604–12.e3.

92. Gonzalez-Cervera J, Arias A, Redondo-Gonzalez O, et al. Association between atopic manifestations and eosinophilic esophagitis: a systematic review and meta-analysis. Ann Allergy Asthma Immunol 2017;118(5):582–90.e2.

93. Nankervis H, Pynn EV, Boyle RJ, et al. House dust mite reduction and avoidance measures for treating eczema. Cochrane Database Syst Rev 2015;(1):CD008426.

94. Tam HH, Calderon MA, Manikam L, et al. Specific allergen immunotherapy for the treatment of atopic eczema: a Cochrane systematic review. Allergy 2016;71(9):1345–56.

95. Bremmer SF, Simpson EL. Dust mite avoidance for the primary prevention of atopic dermatitis: A systematic review and meta-analysis. Pediatr Allergy Immunol 2015;26(7):646–54.

96. Robison RG, Singh AM. Controversies in allergy: food testing and dietary avoidance in atopic dermatitis. J Allergy Clin Immunol Pract 2019;7(1):35–9.

97. Bath-Hextall F, Delamere FM, Williams HC. Dietary exclusions for improving established atopic eczema in adults and children. Syst Rev Allergy 2009;64(2):258–64.

98. Schneider L, Tilles S, Lio P, et al. Atopic dermatitis: a practice parameter update 2012. J Allergy Clin Immunol 2013;131(2):295–9.

99. Ronnstad ATM, Halling-Overgaard AS, Hamann CR, et al. Association of atopic dermatitis with depression, anxiety, and suicidal ideation in children and adults: a systematic review and meta-analysis. J Am Acad Dermatol 2018;79(3):448–56.e30.

100. Patel KR, Immaneni S, Singam V, et al. Association between atopic dermatitis, depression and suicidal ideation: a systematic review and meta-analysis. J Am Acad Dermatol 2019;80(2):402–10.

101. Yu SH, Silverberg JI. Association between atopic dermatitis and depression in US adults. J Invest Dermatol 2015;135(12):3183–6.

102. Silverberg JI, Gelfand JM, Margolis DJ, et al. Symptoms and diagnosis of anxiety and depression in atopic dermatitis in U.S. adults. Br J Dermatol 2019. [Epub ahead of print].

103. Silverberg JI, Becker L, Kwasny M, et al. Central obesity and high blood pressure in pediatric patients with atopic dermatitis. JAMA Dermatol 2015;151(2): 144–52.

104. Silverberg JI, Silverberg NB, Lee-Wong M. Association between atopic dermatitis and obesity in adulthood. Br J Dermatol 2012;166(3):498–504.

105. Silverberg JI, Greenland P. Eczema and cardiovascular risk factors in 2 US adult population studies. J Allergy Clin Immunol 2015;135(3):721–8.e6.

106. Hida T, Tano Y, Okinami S, et al. Multicenter retrospective study of retinal detachment associated with atopic dermatitis. Jpn J Ophthalmol 2000;44(4):407–18.

107. Chen JJ, Applebaum DS, Sun GS, et al. Atopic keratoconjunctivitis: A review. J Am Acad Dermatol 2014;70(3):569–75.

108. Bair B, Dodd J, Heidelberg K, et al. Cataracts in atopic dermatitis: a case presentation and review of the literature. Arch Dermatol 2011;147(5):585–8.

109. Garg N, Silverberg JI. Association between eczema and increased fracture and bone or joint injury in adults: a US population-based study. JAMA Dermatol 2015;151(1):33–41.

110. Silverberg JI, Simpson EL. Association between severe eczema in children and multiple comorbid conditions and increased healthcare utilization. Pediatr Allergy Immunol 2013;24(5):476–86.

111. Silverberg JI, Silverberg NB. Childhood atopic dermatitis and warts are associated with increased risk of infection: a US population-based study. J Allergy Clin Immunol 2014;133(4):1041–7.

112. Hanifin J, Rajka G. Diagnostic features of atopic eczema. Acta Derm Venereol (stockh) 1980;92(Suppl):44–7.

113. Vakharia PP, Chopra R, Silverberg JI. Systematic review of diagnostic criteria used in atopic dermatitis randomized controlled trials. Am J Clin Dermatol 2018;19(1):15–22.

114. Elston DM, Stratman EJ, Miller SJ. Skin biopsy: biopsy issues in specific diseases. J Am Acad Dermatol 2016;74(1):1–16 [quiz: 17–8].

115. Chen JK, Jacob SE, Nedorost ST, et al. A pragmatic approach to patch testing atopic dermatitis patients: clinical recommendations based on expert consensus opinion. Dermatitis 2016;27(4):186–92.

116. Bonamonte D, Foti C, Vestita M, et al. Nummular eczema and contact allergy: a retrospective study. Dermatitis 2012;23(4):153–7.

117. Krupa Shankar DS, Shrestha S. Relevance of patch testing in patients with nummular dermatitis. Indian J Dermatol Venereol Leprol 2005;71(6):406–8.

118. Rastogi S, Patel KR, Singam V, et al. Allergic contact dermatitis to personal care products and topical medications in adults with atopic dermatitis. J Am Acad Dermatol 2018;79(6):1028–33.e6.

119. Hamann CR, Hamann D, Egeberg A, et al. Association between atopic dermatitis and contact sensitization: A systematic review and meta-analysis. J Am Acad Dermatol 2017;77(1):70–8.

120. Owen JL, Vakharia PP, Silverberg JI. The role and diagnosis of allergic contact dermatitis in patients with atopic dermatitis. Am J Clin Dermatol 2018;19(3): 293–302.

121. Wang B, Li J, Shi W. A case of Churg-Strauss syndrome misdiagnosed as dermatitis. J Xiangya Med 2017;2(7).

122. Dlova NC, Mosam A. Inflammatory noninfectious dermatoses of HIV. Dermatol Clin 2006;24(4):439–48, vi.
123. Schnirring-Judge M, Gustaferro C, Terol C. Vesiculobullous syphilis: a case involving an unusual cutaneous manifestation of secondary syphilis. J Foot Ankle Surg 2011;50(1):96–101.
124. Boguniewicz M, Fonacier L, Guttman-Yassky E, et al. Atopic dermatitis yardstick: Practical recommendations for an evolving therapeutic landscape. Ann Allergy Asthma Immunol 2018;120(1):10–22.e12.
125. Eichenfield LF, Tom WL, Berger TG, et al. Guidelines of care for the management of atopic dermatitis: Section 2. Management and treatment of atopic dermatitis with topical therapies. J Am Acad Dermatol 2014;71(1):116–32.
126. Chopra R, Vakharia PP, Sacotte R1, et al. Efficacy of bleach baths in reducing severity of atopic dermatitis: A systematic review and meta-analysis. Ann Allergy Asthma Immunol 2017;119(5):435–40.
127. Eichenfield LF, Tom WL, Berger TG, et al. Guidelines of care for the management of atopic dermatitis: section 2. Management and treatment of atopic dermatitis with topical therapies. J Am Acad Dermatol 2014;71(1):116–32.

Mast Cell Activation
When the Whole Is Greater than the Sum of Its Parts

Dilawar Khokhar, MD, Cem Akin, MD, PhD*

KEYWORDS

- Mast cell activation • MCAS • Mast cell disorder • Mastocytosis
- Idiopathic anaphylaxis • Tryptase • Mast cell mediators

KEY POINTS

- Mast cell activation syndrome (MCAS) is a rare, distinct clinical entity with severe episodic symptoms of mast cell activation associated with elevated mast cell mediators.
- Idiopathic anaphylaxis should be viewed as the prototypical manifestation of MCAS and can be used to establish a framework for evaluation.
- No single sign, symptom, or laboratory test is sufficient for the diagnosis of MCAS.
- Therapy for MCAS is based on avoidance of triggers and antimediator therapy.

INTRODUCTION

Mast cells are important immunomodulatory cells that are located at the junction of the internal and external environment and release a host of mediators that have significant downstream effects.[1,2] When they are dysfunctional, their location and mediator release result in a broad range of symptoms. One entity that highlights this is mast cell activation syndrome (MCAS). MCAS is a heterogeneous and rare disorder with episodic and severe activation of mast cells.[3–9] Because symptoms of mast cell activation (MCA) are nonspecific, it is important to base the diagnosis on the best available clinical and scientific evidence, and not make it one of exclusion. MCAS, much like the mast cell itself, as a whole is greater than the sum of its proposed diagnostic criteria. When each component is considered in isolation, criteria can seem nonspecific, and thus, a broad constellation of symptoms can be attributed to MCAS when they may be due to other disease processes. Nonspecific symptoms can make it challenging for clinicians to correctly identify MCAS and is equally frustrating for patients who may undergo expensive and unnecessary workups or receive ineffective treatment of their symptoms as a result of

Department of Internal Medicine, Division of Allergy and Clinical Immunology, University of Michigan, 24 Frank Lloyd Wright Drive, Lobby H Suite H-2100, Ann Arbor, MI 48106, USA
* Corresponding author.
E-mail address: cemakin@med.umich.edu

Med Clin N Am 104 (2020) 177–187
https://doi.org/10.1016/j.mcna.2019.09.002
0025-7125/20/© 2019 Elsevier Inc. All rights reserved.

medical.theclinics.com

misdiagnosis.[10,11] It is thus essential to develop a systematic approach when considering the diagnosis of MCAS.

THE MAST CELL AND ITS DISORDERS

The mast cell is a granulocytic cell first described by Paul Ehrlich in 1877.[12] Since their discovery, mast cells have been implicated in several physiologic and pathogenic processes. Although they are best known for their role as the effector cells of immediate type hypersensitivity reactions, they play an important role as immunomodulatory cells, releasing a host of proinflammatory as well as anti-inflammatory mediators affecting the interaction of the immune system with the surrounding microenvironment.[12,13] Their location in connective tissue, the gastrointestinal (GI) tract, and the respiratory tract allows them to often be a first responder when there is a change in environment.[12,13] Dysfunction of mast cells thus can manifest across several different organ systems. MCA may occur at the local level (such as in urticaria) or systemically (as is the case in anaphylaxis).[14] There is no specific symptom or afflicted organ system for mast cell dysfunction, so it is important to establish a systematic approach or framework when considering a mast cell disorder (MCD) in a given patient.

MCDs can be thought of as primary, secondary, or idiopathic.[7,9] In primary MCDs, there is an intrinsic defect within the mast cell or its progenitors resulting in pathologic condition (Table 1). Because these disorders are due to an intrinsic cell defect, they are typically clonal disorders that are associated with KIT mutation and include conditions such as systemic mastocytosis.[8,15–17] In secondary MCDs, there is a primary disease process, such as immunoglobulin E (IgE)-mediated hypersensitivity, that results in mast cell degranulation (nonclonal MCA).[7,9] Finally, there are idiopathic MCDs whereby no specific mast cell deficiency or systemic disease triggering MCA is identified, but MCA occurs.[7,9] MCAS is a severe form of episodic MCA that may be associated with primary, secondary, or idiopathic MCD.

DEFINING MAST CELL ACTIVATION SYNDROME

Various criteria have been proposed for the diagnosis of MCAS.[4,18] The authors strongly recommend the following criteria, which have been accepted by an international group of experts and is based on best available evidence[3–9]:

1. Episodic and recurrent symptoms of mast cell mediator release affecting 2 or more organ systems
2. Complete resolution of symptoms or decrease in the frequency or severity of symptoms with antimast cell mediator therapy (antihistamines, leukotriene modifiers, and mast cell stabilizer agents)
3. Evidence of an increase in a validated urinary or serum marker of MCA (ideally with reproducible results obtained during more than 1 symptomatic episode)

Table 1 Examples of mast cell disorders	
MCD Type	**Examples**
Primary	Mastocytosis, monoclonal mast cell activation syndrome (MMAS), mast cell sarcoma, mastocytoma
Secondary	IgE-mediated hypersensitivity, physical urticarias, mast cell hyperplasia (owing to systemic disease such as chronic infection or autoimmune disease)
Idiopathic	MCAS, idiopathic anaphylaxis, chronic idiopathic urticaria/angioedema

It is important to remember that such criteria may apply to primary, secondary, or idiopathic MCA, and the workup for primary and secondary causes may be pursued concurrently. There is no single pathognomonic clinical presentation for MCAS, and thus, it is essential that all 3 consensus criteria be fulfilled before the diagnosis of MCAS is established. An important consideration when assessing for idiopathic MCAS is whether the patient meets criteria for idiopathic anaphylaxis. Idiopathic anaphylaxis is defined as anaphylaxis that is not explained by a presumed or proven cause or stimulus.[12] It is considered a distinct clinical entity, but in the authors' point of view, it should be considered a subtype of MCAS that meets the diagnostic criteria for anaphylaxis because the only effector cells of anaphylaxis in humans are mast cells.[3,15,19] Thus, idiopathic MCAS is a broader entity that includes idiopathic anaphylaxis (IA) and may be a more appropriate term for the patients whose episodes may not meet the clinical definition of anaphylaxis, or who may experience idiopathic episodes mixed with episodes owing to particular triggers. This may be difficult to differentiate from patients with chronic urticaria and angioedema who may also experience extracutaneous symptoms, which can be features of both secondary and idiopathic MCA.[3] This is where the paradigm of IA as the archetypal form of MCAS is helpful because patients with anaphylactic features in which the symptoms involving multiple organ systems occur in distinct episodes are more likely to have an underlying MCAS.[3]

MAST CELL MEDIATORS AND CLINICAL MANIFESTATIONS

In order to gain a better understanding of MCA, one must first characterize mast cell mediators as well as their clinical manifestations (**Table 2**). Perhaps the most well-studied mast cell mediator is histamine. Histamine is a biogenic amine compound that was first described by Henry H. Dale and P.P. Laidlaw in 1910.[20] It is predominantly stored in mast cells and in basophil granules.[21] Histamine exerts its effects in the human body via G-coupled protein receptors.[20] It has a multitude of effects, including modulation of local immune responses, itching, the sleep-wake cycle, body temperature, bronchoconstriction, and vasodilation, to name a few.[20] This underscores the importance of mast cells in maintaining homeostasis and is perhaps one of the reasons that disorders of mast cells manifest with such nonspecific symptoms across a host of different organ systems. Despite its central role in the generation of symptoms of MCDs, assessment of histamine in the clinical setting remains of limited utility. This is due to the variability of blood and urine levels because histamine is influenced by several extrinsic factors, including the method by which samples are obtained and stored, as well as diet.[3,22] Elevated urinary histamine metabolites (eg, N-methylhistamine) may support the diagnosis of a MCD,[3,22] especially when associated with other mediator elevations, but age and disease-specific cutoffs in MCAS

Table 2	
Common manifestations of mast cell mediator release	
System	**Symptoms**
Skin	Urticaria, angioedema, flushing
GI	Nausea, vomiting, diarrhea, abdominal cramping
Respiratory	Wheezing
Nasal/ocular	Conjunctival injection, pruritus, nasal congestion
Vascular	Hypotension

have not been extensively studied, and a single elevated level should be evaluated in the appropriate clinical context and in the presence of other criteria supporting the diagnosis. Available data on patient perceptions of MCDs suggest that patients perceive significant difficulty with establishing a diagnosis of MCD,[10] 1 factor that likely contributes to this variance in interpretation of mast cell mediator studies.[10] In the authors' clinical experience, isolated elevations in a single mediator are generally insufficient to establish a diagnosis. If elevations in mast cell mediators are identified, patients should be referred to a specialist with experience in diagnosing and treating MCDs because MCA markers may need to be repeated to verify the diagnosis.

Prostaglandin D2 is an eicosanoid synthesized and released by mast cells[23,24] within a few minutes of MCA. It plays an important role in the generation of immune responses, including recruitment of T lymphocytes, eosinophils, and basophils.[25,26] One of its primary clinical effects is bronchial airway constriction, particularly in asthma after contact with aeroallergens.[25,26] Metabolites of prostaglandin D2, including 11-β-prostaglandin F2α, can be measured in the urine.[27] Prostaglandin D2, while primarily released by mast cells, is also found in other immune and nonimmune cell types, including macrophages, T lymphocytes, platelets, and the central nervous system.[25,27] This is important to recognize because elevations in prostaglandin D2 may be due to processes independent of MCA.

Leukotrienes have long been known to play a central role in inflammation and many allergic diseases.[20] Leukotriene C4 (LTC4) is an arachidonic acid derivative that is released by mast cells[22] and undergoes metabolism into leukotriene D4 and then to E4.[29,30] LTC4 has been implicated in several disease states, including asthma, allergic rhino-conjunctivitis, and atopic dermatitis.[29] LTE4 can be detected in the urine and thus can be used as a potential marker of MCA, although the degree of elevation correlating with various MCDs has not been well defined. Patients with predominant respiratory, nasal, or ocular symptoms may have a greater release of leukotrienes and thus represent a target phenotype in MCDs for antileukotriene therapies.

The most specific marker of MCA is tryptase, a serine protease predominantly associated with mast cells.[31–33] Mast cell tryptase can be categorized into 2 major groups, a protryptase (mainly encoded by the α-tryptase gene in TPSAB1 locus), which lacks enzymatic activity, and mature tryptase (predominantly encoded by the β-tryptase gene at the same locus).[33–36] β-Tryptase is the form stored in mast cell granules and is increased after MCA, whereas α-tryptase is a proenzyme that is secreted outside of the cells and thus is the form of tryptase detected in the blood at baseline conditions.[33–35] There is an increase in β-tryptase when mast cell granulation occurs with peak levels occurring at approximately 1 hour and mostly returning to baseline levels by 4 hours.[33–35] A normal tryptase level is typically considered 5 ng/mL or less. A level greater than 11.4 ng/mL is considered elevated by most clinical diagnostic laboratories. An elevated baseline tryptase level can be indicative of increased mast cell burden, and a level of greater than 20 ng/mL is a minor diagnostic criterion for the diagnosis of systemic mastocytosis.[37] A change of 20% of baseline tryptase plus 2 ng/mL is indicative of a MCA episode.[37] Thus, a normal tryptase level at baseline does not exclude MCA. Many patients may have baseline normal tryptase levels that increase acutely with MCA episodes, especially with systemic symptoms, such as hypotension. It is paramount to obtaining more than 1 tryptase level when assessing for MCAS, ideally a baseline level and level drawn shortly after onset of symptoms (preferably 1 hour or less after onset of symptoms).

The biological activities of tryptase include cleaving of extracellular substrates, such as vasoactive intestinal peptide, kininogens, and fibronectin, as well as stimulating the release of various inflammatory mediators, such as interleukin-8 (IL-8).[31–33] It has been implicated in the upregulation of intercellular adhesion molecule-1 as well as increased messenger RNA expression for IL-1β.[32] In addition, tryptase release from activated mast cells may stimulate secretion from neighboring mast cells.[32] These constellations of findings support tryptase as more than just a marker of MCA, but an enzyme that plays an important role in the immunologic cascade that occurs after mast cell degranulation.

Although tryptase is the most specific marker for MCA, it can be elevated by other processes, including chronic kidney disease, myeloid neoplasms, hypereosinophilic syndromes, and hereditary αhypertryptasemia (HAT).[32,34,38] HAT is important to consider because it represents a pitfall for clinicians in the evaluation of MCAS. It is a recently described condition whereby there is overproduction of α-tryptase owing to copy number variations of the α-tryptase gene encoded at the TPSAB1 locus and is estimated to be present in 6% of the population.[38] The clinical significance of HAT is currently investigated, but mast cells from individuals with HAT do not seem to have a hyperreleasable phenotype. The genetic test for tryptase copy number variation is available clinically (genebygene.com), but may not be covered by insurance.

Historically, another important consideration when evaluating elevated tryptase levels has been laboratory interference.[39] Heterophilic antibodies, such as rheumatoid factor and human antimurine antibodies, have been reported to interfere with immunoassays, such as the tryptase laboratory assay.[39,40] Since the recognition of this phenomenon, commercial tryptase laboratory assays have introduced heterophilic blocking agents to resolve this laboratory interference. This again demonstrates the importance of interpreting laboratory results in the proper clinical context. In the authors' clinical experience, laboratory interference is now an uncommon occurrence, but any suspicious results should be repeated. Providers may need to contact specific laboratories directly to verify if heterophilic blocking agents are used when the tryptase assay is run. It is critical to correctly identify significant tryptase elevation, because bone marrow biopsy may be indicated for evaluation for systemic mastocytosis and other clonal MCDs.[9]

DIFFERENTIAL DIAGNOSIS

The symptoms attributed to MCA, such as flushing, are nonspecific and can be attributed to several different diagnoses, thus leading to a broad differential.[41] Conditions not carrying the typical hallmark symptom of anaphylaxis and those with chronic daily rather than episodic presentation represent a particular challenge for clinicians because it is difficult to ascribe these to MCA with any degree of certainty (**Box 1**).

The differential diagnosis for MCAS can be overwhelming to the point where it may seem any collective of symptoms is attributable to MCAS. In the authors' opinion, it is helpful to view MCAS from the perspective of anaphylaxis as the quintessential presentation. MCAS, like anaphylaxis, should be seen as a severe systemic reaction that is the result of mast cell mediator release. Most cases should have clinical features of anaphylaxis. The authors recognize that this view does not address patients with less severe or localized forms of MCA, and further investigation to categorize these patients is needed.

MANAGEMENT OF MAST CELL ACTIVATION SYNDROME

The cornerstones of MCAS management are avoidance of triggers (exposures that result in direct mast cell degranulation; **Table 3**) and pharmacologic therapies targeting mast cell mediators. A broad array of exposures has been described as direct mast cell triggers.[3,4] One of the most common triggers identified by

---

Box 1
Selected diagnoses considered in differential diagnosis of mast cell activation syndrome

Dysautonomia, including POTS and vasovagal syncope

Endocrine: Carcinoid syndrome, pheochromocytoma, medullary thyroid tumor, adrenal insufficiency

Skin: Rosacea, benign idiopathic flushing, contact or atopic dermatitis, chronic urticaria, dermatomyositis

Neuropsychiatric: Anxiety or panic attacks, seizure disorder, multiple sclerosis, somatoform disorder, eating disorders

Hereditary α tryptasemia

Hereditary or acquired angioedema

Gastrointestinal: Irritable bowel syndrome, inflammatory bowel disease, cyclic vomiting, peptic ulcer disease, eosinophilic gastrointestinal disorders

Cardiac: Arrythmias, coronary artery disease

Drug adverse effects: Niacin-induced flushing, steroid toxicity, withdrawal of adrenergic medications, exposure to sympathomimetics, anticholinergic toxicity, caffeine effect, alcohol use/withdrawal

Abbreviation: POTS, postural orthostatic tachycardia syndrome.

---

patients for symptoms is food.[10] IgE-mediated food reactions are known secondary MCDs,[7,9] but there are limited data on the role of histamine-containing foods in MCAS, and to date, there are no trials demonstrating the benefit of low-histamine diets in MCAS.[3]

It is in the context of history and reported triggers that an allergic evaluation may be appropriate to help guide avoidance strategies. Different patients may have different triggers; thus, counseling on avoidance should be individualized.

Because mast cells release a plethora of mediators, several different antimediator therapies have been used for the treatment of MCAS.[14,42] Perhaps the most common therapy used in MCAS is antihistamines.[43] This is likely due to clinical experience with these agents, low cost, and favorable side-effect profile. The most common second-generation H1 blockers include cetirizine/levocetirizine, fexofenadine, and loratadine/desloratadine. The authors prefer second-generation H1 blockers because they are of equal or greater efficacy as first-generation antihistamines, are less sedating, have less anticholinergic properties, and have a longer duration of action. First-generation antihistamines, such as diphenhydramine, may be useful for breakthrough symptoms on an as-needed basis. Special consideration should be given to the H1 blocker Ketotifen, which also functions as a mast cell stabilizer. It has been shown

---

Table 3
Exposures that have been implicated in direct mast cell degranulation

Venoms	Hymenoptera stings, jellyfish, snakes
Drugs	Narcotics, radiocontrast, aspirin/NSAIDs, muscle relaxants, antibiotics
Temperature	Heat or cold
Mechanical stimuli	Friction, pressure, or tissue trauma (surgery, biopsy, or endoscopy)
Miscellaneous	Alcohol, emotional stress, exercise, infections

to be helpful in steroid-dependent idiopathic anaphylaxis,[12] and in the authors' experience, is often helpful as a step-up therapy in MCAS. Ketotifen is not Food and Drug Administration approved in oral form in the United States, but can be obtained through compounding pharmacies.

H2 blockers, such as ranitidine or famotidine, have been used as adjunctive medications for patients with MCAS.[14,42] Given that H2 receptors are primarily present in the GI tract, H2 blockers may have greater effect for patients with GI-predominant symptoms. They may also help alleviate skin symptoms in conjunction with H1 antihistamines.

Leukotriene antagonists and 5-lipoxygenase inhibitors have also been used as adjunctive medications.[14,42] Available agents in clinical practice include montelukast, zafirlukast, and zileuton. Given the role leukotrienes play in airway inflammation and the generation of bronchospasm, these agents may be of greater benefit in patients with wheezing or respiratory predominant symptoms.

Cromolyn is a mast cell stabilizer that has been used for the treatment of mastocytosis in oral formulation.[14,42] Oral form has poor GI absorption and thus has limited systemic effects. Given that it remains primarily in the GI tract, it may have potential benefit in patients with primary GI symptoms as an adjunctive medication.

Glucocorticoids have been used as therapy for MCDs, including MCAS.[14,42] Their primary role is as a therapy for patients with severe refractory symptoms. There are no controlled trials evaluating the efficacy of steroids in acute treatment of anaphylaxis. Glucocorticoid medications have a significant side-effect profile and many negative long-term effects. Side effects, including flushing, and GI irritation may be confused as symptoms of MCA. They should not be used as a first-line therapy for MCAS, and if used, should be tapered to the lowest dose that controls the patient's symptoms.

Aspirin has been used as a medication for the treatment of MCAS.[44] Aspirin is a cyclooxygenase inhibitor and thus reduces the production of prostaglandins, including PGD2 implicated in MCA pathologic condition. It has been suggested that patients with high urinary prostaglandin metabolite levels may benefit from aspirin therapy the most.[44] The patient's tolerance of aspirin and nonsteroidal anti-inflammatory drugs (NSAIDs) should be known before considering treatment because severe allergic or idiosyncratic reactions occur in some patients.

Omalizumab is an anti-IgE monoclonal antibody that is currently approved for treatment of allergic asthma and chronic spontaneous urticaria, but also has been used off-label in cases of MCAS recalcitrant to other medical therapies.[13,14,42] Omalizumab binds to free IgE and reduces the density of IgE receptors on mast cells (FCeR1) and thus may reduce stimuli for mast cell mediator release.[13] In addition to its use for patients with severe recalcitrant disease, it may be helpful in liberating steroid-dependent patients from steroids.

There are no randomized clinical trials to demonstrate which medication regimen is superior for MCAS. Several different approaches may be taken, including combination therapy, with gradual tapering once symptom control has been achieved versus a step-up approach whereby patients are started on 1 or 2 agents with additional agents considered if adequate symptom control is not achieved. Factors that may help select 1 agent over another include patient symptoms and measured mediator levels as previously mentioned. Other considerations include cost, insurance coverage, and patient tolerability. In the authors' experience, most patients require at least a daily H1 blocker.

Cytoreductive and signal transduction inhibitor therapies have been used in primary MCDs, such as mastocytosis.[8,42] These treatment modalities are not well studied in nonclonal MCDs, such as MCAS, and are not usually recommended in such settings.

WHEN TO REFER

No discussion of MCAS would be complete without discussing when referral to a specialist is warranted. In the authors' point of view, the following patients would derive the most benefit for evaluation by a specialist for MCDs, including MCAS:

- Patients diagnosed with idiopathic anaphylaxis
- Patients with systemic or cutaneous mastocytosis
- Patients with *severe episodic* symptoms attributable to mast cell release
- Patients with *episodic* symptoms *responsive to antihistamines*
- Patients with persistently elevated or event related increase in tryptase

In the authors' allergy clinical practice, they have also found many patients with a multitude of nonepisodic symptoms referred for MCAS evaluation. More research is clearly needed to evaluate whether there are nonclassical chronic presentations of MCA disorders. The authors' experience is that typically patients presenting with chronic ongoing symptoms of multiple chemical and environmental intolerances, chronic disabling fatigue, multiple food intolerances with negative allergy testing resulting in failure to thrive and severe nutritional deficiencies, and patients whose symptoms do not improve on antimediator (eg, H1 antihistamine therapy) are not likely to substantially benefit from an allergist referral, because there remains no objective evidence to implicate a central primary MCD in pathogenesis of these conditions. Some of these patients with complex presentations involving multiple chronic organ system symptoms may have secondary or reactive MCA, and some symptoms, such as itching and flushing, may respond to H1 antihistamine therapy, but this is usually not the disabling or a life-threatening component of their presentation. It is therefore important to identify the underlying pathologic condition causing secondary mast cell activation, because focusing solely on MCA may delay the appropriate workup and treatment of the underlying disorder. These patients are best approached through a multidisciplinary effort with the primary care physician playing a central role as a team leader and synthesizing the data from multiple subspecialists.

FUTURE DIRECTIONS

When all 3 consensus criteria are fulfilled, MCAS represents a rare distinct clinical entity. Unfortunately, this does not address patients with less severe and more localized symptoms owing to MCA, and more refined diagnostic criteria are needed for less severe or secondary forms of MCA. This requires not only continued efforts in understanding mast cell biology and signal transduction but also clinical identification of more useful surrogate markers of MCA in addition to those discussed above. Ehlers-Danlos syndrome and postural orthostatic tachycardia syndrome have been clinically reported to occur with MCAS, but concrete epidemiologic and pathophysiologic evidence for mast cell involvement is lacking. Finally, clinical phenotype of HAT needs to be studied in larger cohorts to see if it is indeed a susceptibility factor for MCAS. New drug development using new agents targeting known mast cell mediator or signal transduction pathways should be pursued and may help not only with treatment of MCAS but also with more common allergic disorders in which mast cells are involved.

DISCLOSURE

Dr D. Khokhar has nothing to disclose. Dr C. Akin has consultancy agreements with Blueprint Medicines and Novartis.

REFERENCES

1. Da silva EZ, Jamur MC, Oliver C. Mast cell function: a new vision of an old cell. J Histochem Cytochem 2014;62(10):698–738.
2. Krishnaswamy G, Kelley J, Johnson D, et al. The human mast cell: functions in physiology and disease. Front Biosci 2001;6:D1109–27.
3. Akin C. Mast cell activation syndromes. J Allergy Clin Immunol 2017;140(2): 349–55.
4. Akin C, Valent P, Metcalfe DD. Mast cell activation syndrome: proposed diagnostic criteria. J Allergy Clin Immunol 2010;126:1099–104.e4.
5. Theoharides TC, Valent P, Akin C. Mast cells, mastocytosis, and related disorders. N Engl J Med 2015;373(2):163–72.
6. Valent P, Akin C, Bonadonna P, et al. Proposed diagnostic algorithm for patients with suspected mast cell activation syndrome. J Allergy Clin Immunol Pract 2019; 7(4):1125–33.e1.
7. Valent P. Mast cell activation syndromes: definition and classification. Allergy 2013;68(4):417–24.
8. Valent P, Akin C, Metcalfe DD. Mastocytosis: 2016 updated WHO classification and novel emerging treatment concepts. Blood 2017;129:1420–7.
9. Weiler CR, Austen KF, Akin C, et al. AAAAI mast cell disorders committee work group report: mast cell activation syndrome (MCAS) diagnosis and management. J Allergy Clin Immunol 2019;144(4) [pii:S0091-6749(19)31116-9].
10. Jennings SV, Slee VM, Zack RM, et al. Patient perceptions in mast cell disorders. Immunol Allergy Clin North Am 2018;38(3):505–25.
11. Valent P, Akin C. Doctor, I think I am suffering from MCAS: differential diagnosis and separating facts from fiction. J Allergy Clin Immunol Pract 2019;7(4): 1109–14.
12. Greenberger PA, Lieberman P. Idiopathic anaphylaxis. J Allergy Clin Immunol Pract 2014;2(3):243–50.
13. Lemal R, Fouquet G, Terriou L, et al. Omalizumab therapy for mast cell-mediator symptoms in patients with ISM, CM, MMAS, and MCAS. J Allergy Clin Immunol Pract 2019;7(7):2387–95.e3.
14. Cardet JC, Castells MC, Hamilton MJ. Immunology and clinical manifestations of non-clonal mast cell activation syndrome. Curr Allergy Asthma Rep 2013; 13(1):10–8.
15. Akin C, Scott LM, Kocabas CN, et al. Demonstration of an aberrant mast-cell population with clonal markers in a subset of patients with "idiopathic" anaphylaxis. Blood 2007;110:2331–3.
16. Alvarez-twose I, González de olano D, Sánchez-muñoz L, et al. Clinical, biological, and molecular characteristics of clonal mast cell disorders presenting with systemic mast cell activation symptoms. J Allergy Clin Immunol 2010;125(6): 1269–78.e2.
17. Volertas S, Schuler CF, Akin C. New insights into clonal mast cell disorders including mastocytosis. Immunol Allergy Clin North Am 2018;38(3):341–50.
18. Molderings GJ, Brettner S, Homann J, et al. Mast cell activation disease: a concise practical guide for diagnostic workup and therapeutic options. J Hematol Oncol 2011;4:10.
19. Akin C. Mast cell activation syndromes presenting as anaphylaxis. Immunol Allergy Clin North Am 2015;35(2):277–85.
20. Lieberman P. The basics of histamine biology. Ann Allergy Asthma Immunol 2011; 106(2 Suppl):S2–5.

21. Borriello F, Iannone R, Marone G. Histamine release from mast cells and basophils. Handb Exp Pharmacol 2017;241:121–39.
22. Castells M. Mast cell mediators in allergic inflammation and mastocytosis. Immunol Allergy Clin North Am 2006;26(3):465–85.
23. Cho C, Nguyen A, Bryant KJ, et al. Prostaglandin D2 metabolites as a biomarker of *in vivo* mast cell activation in systemic mastocytosis and rheumatoid arthritis. Immun Inflamm Dis 2016;4:64–9.
24. Roberts LJ, Sweetman BJ, Lewis RA, et al. Increased production of prostaglandin D2 in patients with systemic mastocytosis. N Engl J Med 1980;303(24):1400–4.
25. Ricciotti E, Fitzgerald GA. Prostaglandins and inflammation. Arterioscler Thromb Vasc Biol 2011;31(5):986–1000.
26. Smyth EM, Grosser T, Wang M, et al. Prostanoids in health and disease. J Lipid Res 2009;50(Suppl):S423–8.
27. Ravi A, Butterfield J, Weiler CR. Mast cell activation syndrome: improved identification by combined determinations of serum tryptase and 24-hour urine 11β-prostaglandin2α. J Allergy Clin Immunol Pract 2014;2:775–8.
28. Murata T, Maehara T. Discovery of anti-inflammatory role of prostaglandin D. J Vet Med Sci 2016;78(11):1643–7.
29. Hammarström S. Leukotrienes. Annu Rev Biochem 1983;52:355–77.
30. Yonetomi Y, Sekioka T, Kadode M, et al. Leukotriene C4 induces bronchoconstriction and airway vascular hyperpermeability via the cysteinyl leukotriene receptor 2 in S-hexyl glutathione-treated guinea pigs. Eur J Pharmacol 2015;754:98–104.
31. Yu Y, Blokhuis BR, Garssen J, et al. Non-IgE mediated mast cell activation. Eur J Pharmacol 2016;778:33–43.
32. Atiakshin D, Buchwalow I, Samoilova V, et al. Tryptase as a polyfunctional component of mast cells. Histochem Cell Biol 2018;149(5):461–77.
33. Payne V, Kam PC. Mast cell tryptase: a review of its physiology and clinical significance. Anaesthesia 2004;59(7):695–703.
34. Schwartz LB. Tryptase, a mediator of human mast cells. J Allergy Clin Immunol 1990;86(4 Pt 2):594–8.
35. Schwartz LB. Clinical utility of tryptase levels in systemic mastocytosis and associated hematologic disorders. Leuk Res 2001;25(7):553–62.
36. Schwartz LB, Sakai K, Bradford TR, et al. The alpha form of human tryptase is the predominant type present in blood at baseline in normal subjects and is elevated in those with systemic mastocytosis. J Clin Invest 1995;96:2702–10.
37. Valent P, Bonadonna P, Hartmann K, et al. Why the 20% + 2 tryptase formula is a diagnostic gold standard for severe systemic mast cell activation and mast cell activation syndrome. Int Arch Allergy Immunol 2019;180(1):44–51.
38. Lyons JJ, Yu X, Hughes JD, et al. Elevated basal serum tryptase identifies a multisystem disorder associated with increased TPSAB1 copy number. Nat Genet 2016;48:1564–9.
39. Sargur R, Cowley D, Murng S, et al. Raised tryptase without anaphylaxis or mastocytosis: heterophilic antibody interference in the serum tryptase assay. Clin Exp Immunol 2011;163(3):339–45.
40. Bolstad N, Warren DJ, Nustad K. Heterophilic antibody interference in immunometric assays. Best Pract Res Clin Endocrinol Metab 2013;27(5):647–61.
41. Murali MR, Castells MC, Song JY, et al. Case records of the Massachusetts General Hospital. Case 9-2011. A 37-year-old man with flushing and hypotension. N Engl J Med 2011;364(12):1155–65.

42. Molderings GJ, Haenisch B, Brettner S, et al. Pharmacological treatment options for mast cell activation disease. Naunyn Schmiedebergs Arch Pharmacol 2016; 389(7):671–94.
43. Nurmatov UB, Rhatigan E, Simons FE, et al. H1-antihistamines for primary mast cell activation syndromes: a systematic review. Allergy 2015;70(9):1052–61.
44. Butterfield JH, Weiler CR. Prevention of mast cell activation disorder-associated clinical sequelae of excessive prostaglandin D(2) production. Int Arch Allergy Immunol 2008;147(4):338–43.

Moving?

Make sure your subscription moves with you!

To notify us of your new address, find your **Clinics Account Number** (located on your mailing label above your name), and contact customer service at:

Email: journalscustomerservice-usa@elsevier.com

800-654-2452 (subscribers in the U.S. & Canada)
314-447-8871 (subscribers outside of the U.S. & Canada)

Fax number: 314-447-8029

Elsevier Health Sciences Division
Subscription Customer Service
3251 Riverport Lane
Maryland Heights, MO 63043

*To ensure uninterrupted delivery of your subscription, please notify us at least 4 weeks in advance of move.

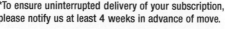

Printed and bound by CPI Group (UK) Ltd, Croydon, CR0 4YY

03/10/2024

01040403-0017